Targets of Treatment in Chronic Inflammatory Bowel Diseases

FALK SYMPOSIUM 131

Targets of Treatment in Chronic Inflammatory Bowel Diseases

Edited by

H. Herfarth
Innere Medizin I
Klinikum der Universität Regensburg
Regensburg
Germany

J. Schölmerich
Innere Medizin I
Klinikum der Universität Regensburg
Regensburg
Germany

B.G. Feagan
University of Western Ontario
Robarts Research Institute
London, Ontario, Canada

M.H. Vatn
University of Oslo
Rikshospital
Medical Department A
Oslo
Norway

U.R. Fölsch
Innere Medizin I
Klinikum der Universität
Kiel
Germany

M. Zeitz
Innere Medizin I
Universitätsklinikum Benjamin
Franklin der Freien Universität Berlin
Berlin
Germany

Proceedings of Falk Symposium 131 (Part II of the Gastroenterology Week Freiburg 2002) held in Freiburg, Germany, October 6–8, 2002

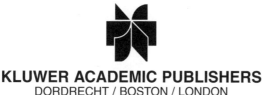

KLUWER ACADEMIC PUBLISHERS
DORDRECHT / BOSTON / LONDON

Library of Congress Cataloging-in-Publication Data is available.

ISBN 0–7923–8784–8

Published by Kluwer Academic Publishers, BV
P.O. Box 17, 3300 AA Dordrecht, The Netherlands.

Sold and distributed in North, Central and South America
by Kluwer Academic Publishers,
101 Philip Drive, Norwell, MA 02061, USA.

In all other countries, sold and distributed
by Kluwer Academic Publishers, Distribution Center,
P.O. Box 322, 3300 AH Dordrecht, The Netherlands.

Printed on acid-free paper

Printed and bound in Great Britain by MPG Books, Bodmin, Cornwall.

Contents

CONTENTS

List of principal contributors

S Bauer
Institut für Mikrobiologie und Hygiene
der TU München
Klinikum rechts der Isar
Trogerstr. 9
D-81675 München
Germany

SM Collins
McMaster University
Health Sciences Centre – Rm 4W8
1200 Main Street West
Hamilton, ON L8N 3Z5
Canada

J-F Colombel
Hôpital Claude Huriez
CHRU Lille
Hépato-Gastroentérologie
1, Place De Verdun
F-59037 Lille
France

M de Vos
Universiteit Gent
Universitair Ziekenhuis
Gastro-enterologie
De Pintelaan 185
B-9000 Gent
Belgium

A Ekbom
Karolinska Institutet
Dept of Medical Epidemiology
PO Box 281
17177 Stockholm
Sweden

CO Elson
University of Alabama at Birmingham
Division of Gastroenterology and
 Hepatology

1530 3rd Avenue South
ZRB 636
Birmingham, AL 35294-0007
USA

BG Feagan
University of Western Ontario
Robarts Research Institute
London, ON N6A 5K8
Canada

S Feuerbach
Röntgendiagnostik
Klinikum der Universität Regensburg
Franz-Josef-Strauss-Allee 11
D-93053 Regensburg
Germany

UR Fölsch
Innere Medizin I
Klinikum der Universität
Kiel
Germany

C Gasché
Allgemeines Krankenhuis
Klinik für Innere Medizin IV
Währinger Gürtel 18-20
A-1090 Wien
Austria

H Herfarth
Innere Medizin I
Klinikum der Universität Regensburg
D-93042 Regensburg
Germany

HJF Hodgson
Royal Free and University College
School of Medicine
Pond Street
London
NW3 2QG
UK

AF Hofmann
University of California, San Diego
Department of Medicine (0813)
Division of Gastroenterology
9500 Gilman Drive
La Jolla, CA 92093-0813
USA

EJ Irvine
McMaster University
Health Science Centre
Department of Gastroenterology
Rm 4W8
1200 Main Street West
Hamilton, ON L8N 3Z5
Canada

W Kruis
Innere Medizin
Evang. Krankenhaus Kalk
Buchforststr. 2
D-51103 Köln
Germany

J Minchew
104 Ellsworth Place
Chapel Hill, NC 27516
USA

U Müller-Ladner
Innere Medizin I
Klinikum der Universität Regensburg
D-93042 Regensburg
Germany

J Müller-Quernheim
Pneumologie
Universitätsklinik Freiburg
Killianstr. 5
D-79106 Freiburg
Germany

P Riis
Nerievej 7
DK-2900 Hellerup
Denmark

G Rogler
Innere Medizin I
Klinikum der Universität Regensburg
D-93042 Regensburg
Germany

DB Sachar
Mount Sinai School of Medicine
Division of Gastroenterology
Box 1069
One Gustave L. Levy Place
New York, NY 10029-6574
USA

WJ Sandborn
Mayo Clinic
Division of Gastroenterology and
  Hepatology
E 19B
200 First Street SW
Rochester, MN 55905
USA

RB Sartor
University of North Carolina
School of Medicine
Division of Digestive Diseases
CB #7038, Room 032 Glaxo Building
Chapel Hill, NC 27599-7038
USA

J Schölmerich
Innere Medizin I
Klinikum der Universität Regensburg
D-93042 Regensburg
Germany

S Schreiber
Innere Medizin I
Klinikum der Universität
Schittenhelmstr. 12
D-24105 Kiel
Germany

J-D Schulzke
Innere Medizin I
Universitätsklinikum Benjamin Franklin
  der Freien Universität Berlin
Hindenburgdamm 30
D-12203 Berlin
Germany

F Tavarela-Veloso
Serviço de Gastrenterologia
Hospital S. João
Porto 4200-319
Portugal

G Van Assche
Univ. Ziekenhuis Gasthuisberg
Department of Gastroenterology
Herestraat 49
D-3000 Leuven
Belgium

S Werner
Institut für Zellbiologie
ETH Zürich Hönggerberg
HPM D42
CH-8093 Zürich
Switzerland

M Zeitz
Innere Medizin I
Universitätsklinikum Benjamin
  Franklin der Freien Universität
  Berlin
Hindenburgdamm 30
D-12203 Berlin
Germany

Preface

While the prevalence of inflammatory bowel disease is still increasing, the aetiology of Crohn's disease as well as ulcerative colitis still remains elusive. However, in recent years our understanding of the pathophysiological processes has strikingly increased. The underlying genetic susceptibility, the molecular cross-talk of mucosal pro- and anti-inflammatory mediators and the role of the intestinal flora in the perpetuation of acute relapsing gut inflammation have been clearly defined in animal models. Nevertheless, a recognisable gap still exists in inflammatory bowel disease between success at the benchside and clinical application at the bedside. This is illustrated by the exciting progress in studying the pathophysiological role of many cytokines and other inflammatory mediators in a still-increasing number of animal models, as well as the discovery of the first gene in inflammatory bowel disease, CARD15, which is at least partly responsible for the development of Crohn's disease in about 25% of all patients. However, the imminent clinical and therapeutic values of these scientific advances have not been achieved but will hopefully occur in the near future.

The aim of this symposium held in Freiburg, on 6–8 October 2002, was to delineate potential new targets of treatment in chronic inflammatory bowel disease. The symposium was laid out in such a way that the aim was approached in two settings. In the first part, targets of treatment were defined by embedding the most recent knowledge of genetic analyses, mucosal immunity and *in vitro* and *in vivo* models of inflammatory bowel disease into new potential therapeutical concepts. In addition an attempt was made to learn from experts of other fields such as dermatology, pulmonology and rheumatology. The second part defined the therapeutic targets by characterizing and solving problems encountered in daily clinical practice as well as by implementing the quality of life and the wishes of patients suffering from Crohn's disease or ulcerative colitis.

The editors wish to thank Dr Herbert Falk and the Falk Foundation, Freiburg, for their generous support and the exceptional organization of the meeting, which surely stimulated new approaches and insights into chronic inflammatory bowel disease. The editors also thank Mr. Phil Johnstone from Kluwer Academic Publishers for his help and cooperation in preparing this volume.

The Editors

Defining targets of treatment by analysis of gut inflammation

1
State of the art lecture: Theories of inflammatory bowel disease aetiology from the 1930s to the 1960s

D. B. SACHAR

The mandate of this chapter is to review the aetiological theories of inflammatory bowel disease (IBD) of previous generations, roughly during the half-century from the 1930s to the 1980s. Clearly, the simplest and most straightforward route to fulfilling this assignment would be to reproduce the best or at least the most comprehensive tabulation of those theories as they existed in or about 1980. In fact, this is precisely what I have done in reprinting below our 221-reference review article, 'Aetiological theories of inflammatory bowel disease', from the 1980 volume of *Clinics in Gastroenterology*. In that paper my colleagues and I surveyed and critiqued the published aetiopathogenetic data and hypotheses from the first Crohn, Ginzburg, and Oppenheimer papers of 1932 and 1933 up to what was then the present day.

However, simply revisiting that retrospective could serve little purpose today unless we were to provide some modern perspective on those early theories. In particular it should prove most useful to reflect upon those avenues that might have led us astray and, perhaps even more important, to consider which pathways are still promising in the light of new insights in the 21st century.

Therefore, as a prologue to our reprint, let me first call attention to the warnings we issued at that time against over-interpretation of the existing data. Even though then, as now, the favoured theories focused on immunological mechanisms and infectious agents, we cautioned then, as we still do today, that 'it has often proved impossible to differentiate between primary pathogenetic mechanisms and secondary consequences of disease'. In fact, at the conclusion of our 1980 review of the putative causative role of immune mechanisms in tissue damage, we were forced to acknowledge that 'the case for any primary pathogenetic role of immunological factors in IBD remains unproved'.

Similarly, and with equal frustration, we recognize now that many of the 'defects in cell-mediated immunity' that we thought we were identifying in the 1970s were nonspecific. We cautioned even then that there was as yet 'no evidence that the [array of microbial antibodies found in IBD] are elicited by any specific environmental agent'. And likewise with reluctant scepticism, we declared that the multiple findings of particular infectious or transmissible agents in IBD tissues 'fall short of demonstrating [any] putative agent's specificity or its aetiological significance'.

However, lest it be thought that we were wallowing in unmitigated negativism in 1980, we hoped then as we do now that a combination of interdisciplinary collaborations, a continued focus upon 'an important genetic role in predisposition to IBD', an unflagging pursuit of those environmental factors that must also play a role in aetiology, open-mindedness to unconventional ideas, and perhaps above all serendipity, would ultimately 'produce the key to the mystery of IBD'. The remainder of this volume represents the true 'state of the art' in all those efforts as they stand in 2002.

Aetiological theories of inflammatory bowel disease*

DAVID B. SACHAR, MILES O. AUSLANDER and JACOB S. WALFISH

While generations of investigators have come and gone, the worldwide search for the aetiology of ulcerative colitis and Crohn's disease has remained unrequited. There has been no lack of provocative hypotheses and tantalizing leads. So far, however, exploration of all these various avenues has not yielded any conclusive answers.

The difficulties in tracking down aetiological agents in ulcerative colitis and Crohn's disease are at least threefold. First, there are no reliable pathognomonic features that define these diseases, that can distinguish them from each other in every case, or that have identified different pathogenetic subgroups among them. Second, there is no firm handle by which to grasp even the fundamental nature of ileitis and colitis. Aetiological theories have invoked allergic, dietary, infectious, autoimmune, vascular, neuromotor and psychosomatic factors, but it has still not been clearly established into which, if any, of these categories the inflammatory bowel diseases fall. Finally, it is difficult to document the pathogenetic significance or specificity of many of the epiphenomena which these disorders manifest. There are, for example, a profusion of immunological derangements demonstrable in the blood and tissues of ileitis and colitis patients, but the selection and availability of appropriate controls are problematical; hence, it has often proved impossible to differentiate between primary pathogenetic mechanisms and secondary consequences of disease.

Throughout the course of this century, as one research fashion after another has had its heyday, two related avenues of investigation have proved more durable than most: immunological mechanisms and infectious agents. This review of the aetiological theories of inflammatory bowel disease will therefore focus most of its attention on immunological and microbiological studies, but it will explore some other arenas of research activity as well.

---

* Reprinted from *Clinics in Gastroenterology* Vol. 9, No. 2, May 1980, with permission of W.B. Saunders Company.

IMMUNOLOGICAL FACTORS

For all the complexity of the hundreds of studies of immunological aspects of inflammatory bowel disease (IBD), they are all basically looking for the answers to three simple questions.

1. Do immunological mechanisms play a role in the initiation or perpetuation of tissue damage in IBD?
2. Are immunological factors involved in rendering certain individuals susceptible to IBD?
3. Can immunological markers provide a clue to the aetiological agent(s) of IBD?

Since we and others have rather exhaustively reviewed immunological aspects of IBD elsewhere (Strickland and Sachar, 1977), we will confine ourselves here to surveying the major pieces of evidence that bear on the three principal questions we have posed above.

Role of immune mechanisms in tissue damage

Immunological mechanisms that induce pathological lesions fall into either of two broad categories: (a) reactions mediated by antibodies or immune complexes without direct participation of mononuclear cells, (b) reactions mediated by activated lymphocytes. Both types of mechanism have been studied extensively in inflammatory bowel disease.

Antibody-mediated reactions

Autoantibodies. The earliest and simplest concept of 'autoimmunity' in these diseases was the idea that circulating antiepithelial antibodies combined with antigens on the intestinal cell surface and thus directly damaged the cells. Indeed, circulating anticolon antibodies have been recognized in the sera of patients with ulcerative colitis for 20 years (Broberger and Perlmann, 1959). Their presence was subsequently demonstrated in Crohn's disease as well (Lagercrantz et al., 1968). In the past two decades, substantial information has accumulated concerning the epithelial antigenic specificities and heterogeneous immunoglobulin composition of these circulating autoantibodies (Broberger and Perlmann, 1962; Nairn et al., 1962; Broberger, 1964; Harrison, 1965; Perlmann, Lagercrantz and Gustafsson, 1965; Lagercrantz et al., 1968; Wright and Truelove, 1966a; McGivan, Datta and Nairn, 1967; Zeromski et al., 1970; Marcussen and Nerup, 1973; Marcussen, 1978). A clue to their possible origin in response to cross-reacting bacterial antigens has been provided by the longstanding observation that the circulating autoantibodies in patients with IBD may not only be directed against colon (and buccal mucosa – Walker, 1978; Matthews et al., 1979) epithelial cell antigens but also cross-react with lipopolysaccharide antigens extracted from E. coli (Broberger, 1964; Perlmann et al., 1967; Lagercrantz et al., 1968; Thayer et al., 1969; Lagercrantz, Perlmann and Hammerstrom, 1971; Marcussen, 1978). These findings gave rise to the hypothesis, popular in the 1960s, that IBD was an 'autoimmune' disorder in which antibodies that developed in response to coliform bacterial antigens reacted against

6

intestinal epithelial cells that shared lipopolysaccharide antigenic determinants with the inciting bacteria.

In the last decade, efforts to demonstrate the presence of anticolon antibodies at the tissue level had been unsuccessful (Wright and Truelove, 1966a), although local deposition of complement components, immunoglobulins, and antibacterial antibodies had been described (Koffler *et al.*, 1962; Monteiro *et al.*, 1971; Ballard and Shiner, 1974). More recently, however, Das *et al.* (1978) have reported the isolation and characterization of a specific colonic tissue-bound antibody from patients with ulcerative colitis. This antibody is an IgG which apparently does not cross-react with *E. coli* antigen, and which is quite distinct from the circulating anticolon antibodies described above. Also, Bookman and Bull (1979) have observed a ten-fold increase in IgG synthesis by mucosal lymphoid cells isolated from intestine affected by IBD.

Despite the demonstration of anticolon antibodies in both blood and tissue of IBD patients, the weight of current evidence militates against the likelihood that they play any primary pathogenetic role in the disease. Titres of circulating anticolon antibody bear no clear correlation with the activity, duration, or extent of the underlying disease (Koffler *et al.*, 1962; Wright and Truelove, 1966a). Moreover, these anticolon antibodies are extremely non-specific, with elevated titres found not only in Crohn's disease and ulcerative colitis, but also in urinary tract infections, cirrhosis, polyposis coli, salmonellosis, and irritable bowel syndrome (Carlsson, Lagercrantz and Perlmann, 1977). Also, inflammatory bowel disease has been described in the presence of both agammaglobulinaemia (Kirk and Freedman, 1967; Soltoft, Peterson and Kruse, 1972) and selective IgA deficiency (Hodgson and Jewell, 1977). Most important, anticolon antibodies have failed to exert significant cytopathogenetic effects either in tissue culture in vitro (Broberger and Perlmann, 1963) or in experimental animal models in vivo (Rabin and Rogers, 1976).

Immune complexes. If circulating antibody per se has no demonstrable pathogenetic action in IBD, another closely related immune mechanism of tissue injury could be the deposition of antigen-antibody complexes (Thayer, 1976). Koffler *et al.* (1962) first raised the possibility that local immune complexes might play a role in IBD when they demonstrated the presence of both the C3 component of complement and gamma globulin in colon tissue from patients with ulcerative colitis. A number of subsequent studies of serum levels of complement components and anticomplementary activity have provided some indirect evidence for the presence of circulating immune complexes in Crohn's disease and ulcerative colitis (Doe, Booth and Brown, 1973; Jewell and MacLennan, 1973; Ballard and Shiner, 1974; Hodgson, Potter and Jewell, 1977a and b; Fiasse *et al.*, 1978; Nielson, Petersen and Svehag, 1978; Nielson *et al.*, 1978). As another measure of immune complex formation and clearance, Eckhardt *et al.* (1978) have reported in vivo fixation of IgG onto the hepatocellular membranes of 93 per cent of patients with active Crohn's disease, but not of patients with inactive disease. More significantly, some investigators have provoked an acute experimental proctitis in rabbits by first inducing mild non-specific inflammation with intrarectal formalin, followed two hours later by intravenous inoculation of albumin-based antigen-antibody complexes (Hodgson *et al.*, 1978). When rabbits were pre-sensitized with colonic bacterial antigen, this same experimental procedure reportedly produced a chronic proctitis persisting at least six months (Mee *et al.*, 1979).

However, the case for immune complex mediation of IBD is still weak at best. The complement aberrations demonstrated in the sera of patients are not very consistent, and may represent little more than non-specific markers of acute inflammation (Hodgson, Potter and Jewell, 1977c; Lake *et al.*, 1979). Moreover, the assays heretofore applied have been unreliable measures of immune complex formation. Recent studies utilizing more specific techniques have failed to corroborate significantly increased frequency or concentration of circulating immune complexes in patients with IBD, regardless of disease activity or extra-intestinal manifestations (Soltis *et al.*, 1979).

Immediate hypersensitivity. Besides autoantibodies and immune complexes, a third antibody-mediated mechanism of tissue injury has been proposed for IBD, namely an immediate hypersensitivity reaction, in which IgE causes degranulation of mast cells in the bowel wall. Most studies of IgE concentrations in serum (Brown, Lansford and Hornbrook, 1973) and intestinal fluid (Brown, Borthistle and Chen, 1975; Heatley *et al.*, 1975) have agreed that these levels are not conspicuously altered in IBD. Immunofluorescent studies of IgE-containing immunocytes in the bowel wall have yielded more variable results, from decreased (Lloyd *et al.*, 1975) to normal (Baklien and Brandtzaeg, 1975; Green and Fox, 1975; Strickland *et al.*, 1975) to increased (Brown, Borthistle and Chen, 1975; Heatley *et al.*, 1975a; Rimpila *et al.*, 1976; O'Donoghue and Kumar, 1979). With respect to mucosal mast cells, there is at least some consensus that counts are increased in ulcerative colitis (Sommers, 1966; Lloyd *et al.*, 1975; Sommers and Korelitz, 1975); but for Crohn's disease, reports once again run the gamut from increased (Hiatt and Katz, 1962; Rao, 1973) to decreased (Lloyd *et al.*, 1975). This variability of results need not trouble ardent proponents of immediate hypersensitivity theories of IBD, since they can cite *increased* IgE cells and mast cells as indicative of a heightened capacity for immediate hypersensitivity, or else point to *decreased* IgE cells and mast cells as evidence for IgE consumption and mast cell degranulation! Perhaps more germane to the issue are ultra-structural studies that have directly observed an abundance of degranulating mast cells in the bowel walls of patients with Crohn's disease (Dvorak *et al.*, 1978b; Levo and Livni, 1978). In any event, the concept that immediate hypersensitivity plays any primary pathogenetic role in IBD still remains speculative. Early reports of the efficacy of disodium cromoglycate in the treatment of Crohn's disease (Henderson and Hishon, 1978) and ulcerative colitis (Heatley *et al.*, 1975b; Mani *et al.*, 1976) have not been recently confirmed (Buckell *et al.*, 1978; Dronfield and Langman, 1978).

Lymphocyte-mediated reactions

So far, we have examined the ways in which specific antibodies, immune complexes, or IgE may directly initiate tissue damage. There are also several mechanisms whereby antigens and antibodies may play indirect roles in tissue injury that is mediated by lymphocytes. An antigen may stimulate a specifically sensitized lymphocyte (T cell) to destroy a target cell that carries the same antigen. Another species of lymphocyte (K cell, or null cell), which carries Fc receptors on its surface, may attach to the Fc portion of an antibody that is coating a target cell and kill the target cell (antibody-dependent cell-mediated cytotoxicity, ADCC). Either the same or a closely related variety of lymphocyte can destroy target cells without the participation of antibody or Fc receptors (NK-activity, spontaneous cell-mediated cytotoxicity, SCMC). All three of these mechanisms have been examined for clues to the pathogenesis of IBD.

T-cell cytotoxicity. The literature is replete with studies showing that patients with IBD have circulating T lymphocytes which have been sensitized to a multiplicity of colon and bacterial antigens, including the enterobacterial common antigen of Kunin. These data have been extensively discussed by us and others (Strickland and Sachar, 1977; Meuwissen, Nadorp and Tytgat, 1977) so we will not review them in detail here. The point is that immuno-fluorescently and functionally identifiable T cells have been identified not only in the circulation but also in the bowel wall of patients with and without IBD (Breucha and Riethmuller, 1975; Meuwissen *et al.*, 1976; Bull and Bookman, 1977; Clancy, 1978; Falchuk, Barnhard and Machado, 1979; MacDermott *et al.*, 1979). In fact, experimental colitis induced in sensitized guinea pigs by dinitrochlorobenzene (DNCB) enemas is associated with a significant increase in T cells in the lamina propria (Glick and Falchuk, 1979). Moreover, heightened responsiveness to PHA-stimulation has been reported for lamina propria lymphocytes from IBD-affected colon (Machado and Falchuk, 1978). No one has yet demonstrated, however, that the intestinal T cells in human or experimental IBD exert significantly heightened cytotoxicity against either intestinal or other target cell lines. Moreover, this phenomenon of T lymphocyte sensitization, at least to the Kunin antigen, is not specific to IBD, but appears to occur with equal frequency among patients with cirrhosis of the liver (Eckhardt, Heinisch and Buschenfelde, 1976).

ADCC (K-cell activity). Whereas increased cytotoxicity of classical T cells in IBD has not yet been demonstrated, Shorter *et al.* have accumulated impressive evidence that there is a class of circulating lymphocytes in IBD patients which exerts specific cytotoxicity against colon epithelial cells in culture (Shorter, Spencer and Huizenga, 1968; Shorter *et al.*, 1969a and b, 1970a and b, 1971, 1972, 1973). Their studies have indicated that this cytotoxicity can be conferred even upon normal lymphocytes by incubation either with the IgM fraction of serum from patients with colitis or with a crude extract of *E. coli* lipopolysaccharide. Careful analysis of the effector cells in Shorter's cytotoxicity assay suggests that they may be Fc-receptor-bearing K cells, which mediate ADCC (Stobo *et al.*, 1976). Similar observations have recently been reported by Kemler and Alpert (1979). There are, however, three lines of evidence that militate somewhat against the primary importance of ADCC. One is Shorter's own observation that the cytotoxicity of ileitis and colitis patients' lymphocytes, as well as the capacity of their sera to confer cytotoxicity upon normal lymphocytes, both disappear within two to ten days after resection of diseased bowel (Shorter *et al.*, 1969a). The second line of evidence is that increased K cell activity may be a relatively non-specific phenomenon, occurring in acute viral hepatitis and other diseases as well as in IBD (Eckhardt *et al.*, 1977). The third line of evidence comprises several studies suggesting that the cell type necessary for ADCC, while

9

possibly present in mesenteric lymph nodes (Britton, Eklund and Bird, 1978), is absent from the normal intestinal tissues of mice and humans (Kagnoff and Campbell, 1976a and b; Bull and Bookman, 1977; Falchuk, Barnhard and Machado, 1979) and even from human colonic mucosa affected by Crohn's disease or ulcerative colitis (Clancy and Pucci, 1978). Even the rare observation of K-cell activity in gut mucosal lymphocytes appears to show more ADCC against red blood cells than against tissue cell lines and, in any event, indicates no difference between normal and IBD intestinal lymphocytes (MacDermott et al., 1979).

SCMC (NK-activity). Little or no SCMC activity is demonstrable in human colonic lamina propria lymphocytes, and no differences are discernible in SCMC between lymphocytes from normal and IBD colons (Falchuk, Barnhard and Machado, 1979; MacDermott et al., 1979).

With respect to the evidence implicating immune mechanisms in the tissue damage of ileitis and colitis, we can conclude that the disease process probably induces immune aberrations in the host, and that the inflammatory reaction may even be mediated in part via immune effector pathways. To date, however, the case for any primary pathogenetic role of immunological factors in IBD remains unproven.

Role of immune mechanisms in susceptibility to IBD

There are two related immune mechanisms which could potentially predispose people to chronic progressive inflammatory diseases like Crohn's disease and ulcerative colitis. One is a defect in cell-mediated immunity; the other is an immunogenetic vulnerability linked to the major histocompatibility (HLA) system on the sixth human chromosome. Both mechanisms have been extensively studied in IBD.

Defective cell-mediated immunity

Evaluations of the cellular immune status of patients with IBD remain shrouded in controversy. Between 1939 and 1976, at least 29 studies assessed various indices of cellular immunity in Crohn's disease and ulcerative colitis, with conflicting conclusions. One school of thought has held that cellular immunity is depressed in Crohn's disease but not in ulcerative colitis. Another viewpoint has been that there is no cellular immune defect in either Crohn's disease or ulcerative colitis. In 1976, one of us reviewed the available data (Strickland and Sachar, 1977) and concluded on the basis of our own and others' studies that some impairments of cellular immunity were demonstrable in most patients with Crohn's disease and ulcerative colitis alike, irrespective of their clinical status (Sachar et al., 1973; Ramachandar et al., 1974; Meuwissen et al., 1975; Meyers et al., 1976; Sachar et al., 1976). These impairments included lymphocyte hyporesponsiveness to mitogen stimulation (Sachar et al., 1973), depressed T-lymphocyte counts, and cutaneous anergy (Ramachandar et al., 1974; Meuwissen et al., 1975; Meyers et al., 1976; Sachar et al., 1976). Since the publication of our review article in 1976, at least three other groups of investigators have reported studies of lymphocyte functions and subpopulations in IBD (Sorensen and Hoj, 1977; Auer, Buschmann and Ziemer, 1978; Auer et al., 1978; Engstrom et al., 1978). While some lymphocyte aberrations were observed in certain subgroups of patients, results were still inconsistent. Our own most recent investigations (Meyers *et al.*, 1978) have demonstrated cutaneous anergy among 70 per cent of patients with Crohn's disease and 48 per cent of those with ulcerative colitis, but no increased incidence of anergy among patients' first-degree relatives or spouses. Anergy tended to persist among postoperative patients with Crohn's disease but to disappear after colectomy for ulcerative colitis. The immune defect in IBD seems therefore to be a secondary phenomenon, reversible upon removal of the target organ in ulcerative colitis but not after resection of grossly diseased tissue in Crohn's disease. The possible role of increased suppressor cell function, as recently described in sarcoidosis (Goodwin *et al.*, 1979) and other diseases, has yet to be thoroughly studied in IBD. Preliminary evidence suggests, however, that suppressor cell activity in IBD is, if anything, decreased (Hodgson, Wands and Isselbacher, 1978).

Besides depressed lymphocyte function, three other areas of potential immune deficiency have been investigated in IBD. The first area represents neutrophil dysfunction. Impaired neutrophil migration in vivo (Segal and Loewi, 1976) and decreased phagocytic capacity in vitro (Krause, Michaelsson and Juhlin, 1978) have both been observed in Crohn's disease, although the relation of these defects to disease pathogenesis remains entirely speculative. Another variety of immune deficiency that could potentially contribute to the pathogenesis of IBD is monocyte-macrophage dysfunction. Two recent studies, however, have shown that in both Crohn's disease and ulcerative colitis there is appropriate monocytopoietic hyperproliferation (Meuret, Bitzi and Hammer, 1978), as well as normal bacterial phagocytosis and intracellular killing by monocytes (Mee, Szalvatkowski and Jewell, 1978). A final category of immune impairment that could conceivably compromise host defences in IBD is a deficiency of the mucosal secretory immune system. Engstrom *et al.* (1978) have described low or absent levels of the secretory component of salivary IgA in five of eight patients with ulcerative colitis; the significance and general applicability of this finding have yet to be determined.

Immunogenetic vulnerability

The HLA-A and B distributions in patients with IBD have been extensively studied, with no important associations identified. (For a review of these data, see Strickland and Sachar (1977).) Schwartz *et al.* have very recently reported concordance for both HLA-A and B haplotypes among four of five sibling pairs with Crohn's disease, as opposed to similar HLA identity among only one of 17 sibling pairs in which just one member of the pair had the disease (Siegelbaum *et al.*, 1979). This observation could suggest an important genetic role in predisposition to IBD. On the other hand, no particular HLA haplotype was associated with IBD among the different kindred's in Schwartz's study. Moreover, Engstrom's HLA family data are less impressive, with concordance for both A and B haplotypes observed among three of four ulcerative colitis patients in one family and among four of six of their unaffected relatives (Engstrom *et al.*, 1978). If any particular HLA phenotype is likely to be linked to an immunological vulnerability to IBD, however, the HLA-D type would appear to be a leading candidate. Studies of the HLA-D associations with IBD are currently underway in New York City.

Immune markers of potential aetiological agents

If our current state of knowledge still does not permit definite implication of immune mechanisms either in producing tissue damage or in causing host susceptibility in IBD, perhaps immunological techniques can at least help identify potential aetiological agents. We have already seen that T lymphocytes in patients with IBD often appear to be sensitized to certain bowel- and/or bacteria-related antigens. It is still likely, however, that these antigenic sensitizations are secondary consequences of IBD, rather than indicators of primary aetiological agents.

Serological markers of infectious agents have also been widely sought. Korsmeyer *et al.* (1974, 1975) have described a high prevalence of lymphocyto-toxic antibodies among patients with IBD, their first-degree relatives, and especially their non-consanguineous household contacts. These findings have been taken as evidence for common exposure to a potentially aetiological environmental agent. What makes these data hard to interpret, however, is the observation that the antilymphocyte antibodies seen among these patients and their families are an exceedingly heterogeneous conglomeration of proteins (Henderson *et al.*, 1976). There is as yet no evidence that these antibodies are elicited by any specific environmental agent, nor even that the antibodies present among the different members of a single family share the same immunological characteristics.

Other studies of IBD patients have sought immunological evidence for infection with particular organisms such as rotavirus, Epstein-Barr virus, *Chlamydia*, mycobacteria, and others. These investigations will be considered in the next section, 'Infectious Agents'.

INFECTIOUS AGENTS

The idea that idiopathic inflammatory bowel disease might in fact be the result of an infection of the intestines dates back to the earliest scientific investigation of these diseases. Ulcerative colitis has long been recognized to be both clinically and histologically very similar to the acute dysentery produced by the shigella bacterium (Felsen, 1936). Similarly, the striking resemblance of Crohn's disease to tuberculous involvement of the gut has long suggested that this disease might be caused by a mycobacterial agent (Crohn, Ginzburg and Oppenheimer, 1932). Therefore, it is not surprising that much aetiological research has focused on animal transmission experiments and other studies of putative infectious agents.

Animal transmission studies

An experimental approach which had succeeded in isolating the bacterium responsible for leprosy was applied to Crohn's disease by Mitchell and Rees in 1970. This study suggested that a granulomatous inflammatory response could be transmitted by crude homogenates of Crohn's disease tissue using the mouse footpad as an assay model. This early study led to a number of subsequent reports using various techniques and animal models to confirm and characterize the transmissibility of inflammatory bowel disease. Taub *et al.* (1974, 1976) reproduced the granuloma-transmission phenomenon in the mouse footpad, but questioned its specificity.

Additional studies by Mitchell, Cave, and their associates demonstrated more specificity for granuloma transmission to mice, using 0.2 micron filtrates of Crohn's disease tissue homogenates. They also showed a tendency for systemic dissemination of granulomas, as well as their serial passage through several generations of murine hosts (Mitchell, Rees and Goswami, 1976; Cave, Mitchell and Brooke, 1978). These data were interpreted as evidence for the presence in Crohn's disease tissue of a virus-sized replicating agent. Even these extensive studies, however, cannot be taken as firm proof of the existence of a transmissible agent. We have previously reviewed some of the grounds for scepticism (Sachar and Auslander, 1978). Bolton *et al.*, for example, have reported uniformly negative findings using homogenates of Crohn's disease tissue inoculated into rats, guinea pigs and mice (Bolton *et al.*, 1973; Heatley *et al.*, 1975c). Others have reported negative results too (Ahlberg *et al.*, 1978; Bergstrand, Holmstrom and Gustafsson, 1978). Moreover, even in the hands of Cave and Mitchell (Cave, Mitchell and Brooke, 1978), granuloma transmission occurs with an exceedingly low frequency. Finally, at a recent Workshop on Infectious Agents in IBD (1978), Dr John Yardley independently reviewed the histological slides which purportedly demonstrated granulomas in the mouse footpad assays. Many of the supposed granulomas were relatively non-specific accumulations of inflammatory cells, while others were actually spontaneous murine neoplasms; most of the true granulomas showed evidence of foreign bodies such as hair, bone, and non-specific refractile material. The relevance of granuloma transmission to the aetiology of IBD therefore remains in considerable doubt.

Another animal model used to study the transmissibility of an agent in IBD is the rabbit. Cave *et al.* have published two reports of granulomatous bowel lesions in New Zealand White rabbits incoculated intraserosally with crude homogenates and fine filtrates of Crohn's disease tissues (Cave *et al.*, 1973; Cave, Mitchell and Brooke, 1975). Once again, serial passage of the histological lesions from animal to animal was demonstrated.

Other studies of the rabbit transmission model have been less specific in their findings, however. Simonowitz *et al.* (1977) reported gross pathology including bowel wall thickening, creeping mesenteric fat, thickening of the mesentery, and enlargement of mesenteric lymph nodes in rabbits inoculated with Crohn's homogenates. Microscopic examination, however, revealed only non-specific findings; no granulomas were found in the bowels of these rabbits. The phenomenon of granuloma transmission in both mice and rabbits has been observed as regularly with ulcerative colitis tissues as with Crohn's disease homogenates (Cave *et al.*, 1973; Taub *et al.*, 1974; Cave, Mitchell and Brooke, 1975). Another study demonstrating the possible non-specificity of the transmission of histological changes in rabbits was reported by Donnelly, Delaney and Healy (1977). In this study, seven of 11 rabbits inoculated with normal human bowel homogenate and four of 16 inoculated with human Crohn's disease tissue homogenate developed Crohn's-like changes, including nine animals with epithelioid granulomas. These changes were therefore produced even more frequently by control than by Crohn's disease homogenates.

In summary, then, the animal transmission studies reported to date suggest that a transmissible agent may indeed be present in Crohn's disease tissues, but they fall short of demonstrating this putative agent's specificity or its aetiological significance.

Enteric bacterial flora

The concept of an enteric bacterial agent producing idiopathic inflammatory bowel disease has a long history. Early reports of organisms such as Bargen's Diplococcus (Bargen, 1924) or the bacterium necrophorum of Dragstedt, Dack and Kirsner (1941) were not confirmed. More recently, interest in the variability of *E. coli* subtypes producing intestinal disease in man led to many immunological experiments that sought to implicate an enterobacterial antigen in the pathogenesis of IBD. These efforts have been described in the preceding section on Immunological Factors.

In brief, despite circumstantial data that point to enteric bacteria in the aetiology of IBD, no specific organism has consistently been isolated from patients, nor produced disease in experimental animals. The possibility that a transient enteric infection might induce a change which then continues in a self-perpetuating fashion despite the absence of continued infection has been suggested (Shorter, Huizenga and Spencer, 1972). It has been noted that there is a 10 to 15 per cent incidence of ulcerative colitis following shigella dysentery (Felsen, 1936). Damage to the colonic epithelium by shigella or other bacterial flora inducing a chronic inflammatory response remains tenable but unproved.

A subclass of enteric bacterial flora, the cell wall-defective variant, has more recently been implicated in the aetiology of inflammatory bowel disease. In 1971 Aluwihare described an electron microscopic study in which intramural bacteria were identified in the lamina propria and submucosa of intestinal tissue from a patient with Crohn's disease. It was suggested that, as in Whipple's disease, a cell wall-deficient or variant bacteria might be present in these specimens. To support the ability of a cell wall-deficient bacteria to produce the pathophysiological abnormality of inflammatory bowel disease, Orr reported that direct inoculation of the terminal ileum of rabbits with a stable L-form of *Streptococcus faecalis*, but not with the parent organism, produced focal granulomatous lesions (Orr, 1975).

In an attempt to explain the chronic and recurrent course of inflammatory bowel disease as well as the inability to culture routine enteric flora from specimens with inflammatory bowel disease, Parent and Mitchell (1976, 1978) used laboratory methods designed specifically to isolate bacterial variants. They obtained a bacterium classified by the Center for Disease Control as a *Pseudomonas*-like Va from eight consecutive patients with Crohn's disease. None of five ulcerative colitis nor 20 control tissues yielded this organism. Parent and Mitchell have subsequently reported that patients with Crohn's disease often have high titres of serum antibody directed against this *Pseudomonas* Va bacterium, while patients with ulcerative colitis or other gastrointestinal diseases do not (Parent, Mitchell and Krueger, 1978). On the basis of their cultural isolation and antibody studies, they suggest that this cell wall variant may be the aetiological agent of Crohn's disease, but their provocative work has not yet been confirmed.

14

Other serological data have recently sought to implicate *Chlamydia*, an intracellular parasite closely resembling a bacterium, in the aetiology of Crohn's disease (Schuller *et al.*, 1979). This work too is unconfirmed at present, and has been disputed from several sources (Munro *et al.*, 1979; Swarbrick *et al.*, 1979; Taylor-Robinson *et al.*, 1979).

Mycobacteria

The concept of mycobacteria producing an inflammatory reaction in the gut dates back to the classical description of Crohn's disease as a specific entity by Crohn, Ginzburg and Oppenheimer in 1932. They described a disease which was grossly and histologically similar to intestinal tuberculosis but in which mycobacteria could not be cultured. All attempts to identify *M. tuberculosis* and later atypical mycobacteria produced negative results. But in 1975 Watson and Martucci reported that lymphocytes from patients with Crohn's disease demonstrated a specifically increased sensitivity to mycobacterial antigens. More recently, Burnham *et al.* (1978) have described renewed efforts to identify a mycobacterial agent in Crohn's disease tissues. Long-term cultures of lymph node material, after eight months of cultivation, revealed the growth of an acid-fast organism of the *Mycobacterium kansasii* group in one out of 27 patients with Crohn's disease. Neither electron microscopic studies nor skin tests with *M. kansasii* antigen, however, lent strong support to the specific association of this organism with Crohn's disease, and further verification of the original work has proved difficult (Stanford *et al.*, 1979).

Viruses

Early studies were unable to demonstrate a specific virus associated with inflammatory bowel disease. In 1961, Syverton reported a negative study with rectal biopsies and colonic washing as the human source injected into various tissue culture lines. A more extensive study by Schneierson *et al.* in 1962 studied specimens from 74 patients with Crohn's disease, 18 with ulcerative colitis, and 20 controls. Homogenates of these specimens were injected in various human and animal tissue culture lines as well as into the brains of suckling mice and into the terminal ileums of guinea pigs. This very meticulous study identified the presence of several viruses, including three types of Coxsackie and several contaminant mouse viruses, but it was unable consistently to identify any single human virus from the Crohn's disease or ulcerative colitis tissue.

In 1973 Farmer *et al.* surveyed 57 patients with ulcerative colitis, 15 with Crohn's disease, and 65 matched controls, searching for the presence of antibodies to a battery of 12 common viral antigens. The only significant serological finding was a greater frequency of antibody to cytomegalovirus in ulcerative colitis patients than in controls. This same study reported tissue culture results positive for the presence of cytomegalovirus in three of six patients tested; one of these tissue cultures demonstrated viral particles by electron microscopy. More recently Cooper *et al.* (1977) reported that electron microscopic studies revealed cytomegalovirus inclusion bodies in six severely inflamed ulcerative colitis specimens out of 46 cases. The significance of this finding in the absence of a control population is difficult to interpret. Other studies have failed to observe histological evidence of cytomegalovirus in surgical colitis specimens and have found no use for antibody titres during acute colitis attacks (Swarbrick et al., 1979).

Further studies on viral aetiologies of inflammatory bowel disease were stimulated by the reports of Mitchell, Cave and others that their purported transmissible agent could pass through a 0.2 micron filter (Mitchell, Rees and Goswami, 1976; Ahlberg et al., 1978; Bergstrand, Holmstrom and Gustafsson, 1978; Cave, Mitchell and Brooke, 1978). In 1975 Aronson et al. used a modified co-cultivation technique for primary isolation of viruses. A cytopathic effect in the feeder layer following inoculation was found using 16 of 24 Crohn's disease tissues, 14 of 20 other gastrointestinal disease tissues, and one of nine normal tissues. The putative virus was clearly not specific for Crohn's disease.

More specific results were reported by Gitnick, Arthur and Shibata in 1976. A variety of tissue culture lines were inoculated with 0.2 micron filtrates obtained from the diseased, resected tissue of four patients with Crohn's disease, and four control tissues. A cytopathic effect was demonstrated by each case of Crohn's disease but not from the control tissue. The contention that this cytopathic effect was indeed of viral cause was supported by the accompanying report by Gitnick and Rosen (1976) demonstrating electron microscopic evidence of a small virus-like particle in the tissue culture material.

In perhaps the strongest case for an IBD-associated virus yet published, these same investigators recently expanded their studies to include tissue filtrates from 21 specimens of Crohn's disease, 12 cases of ulcerative colitis, and 20 controls (Gitnick et al., 1979). They reported cytopathic effects (CPE) in tissue culture in all but one of the IBD specimens and in only 20 per cent of their controls. Roughly half the IBD specimens which produced CPE, but none of the controls, manifested virus-like particles on electron microscopy. Guinea pig antiserum to Crohn's disease and ulcerative colitis tissue-culture fluid reportedly produced specific inhibition of the CPE from the specimens of corresponding disease, with no cross-inhibition among Crohn's disease, ulcerative colitis, or controls. The extremely low titres of cytopathic agent, however, precluded any standard neutralization tests. It was also claimed that the putative viruses were passed through five to 15 tissue culture passages, although no increase in titre was obtained, and no methods or criteria for passage were described.

Positive tissue culture results were also obtained by Whorwell et al. (1977), who demonstrated a cytopathic effect from Crohn's disease tissue which could be passaged to subsequent tissue culture lines. Several groups have now reported the cytopathic agent to be approximately 50 to 60 nm in diameter, to contain RNA, and to be acid- and ether-stable and heat-resistant (Aronson et al., 1975; Gitnick and Rosen, 1976; Gitnick, Arthur and Shibata, 1976; Whorwell et al., 1977; Gitnick et al., 1979; Strickland et al., 1979).

Firm proof that this agent is in fact a virus is still lacking. Despite a claim that virus-like particles have been seen in Crohn's disease tissues (Riemann, 1977), the most meticulous electron microscopic study of diseased tissue has been negative (Dvorak et al., 1978a). An immune electron microscopic study was unable to detect the presence of viral particles in the stool of patients with Crohn's disease, using the patient's sera as a source of agglutinating antibody (Phillpotts et al., 1977). The classification of the proposed virus is also unclear.

Original reports had suggested a picornavirus (Gitnick and Rosen, 1976) or rotavirus (Whorwell *et al.*, 1977) on the basis of the agent's physical characteristics. At least two independent studies, however, have been unable to detect a statistically significant increase of titre against rotavirus or the Norwalk agent in patients with Crohn's disease (DeGroote *et al.*, 1977; Greenberg *et al.*, 1979). A recent report by Kapikian *et al.* (1979) has also cast doubt on Whorwell's early suggestion (Whorwell *et al.*, 1977) of a rotavirus aetiology, and has described evidence of mycoplasma contamination of some of Whorwell's materials.

In other negative studies, Jarnerot and Lantorp (1972) were unable to demonstrate increased titres of antibody to various herpes viruses in Crohn's disease. Others have found no evidence for increased titres of EB virus or mycobacteriophage among patients with Crohn's disease (Grotsky *et al.*, 1971).

In summary, several investigators have reported the presence of cytopathic agents from tissues involved with IBD. There remains considerable controversy concerning the specificity of these findings and whether the cytopathic agents are indeed viruses. Serological studies have been unable to classify the proposed viral agents into a single group, and viral particles have not been convincingly demonstrated on direct electron microscopic examination of diseased tissue.

OTHER AETIOLOGICAL THEORIES

Psychosomatic factors

Among the most controversial issues surrounding IBD has been the role of psychosomatic factors. Since the time of Murray's first paper on the psychological aspects of ulcerative colitis (Murray, 1930), the gamut of opinion has ranged from acceptance of the disorder as the prototype of psychosomatic illness to total rejection of emotional factors in the onset and course of the disease.

Proponents of the psychosomatic theory of ulcerative colitis, although differing in particulars, in general agree that ulcerative colitis patients have a characteristic predisposing personality which renders them vulnerable to particular stressful situations which may precipitate or exacerbate symptoms. Colitis patients, according to these theorists, are emotionally immature, dependent, passive, and restricted in their relationships with others. They are thus felt to be especially sensitive to circumstances which threaten separations from key figures or which demand assumption of responsibilities beyond their emotional capacity (Lindemann, 1950). The literature is replete with papers that describe the antecedence of the 'colitis personality' to the onset of disease, and that demonstrate a close chronological relationship between specific precipitating events and the appearance of bowel symptoms (Sullivan, 1935; Engel, 1955; Groen and Bastiaans, 1955). Further support for the psychosomatic theory is drawn from anecdotal reports of improvement with psychotherapy in cases where medical therapy has failed (Grace, Pinsley and Wolff, 1954; Weinstock, 1962). As pointed out by Latimer (1978) our knowledge of the psychosomatic aspects of Crohn's disease is relatively limited, but at least one report revealed no difference from ulcerative colitis in psychosocial and behavioural characteristics (McKegney, Gordon and Levine, 1970).

Proposed pathophysiological mechanisms to explain the role of emotional factors invoke the long-recognized but poorly understood neural and hormonal relationships between the central nervous system and the bowel. The varied effects of stress on the gastrointestinal tract were extensively studied by Wolf and Wolff (Wolf and Goodell, 1968). With Grace, these pioneer workers made direct observations of hyperaemia and fragility in association with feelings of anger and hostility among patients with ulcerative colitis who had externalized bowel mucosa (Grace, Wolf and Wolff, 1950). Almy (1961) documented abnormal motility with sustained colonic contractions in patients with ulcerative colitis, while Fairburn (1973) suggested that prolonged colonic spasm may compromise mucosal blood flow and thus produce pathological changes.

Opponents of the psychosomatic theory point out that the concept is based on either anecdotal or uncontrolled studies. They cite the controlled studies of Feldman and Mendeloff, which found no evidence of either 'abnormal personalities' or preceding stressful events in ulcerative colitis or Crohn's disease (Feldman et al., 1967a and b; Mendeloff et al., 1970; Monk et al., 1970). Psychosomatic adherents rebut these arguments by contending that they are based on limited interviews which, no matter how well designed, cannot elicit essential psychiatric information which requires a long-cultivated, intimate doctor-patient relationship. Of course, such a stance virtually precludes the possibility of an adequate large-scale controlled study of the problem and thus mirrors the rift between the psychiatric and medical literature, as recently noted by Engel and Salzman (1973). Recently, in an unusual team effort comprising surgeons, internists, and psychiatrists, a group of investigators at Columbia Presbyterian Hospital have described their efforts to clarify the role of psychopathology and psychotherapy in inflammatory bowel disease (Karush et al., 1977). The continuing controversy over psychosomatic factors in inflammatory bowel disease, however, need not obscure the influence of psychological factors on patients' symptoms and on their subjective responses to their disease, nor the important role their physicians must play in providing firm and continuing support.

Dietary factors

One of the earliest pathogenetic theories of ulcerative colitis was that of food allergy, with cow's milk suspected as a primary offender (Anderson, 1942). Supporting this hypothesis were Truelove's studies, which demonstrated remission and exacerbation of symptoms with the respective exclusion and reintroduction of milk in the diets of certain ulcerative colitis patients (Taylor and Truelove, 1961; Truelove, 1961). Wright and Truelove (1965a and b) followed up these observations with a report of elevated milk-protein antibodies in colitis patients as compared to a control population. Later studies, which included blind rectal biopsy interpretation, confirmed the earlier ones and also showed higher levels of milk-protein antibodies in those patients who suffered more frequent relapses (Wright and Truelove, 1966b). No correlation could be made, however, between titres of milk antibodies and clinical response to milk exclusion, and later studies contradicted earlier ones (Jewell and Truelove, 1972).

It is therefore possible that the antibody studies simply reflect the secondary phenomenon of increased milk-protein absorption through a damaged mucosal barrier, rather than a primary pathogenetic mechanism. Indeed, increased absorption of dietary antigens and stimulation of antibody production has been noted as a probable consequence of mucosal damage in coeliac disease as well as in IBD (Falchuk and Isselbacher, 1976).

With the growing recognition of disaccharidase deficiency, investigations were launched into the role of lactose intolerance in colitis. Cady *et al.* (1967) reported an increased incidence of lactase deficiency in ulcerative colitis. Some of the adverse effects of milk may thus be explained on this basis. Although the role of true milk allergy has not been absolutely disproven, the only documented cases of frank 'milk-induced colitis' have been in infants, and these cases have not clinically resembled chronic idiopathic ulcerative colitis (Gryboski, Burkle and Hillman, 1966).

The paucity of documented cases of Crohn's disease before the twentieth century, together with its accelerating incidence in the past few decades, especially in developed populations, has led to speculation that Crohn's disease may be a by-product of dietary and environmental changes which have accompanied modern industrialized civilization (*British Medical Journal*, 1977). Chemical food additives have fallen under particular suspicion (Carstensen and Poulsen, 1971). For example, considerable interest has focused on carrageenan, a seaweed derivative used as a stabilizer in many foods (Melnyk, 1975). Repeated studies have demonstrated that ulcerative colonic lesions can be induced in a number of laboratory animals by ingestion of carrageenan, but there is thus far little evidence for a pathological effect in humans (Melnyk, 1975). Similarly, recent awareness of widespread environmental contamination by mercury has led to speculation about the role of mercury and other heavy metals in the genesis of inflammatory bowel disease (Aaronson and Spiro, 1973). This is an area which has not yet been thoroughly explored.

Epidemiological overlap between diverticular disease and IBD has led to reflection on the possible roles of fibre depletion and refined sugar intake (*British Medical Journal*, 1977), and two recent papers lend some support to the role of processed foods in the diet. A West German study has reported that patients with Crohn's disease had a highly significant increase in intake of refined carbohydrates before the onset of their illness (Martini and Brandes, 1976). Another study from England found increased consumption of cornflakes among patients with Crohn's disease (James, 1977). The latter observation has been confirmed by another report (Thomas, Jarrett and Keen, 1977) but disputed in three subsequent studies (Archer and Harvey, 1978; Mayberry, Rhodes and Newcombe, 1978; Rawcliffe and Truelove, 1978). These conflicting data illustrate the difficulties inherent in dietary surveys which rely on patients' memories of their eating habits many years in the past. Nevertheless, there is a great need for continued investigation of those environmental and dietary factors associated with twentieth-century living which might account for the steadily rising incidence of Crohn's disease.

Vascular factors

Clinical and pathological similarities between inflammatory and ischaemic bowel disease have been recognized for many years. As early as 1933, Ginzburg and Oppenheimer described the occurrence of ulcerative, obstructive, and granulomatous lesions secondary to vascular compromise. Similarly, Bockus and Lee (1935) suggested that intermittent volvulus or intussusception may predispose to insufficiency of the ileo-colic artery and thus give rise to regional ileitis. In a large review of surgical and autopsy cases of ulcerative colitis, Warren and Sommers (1949) found 19 cases (11 per cent) with evidence of local vasculitis, which they felt was of primary aetiological significance.

Marston et al. (1966) stressed the role of ischaemia in cases of segmental colitis which occurred in the older age group. With the recent increasing awareness of the broad spectrum of ischaemic disease of the bowel, there has arisen new interest in a possible vascular aetiology of IBD. Using ^{32}P regional flow studies in patients with ulcerative colitis, Bacaner (1966) demonstrated an insufficient flow pattern possibly characteristic of patients with a later onset of the disease, and increased flow with arterio-venous shunting in other patients suggestive of vasomotor irritability. More recent isotope washout studies correlated blow flow with morphological changes in the bowel and reported significantly increased blood flow associated with severe acute inflammation and reduced perfusion in the late fibrosing stages of disease (Hulten et al., 1977). Allen (1971) called attention to the vascular features of a broad range of intestinal disorders and suggested a common vascular basis for multiple forms of enterocolitis including Crohn's disease and ulcerative colitis. As noted earlier, Fairburn (1973) has suggested that the mucosal damage in ulcerative colitis results from pressure-induced impairment of the microcirculation caused by prolonged, high-amplitude colonic contractions. Numerous reports of extra-intestinal large and small vessel disease, both arterial and venous, may also lend some support to the role of vascular compromise in inducing inflammatory lesions of the bowel (Graef et al., 1966; Salley, Winkleman and Rovelstad, 1975; Yassinger et al., 1976; Wackers et al., 1979).

Besides those studies which have implicated primary vascular disorders, a number of reports have documented a hypercoagulable state associated with inflammatory bowel disease (Lee et al., 1968; Morowitz, Allen and Kirsner, 1968). It is likely, however, that this phenomenon is a secondary event related to chronic inflammation and to the stasis associated with general disability rather than an aetiological mechanism. Again, there may be a subpopulation of patients, especially in the older age peak of IBD, in whom vascular insufficiency plays an intermediary pathogenetic role (Brandt et al., 1979).

Other theories

A handful of other aetiological theories deserve mention. Trauma has been mentioned in the earlier literature as a cause of Crohn's disease, but documented cases are quite rare (Crohn and Yarnis, 1958; Taylor, 1971). Lymphatic obstruction may be an intermediary mechanism in Crohn's disease, explaining its propensity for terminal ileal involvement, and early experimental models gave some support to this mechanism (Reichert and Mathes, 1936). However, underlying causes for lymph node hyperplasia and obstructive lymphoedema would still have to be sought.

Lastly, the role of prostaglandins in the pathogenesis of ulcerative colitis has recently been given attention. After initial reports of elevated prostaglandin levels in the stool, urine, and colonic venous blood in patients with ulcerative colitis (Gould, Brach and Conolly, 1977), Sharon *et al.* (1978) demonstrated the increased synthesis of prostaglandin E by rectal biopsy cultures from patients with ulcerative colitis. Harris, Smith and Swan (1978) further demonstrated increased prostaglandin synthetase activity in rectal biopsy specimens obtained from patients with active colitis as compared with controls who had inactive disease or irritable colon. A similar increase in prostaglandin formation by the rectal mucosa in ulcerative colitis has been reported by Sinzinger, Silberbauer and Seyfried (1979). Nevertheless, as Kimberg (1978) has suggested, prostaglandins may be important not only as mediators of the inflammatory process in the colonic mucosa, but also by alteration of secretory and absorption function in the small and large bowel respectively. Furthermore, the effect of sulphasalazine in inhibiting in vitro synthesis of prostaglandin E by rectal mucosa may play some role in its therapeutic action (Sharon *et al.*, 1978). Further investigation into this area is certain to be forthcoming.

CONCLUSIONS

This review should make it clear to even the most wishful thinkers among us that no aetiological theory has yet produced the key to the mystery of IBD. At this stage of our knowledge, we cannot predict whether the cause of ileitis and colitis will eventually be unearthed by further exploration along the immunological, microbiological, psychosomatic, vascular, dietary, and other avenues outlined in this chapter, or whether – as so often happens in biomedical science – it will be stumbled across serendipitously, perhaps by a veterinary pathologist, food technologist, dental technician, or water pollution control engineer.

For the moment, the only practical approach appears to be to keep working in good faith along all traditional pathways, while keeping our minds receptive to unconventional ideas and our lines of communication open to investigators from many far-flung disciplines.

References

Aaronson, A. & Spiro, H. M. (1973) Mercury and the gut. *American Journal of Digestive Diseases*, **18**, 583–594.

Ahlberg, J., Bergstrand, O., Holmstrom, B., Kronevi, T. & Reiland, S. (1978) Negative findings in search for a transmissible agent in Crohn's disease. *Acta Chirurgica Scandinavica*, Supplement, **482**, 45–47.

Allen, A. C. (1971) A unified concept of the vascular pathogenesis of enterocolitis of varied etiology. A pathophysiologic analysis. *American Journal of Gastroenterology*, **55**, 347–378.

Almy, T. P. (1961) Observations on the pathologic physiology of ulcerative colitis. *Gastroenterology*, **40**, 299–306.

Aluwihare, A. P. (1971) Electron microscopy in Crohn's disease. *Gut*, **12**, 509–518.

Anderson, A. F. R. (1942) Ulcerative colitis – an allergic phenomenon. *American Journal of Digestive Diseases*, **9**, 91–98.

Archer, L. N. & Harvey, R. F. (1978) Breakfast and Crohn's disease – II. *British Medical Journal*, **ii**, 540.

Aronson, M. D., Phillips, C. A., Beeken, W. L. & Forsyth, B. R. (1975) Isolation and characterization of a viral agent from intestinal tissue of patients with Crohn's disease and other intestinal disorders. *Progress in Medical Virology*, **21**, 165–176.

Auer, I. O., Buschmann, Ch. & Ziemer, E. (1978) Immune status in Crohn's disease. 2. Originally unimpaired primary cell mediated immunity in vitro. *Gut*, **19**, 618–626.

Auer, I. O., Wechsler, W., Ziemer, E., Malchow, H. & Sommer, H. (1978) Immune status in Crohn's disease. I. Leukocyte and lymphocyte subpopulations in peripheral blood. *Scandinavian Journal of Gastroenterology*, **13**, 561–571.

Bacaner, M. B. (1966) Quantitative measurement of regional colon blood flow in the normal and pathological human bowel. *Gastroenterology*, **51**, 764–767.

Baklien, K. & Brandtzaeg, P. (1975) Comparative mapping of the local distribution of immunoglobulin-containing cells in ulcerative colitis and Crohn's disease of the colon. *Clinical and Experimental Immunology*, **22**, 197–229.

Ballard, J. & Shiner, M. (1974) Evidence of cytotoxicity in ulcerative colitis from immuno-fluorescent staining of the rectal mucosa. *Lancet*, **i**, 1014–1017.

Bargen, J. A. (1924) Experimental studies on etiology of chronic ulcerative colitis. *Journal of the American Medical Association*, **83**, 332–336.

Bergstrand, O., Holmstrom, B. & Gustafsson, B. G. (1978) Contamination of germfree animals with intestinal Crohn's tissue: a preliminary report. *Acta Chirurgica Scandinavica*, Supplement, **482**, 48–50.

Bockus, H. L. & Lee, W. E. (1935) Regional (terminal) ileitis. *Annals of Surgery*, **102**, 412–421.

Bolton, P. M., Owen, E., Heatley, R. V., Jones Williams, W. & Hughes, L. E. (1973) Negative findings in laboratory animals for a transmissible agent in Crohn's disease. *Lancet*, **ii**, 1122–1123.

Bonfils, S. (1970) Carrageenan and the human gut. *Lancet*, **ii**, 414.

Bookman, M. A. & Bull, D. M. (1979) Characteristics of isolated intestinal mucosal lymphoid cells in inflammatory bowel disease. *Gastroenterology*, **77**, 503–510.

Brandt, L. J., Goldberg, L., Boley, S. J., Mitsudo, S. & Berman, A. (1979) Ulcerative colitis in the elderly (abstract). *Gastroenterology*, **76**, 1106.

Breucha, G. & Riethmuller, G. (1975) Intestinal lymphocytes in Crohn's disease. *Lancet*, **i**, 976.

British Medical Journal (1977) Chasing the cause of Crohn's disease (editorial). *British Medical Journal*, **i**, 929–930.

Britton, S., Eklund, A. E. & Bird, A. G. (1978) Appearance of killer (K) cells in the mesenteric lymph nodes of Crohn's disease. *Gastroenterology*, **75**, 218–220.

Broberger, O. (1964) Immunologic studies in ulcerative colitis. *Gastroenterology*, **47**, 229–240.

Broberger, O. & Perlmann, P. (1959) Autoantibodies in human ulcerative colitis. *Journal of Experimental Medicine*, **110**, 657–674.

Broberger, O. & Perlmann, P. (1962) Demonstration of an epithelial antigen in colon by means of fluorescent antibodies from children with ulcerative colitis. *Journal of Experimental Medicine*, **115**, 13–25.

Broberger, O. & Perlmann, P. (1963) In vitro studies of ulcerative colitis. 1. Reactions of patients' serum with human fetal colon cells in tissue culture. *Journal of Experimental Medicine*, **117**, 705–715.

Brown, W. R., Borthistle, B. K. & Chen, S. T. (1975) Immunoglobulin E (IgE) and IgE-containing cells in human gastrointestinal fluids and tissues. *Clinical and Experimental Immunology*, **20**, 227–237.

Brown, W. R., Lansford, C. L. & Hornbrook, H. (1973) Serum immunoglobulin E (IgE) concentrations in patients with gastrointestinal disorders. *American Journal of Digestive Diseases*, **18**, 641–645.

Buckell, N. S., Gould, S. R., Day, D. W., Lennard-Jones, J. E. & Edwards, A. M. (1978) Controlled trial of disodium cromoglycate in chronic persistent ulcerative colitis. *Gut*, **19**, 1140–1143.

Bull, D. M. & Bookman, M. A. (1977) Isolation and functional characterization of human intestinal submucosal lymphoid cells. *Journal of Clinical Investigation*, **59**, 966–974.

Burnham, W. R., Lennard-Jones, J. E., Stanford, J. L. & Bird, R. G. (1978) Mycobacteria as a possible cause of inflammatory bowel disease. *Lancet*, **ii**, 693–698.

Cady, A. B., Rhodes, J. B., Littman, A. & Crane, R. (1967) Significance of lactose deficit in ulcerative colitis. *Journal of Laboratory and Clinical Medicine*, **70**, 279–286.

Carlsson, H. E., Lagercrantz, R. & Perlmann, P. (1977) Immunological studies in ulcerative colitis. VIII. Antibodies to colon antigen in patients with ulcerative colitis, Crohn's disease and other diseases. *Scandinavian Journal of Gastroenterology*, **12**, 707–714.

Carstensen, J. & Poulsen, E. (1971) Food additives and food contaminants. In *Regional Enteritis (Crohn's Disease)*, Skandia International Symposia, pp. 283–299. Stockholm: Nordiska Bokhandelns Forlag.

Cave, D. R., Mitchell, D. N. & Brooke, B. N. (1975) Experimental animal studies of the etiology and pathogenesis of Crohn's disease. *Gastroenterology*, **69**, 618–624.

Cave, D. R., Mitchell, D. N. & Brooke, B. N. (1976) Preliminary evidence of an agent from ulcerative colitis tissue. *Lancet*, **i**, 1311–1314.

Cave, D. R., Mitchell, D. N. & Brooke, B. N. (1978) Induction of granulomas in mice by Crohn's disease tissue. *Gastroenterology*, **75**, 632–637.

Cave, D. R., Mitchell, D. N., Kane, S. P. & Brooke, B. N. (1973) Further animal evidence of a transmissible agent in Crohn's disease. *Lancet*, **ii**, 1120–1122.

Clancy, E. & Pucci, A. (1978) Absence of K cells in human gut mucosa. *Gut*, **19**, 273–276.

Clancy, R. (1978) Isolation and kinetic characteristics of mucosal lymphocytes in Crohn's disease. *Gastroenterology*, **70**, 177–180.

Cooper, H. S., Raffensperger, E. C., Jonas, L. & Fitts, W. T. (1977) Cytomegalovirus inclusions in patients with ulcerative colitis and toxic dilation requiring colonic resection. *Gastroenterology*, **72**, 1253–1256.

Crohn, B. B. & Yarnis, H. (1958) *Regional Ileitis*. pp. 14–18. New York: Grune and Stratton.

Crohn, B. B., Ginzburg, L. & Oppenheimer, G. D. (1932) Regional ileitis. A pathologic and clinical entity. *Journal of the American Medical Association*, **99**, 1323–1329.

Das, D. M., Dubin, R. & Nagai, T. (1978) Isolation and characterization of colonic tissue-bound antibodies from patients with idiopathic ulcerative colitis. *Proceedings of the National Academy of Sciences*, **9**, 4528–4532.

De Groote, G., Desmyter, J., Vantrappen, G. & Phillips, C. A. (1977) Rotavirus antibodies in Crohn's disease and ulcerative colitis. *Lancet*, **i**, 1263.

Doe, W. F., Booth, C. C. & Brown, D. L. (1973) Evidence for complement-building immune complexes in adult celiac disease, Crohn's disease and ulcerative colitis. *Lancet*, **i**, 402–403.

Donnelly, B. J., Delaney, P. V. & Healy, T. M. (1977) Evidence for a transmissible factor in Crohn's disease. *Gut*, **18**, 360–363.

Dragstedt, L. R., Dack, G. M. & Kirsner, J. B. (1941) Chronic ulcerative colitis: Bacterium necrophorum as etiologic agent. *Annals of Surgery*, **114**, 653–662.

Dronfield, M. W. & Langman, M. J. S. (1978) Comparative trial of sulphasalazine and oral sodium cromoglycate in the maintenance of remission in ulcerative colitis. *Gut*, **19**, 1136–1139.

Dvorak, A. M., Dickersin, G. R., Osage, J. L. & Monahan, R. A. (1978a) Absence of virus structures in Crohn's disease tissues studied by electron microscopy. *Lancet*, **i**, 328.

Dvorak, A. M., Monahan, R. A., Osage, J. E. & Dickersin, G. R. (1978b) Mast-cell degranulation in Crohn's disease. *Lancet*, **i**, 498.

Eckhardt, R., Heinisch, M. & Meyer zum Buschenfelde, K. H. (1976) Cellular immune reactions against common antigen small intestine and colon antigen in patients with Crohn's disease, ulcerative colitis and cirrhosis of the liver. *Scandinavian Journal of Gastroenterology*, **11**, 49–54.

Eckhardt, R., Kloos, P., Dierich, M. P. & Meyer zum Buschenfelde, K. H. (1977) K-lymphocytes (killer cells) in Crohn's disease and acute virus B-hepatitis. *Gut*, **18**, 1010–1016.

Eckhardt, V. R., Hopf, U., Hutteroth, T. H. & Meyer zum Buschenfelde, K. H. (1978) Circulating immune complexes and in vivo fixation of immunoglobulin G, A and C3 onto hepatocytes in patients with Crohn's disease. (In German.) *Zeitschrift für Gastroenterologie*, **12**, 739–744.

Engel, G. L. (1955) Studies of ulcerative colitis. III. The nature of the psychological process. *American Journal of Medicine*, **19**, 231–256.

Engel, G. L. & Salzman, L. F. (1973) A double standard for psychosomatic papers. *New England Journal of Medicine*, **288**, 44–46.

Engstrom, J. F., Arvanitakis, C., Sagawa, A. & Abdou, N. I. (1978) Secretory immunoglobulin deficiency in a family with inflammatory bowel disease. *Gastroenterology*, **74**, 746–751.

Fairburn, R. A. (1973) On the etiology of ulcerative colitis: a vascular hypothesis. *Lancet*, **i**, 697–699.

Falchuk, K. R. & Isselbacher, K. J. (1976) Circulating antibodies to bovine albumin in ulcerative colitis and Crohn's disease. *Gastroenterology*, **70**, 5–8.

Falchuk, Z. M., Barnhard, E. & Machado, I. (1979) Human colonic lamina propria lymphocytes mediate mitogen-induced but not spontaneous cell mediated cytotoxicity (abstract). *Gastroenterology*, **76**, 1129.

Farmer, G. W., Vincent, M. D., Fucillo, D. A., Horta-Barbosa, L., Ritman, S., Sever, J. L. & Gitnick, G. L. (1973) Viral investigations of ulcerative colitis and regional enteritis. *Gastroenterology*, **65**, 8–18.

Feldman, F., Cantor, D., Soll, S. & Bachrach, W. (1967a) Psychiatric study of a consecutive series of 34 patients with ulcerative colitis. *British Medical Journal*, **iii**, 14–17.

Feldman, F., Cantor, D., Soll, S. & Bachrach, W. (1967b) Psychiatric study of a consecutive series of 19 patients with regional ileitis. *British Medical Journal*, **iv**, 711–714.

Felsen, J. (1936) The relationship of bacillary dysentery to distal ileitis, chronic ulcerative colitis, and non-specific intestinal granuloma. *Annual Review of Medicine*, **10**, 645–669.

Fiasse, R., Lurhuma, A. Z., Cambiaso, C. L., Masson, P. L. & Dive, C. (1978) Circulating immune complexes and disease activity in Crohn's disease. *Gut*, **19**, 611–617.

Ginzburg, L. & Oppenheimer, G. D. (1933) Non-specific granulomata of the intestines. *Annals of Surgery*, **98**, 1046–1062.

Gitnick, G. L. & Rosen, V. J. (1976) Electron microscopic studies of viral agents in Crohn's disease. *Lancet*, **ii**, 217–219.

Gitnick, G. L., Arthur, M. H. & Shibata, I. (1976) Cultivation of viral agents from Crohn's disease. *Lancet*, **ii**, 215–217.

Gitnick, G. L., Rosen, V. J., Arthur, M. S. & Hertweck, S. A. (1979) Evidence for the isolation of a new virus from ulcerative colitis patients: comparison with virus derived from Crohn's disease. *Digestive Diseases and Sciences*, **24**, 609–619.

Glick, M. C. & Falchuk, Z. M. (1979) Dinitrochlorobenzene-induced colitis: increased T-cells in the lamina propria (abstract). *Gastroenterology*, **76**, 1139.

Goodwin, J. S., DeHoratius, R., Israel, H., Peake, G. T. & Messner, R. P. (1979) Suppressor cell function in sarcoidosis. *Annals of Internal Medicine*, **90**, 169–173.

Gould, S. R., Brach, A. R. & Conolly, M. E. (1977) Increased prostaglandin production in ulcerative colitis (letter). *Lancet*, **ii**, 98.

Grace, W. J., Pinsley, R. H. & Wolff, H. G. (1954) Treatment of ulcerative colitis. II. *Gastroenterology*, **26**, 462–468.

Grace, W. J., Wolf, S. & Wolff, H. G. (1950) Life situations, emotions and chronic ulcerative colitis. *Journal of the American Medical Association*, **142**, 1044–1048.

Graef, V., Baggenstoss, A. H., Sauer, W. G. & Spittell, J. A. Jr (1966) Venous thrombosis occurring in nonspecific ulcerative colitis. A necropsy study. *Archives of Internal Medicine*, **117**, 377–382.

Green, F. H. Y. & Fox, H. (1975) The distribution of mucosal antibodies in the bowel of patients with Crohn's disease. *Gut*, **16**, 125–131.

Greenberg, H. B., Gebhard, R., McClain, C. J., Soltis, R. D. & Kapikian, A. Z. (1979) Antibodies to viral gastroenteritis viruses in Crohn's disease. *Gastroenterology*, **76**, 349–350.

Groen, J. & Bastiaans, O. (1955) Studies on ulcerative colitis: personality structure, emotional conflict, situations and effects of psychotherapy. In *Modern Trends in Psychosomatic Medicine*. pp. 242ff. London: Butterworth.

Grotsky, H., Hirshaut, Y., Sorokin, C., Sachar, D., Janowitz, H. D. & Glade, P. R. (1971) Epstein-Barr virus and inflammatory bowel disease. *Experientia*, **27**, 1474–1475.

Gryboski, J., Burkle, F. & Hillman, R. (1966) Milk induced colitis in an infant. *Pediatrics*, **38**, 299–302.

Harris, D. W., Smith, P. R. & Swan, H. J. (1978) Determination of prostaglandin synthetase activity in rectal biopsy material and its significance in colonic disease. *Gut*, **19**, 875–877.

Harrison, W. J. (1965) Autoantibodies against intestinal and gastric mucous cells in ulcerative colitis. *Lancet*, **i**, 1346–1350.

Heatley, R. V., Rhodes, J., Calcraft, B. J., Whitehead, R. H., Fifield, R. & Newcombe, R. G. (1975a) Immunoglobulin E in rectal mucosa of patients with proctitis. *Lancet*, **ii**, 1010–1012.

Heatley, R. V., Calcraft, B. J., Rhodes, J., Owen, E. & Evans, B. K. (1975b) Disodium cromoglycate in the treatment of chronic proctitis. *Gut*, **16**, 559–563.

Heatley, R. V., Bolton, P. M., Jones Williams, W., Hughes, L. E. & Owen, E. (1975c) A search for a transmissible agent in Crohn's disease. *Gut*, **16**, 528–532.

Henderson, A. & Hishon, S. (1978) Crohn's disease responding to oral disodium cromoglycate (letter). *Lancet*, **i**, 109–110.

Henderson, C. A., Greenlee, L., Williams, R. G. Jr & Strickland, R. G. (1976) Characterization of antilymphocyte antibodies in inflammatory bowel disease. *Scandinavian Journal of Immunology*, **5**, 837–844.

Hiatt, R. B. & Katz, L. (1962) Mast cells in inflammatory conditions of the gastrointestinal tract. *American Journal of Gastroenterology*, **37**, 541–545.

Hodgson, H. J. F. & Jewell, D. P. (1977) Selective IgA deficiency and Crohn's disease: report of two cases. *Gut*, **18**, 644–646.

Hodgson, H. J. F., Potter, B. J. & Jewell, D. P (1977a) C3 metabolism in ulcerative colitis and Crohn's disease. *Clinical and Experimental Immunology*, **28**, 490–495.

Hodgson, H. J. F., Potter, B. J. & Jewell, D. P. (1977b) Immune complexes in ulcerative colitis and Crohn's disease. *Clinical and Experimental Immunology*, **29**, 187–196.

Hodgson, H. J. F., Potter, B. J. & Jewell, D. P. (1977c) Humeral immune system in inflammatory bowel disease. I. Complement levels. *Gut*, **18**, 749–753.

Hodgson, H. J. F., Wands, J. R. & Isselbacher, K. J. (1978) Decreased suppressor cell activity in inflammatory bowel disease. *Clinical and Experimental Immunology*, **32**, 451–458.

Hodgson, H. J. F., Potter, B. J., Skinner, J. & Jewell, D. P. (1978) Immune-complex mediated colitis in rabbits: an experimental model. *Gut*, **19**, 225–232.

Hulten, L., Lindhagen, J., Lundgren, O., Fasth, S. & Ahren, C. (1977) Regional intestinal blood flow in ulcerative colitis and Crohn's disease. *Gastroenterology*, **72**, 388–396.

James, A. H. (1977) Breakfast and Crohn's disease. *British Medical Journal*, **i**, 943–945.

Jarnerot, G. & Lantorp, K. (1972) Antibodies to EB virus in cases of Crohn's disease. *New England Journal of Medicine*, **286**, 1215–1216.

Jewell, D. P. & MacLennan, I. C. M. (1973) Circulating immune complexes in inflammatory bowel disease. *Clinical and Experimental Immunology*, **14**, 219–226.

Jewell, D. P. & Truelove, S. C. (1972) Circulating antibodies to cow's milk proteins in ulcerative colitis. *Gut*, **13**, 796–801.

Kagnoff, M. F. & Campbell, S. (1976a) Functional characteristics of Peyer's patch lymphoid cells: I. Induction of humoral antibody and cell-mediated allograft reactions. *Journal of Experimental Medicine*, **139**, 398–406.

Kagnoff, M. F. & Campbell, S. (1976b) Antibody-dependent cell-mediated cytotoxicity: comparative ability of murine Peyer's patch and spleen cells to lyse lipopolysaccharide-coated and uncoated erythrocytes. *Gastroenterology*, **70**, 341–346.

Kapikian, A. Z., Barile, M. F., Wyatt, R. G., Yolken, R. H., Tully, J. G., Greenberg, H. B., Kalica, A. R. & Chanock, R. M. (1979) Mycoplasma contamination in cell culture of Crohn's disease material. *Lancet*, **ii**, 466–467.

Karush, A., Daniels, G. E., Flood, C. & O'Connor, J. F. (1977) *Psychotherapy in Chronic Ulcerative Colitis*. pp. 49–50. Philadelphia: W. B. Saunders.

Kemler, B. J. & Alpert, E. (1979) Immunopathogenesis of inflammatory bowel disease: studies of cytotoxicity of [sic] isolated human colon epithelial cells (abstract). *Clinical Research*, **27**, 455A.

Kimberg, D. V. (1978) The ubiquitous prostaglandins and their role in ulcerative colitis (editorial). *Gastroenterology*, **75**, 748–749.

Kirk, B. W. & Freedman, S. O. (1967) Hypogammaglobulinemia, thymoma and ulcerative colitis. *Canadian Medical Association Journal*, **96**, 1272–1277.

Koffler, D., Minkowitz, S., Rothman, W. & Garlock, J. (1962) Immuno-cytochemical studies in ulcerative colitis and regional ileitis. *American Journal of Pathology*, **41**, 733–740.

Korsmeyer, S., Strickland, R. G., Wilson, I. D. & Williams, R. C. Jr (1974) Serum lymphocyto-toxic and lymphocytophilic antibody activity in inflammatory bowel disease. *Gastroenterology*, **67**, 578–583.

Korsmeyer, S. J., Williams, R. G. Jr, Wilson, I. D. & Strickland, R. G. (1975) Lymphocytotoxic antibody in inflammatory bowel disease. A family study. *New England Journal of Medicine*, **293**, 1117–1120.

Krause, U., Michaelsson, G. & Juhlin, L. (1978) Skin reactivity and phagocytic function of neutrophil leucocytes in Crohn's disease and ulcerative colitis. *Scandinavian Journal of Gastroenterology*, **13**, 71–75.

Lagercrantz, R., Perlmann, P. & Hammarstrom, S. (1971) Immunological studies in ulcerative colitis. V. Family studies. *Gastroenterology*, **60**, 381–389.

Lagercrantz, R., Hammarstrom, S., Perlmann, P. & Gustaffsson, B. E. (1968) Immunological studies in ulcerative colitis. III. Incidence of antibodies to colon-antigen in ulcerative colitis and other gastrointestinal diseases. *Clinical and Experimental Immunology*, **1**, 263–276.

Lagercrantz, R., Hammarstrom, S., Perlmann, P. & Gustaffsson, B. E. (1968) Immunological studies in ulcerative colitis. IV. Origin of autoantibodies. *Journal of Experimental Medicine*, **128**, 1339–1352.

Lake, A. M., Stitzel, A. E., Urmson, J. R., Walker, W. A. & Spitzer, R. E. (1979) Complement alterations in inflammatory bowel disease. *Gastroenterology*, **76**, 1374–1379.

Latimer, P. R. (1978) Crohn's disease: a review of the psychological and social outcome. *Psychological Medicine*, **8**, 649–656.

Lee, J. C., Spittell, J. A., Sauer, W. G., Owen, C. A. Jr & Thompson, J. H. Jr (1968) Hyper-coagulability associated with chronic ulcerative colitis: changes in blood coagulation factors. *Gastroenterology*, **54**, 76–86.

Levo, Y. & Livni, N. (1978) Mast-cell degranulation in Crohn's disease (letter). *Lancet*, **i**, 1262.

Lindemann, E. (1950) Modifications in the course of ulcerative colitis in relationship to changes in life situations and reaction patterns. *Proceedings of the Association of Research in Nervous and Mental Disorders*, **29**, 706–723.

Lloyd, G., Green, F. H. Y., Fox, H., Mani, V. & Turnberg, L. A. (1975) Mast cells and immunoglobulin E in inflammatory bowel disease. *Gut*, **16**, 861–866.

MacDermott, R. P., Jenkins, K. M., Franklin, G. O., Weinrieb, I. J., Nash, G. S. & Kodner, I. J. (1979) Antibody dependent (ADCC), spontaneous (SCMC), and lectin induced (LICC) cellular cytotoxicity by human intestinal lymphocytes (abstract). *Gastroenterology*, **76**, 1190.

Machado, I. & Falchuk, Z. M. (1978) Lamina propria lymphocytes: differing responses to mitogenic stimulation between inflammatory bowel disease and other diseases (abstract). *Gastroenterology*, **74**, 1059.

Mani, V., Lloyd, G., Green, F. H. Y., Fox, M. & Turnberg, L. A. (1976) Treatment of ulcerative colitis with oral disodium cromoglycate: a double blind controlled trial. *Lancet*, **i**, 439–441.

Marcussen, H. (1978) Fluorescent anti-colonic and E. coli antibodies in ulcerative colitis. *Scandinavian Journal of Gastroenterology*, **14**, 277–281.

Marcussen, H. & Nerup, J. (1973) Fluorescent anticolon and organ-specific antibodies in ulcerative colitis. *Scandinavian Journal of Gastroenterology*, **8**, 9–14.

Marston, A., Pheils, M. T., Thomas, L. & Morson, B. C. (1966) Ischemic colitis. *Gut*, **7**, 1–15.

Martini, G. A. & Brandes, J. W. (1976) Increased consumption of refined carbohydrates in patients with Crohn's disease. *Klinische Wochenschrift*, **54**, 367–371.

Matthews, N., Tapper-Jones, L., Mayberry, J. F. & Rhodes, R. (1979) Buccal biopsy in diagnosis of Crohn's disease (letter). *Lancet*, **i**, 500–501.

Mayberry, F. J., Rhodes, J. & Newcombe, R. G. (1978) Breakfast and dietary aspects of Crohn's disease. *British Medical Journal*, **ii**, 1401.

McGiven, A. R., Datta, S. P. & Nairn, R. C. (1967) Human serum antibodies against rat colon mucosa. *Nature (London)*, **214**, 288–289.

McKegney, F. P., Gordon, R. O. & Levine, S. M. (1970) A psychosomatic comparison of patients with ulcerative colitis and Crohn's disease. *Psychosomatic Medicine*, **32**, 153–166.

Mee, A. S., Szalvatkowski, M. & Jewell, D. P. (1978) Phagocytosis and intracellular killing in inflammatory bowel disease (abstract). *Gut*, **19**, A456.

Mee, A. J., McLaughlin, J. E., Hodgson, H. J. F. & Jewell, D. P. (1979) Chronic immune colitis in rabbits. *Gut*, **20**, 1–5.

Melnyk, C. S. (1975) Experimental colitis. In *Inflammatory Bowel Disease* (Ed.) Kirsner, J. B. & Shorter, R. G. pp. 23–26. Philadelphia: Lea and Febiger.

Mendeloff, A. I., Mark, M., Siegel, C. I. & Lilienfeld (1970) Illness experience and life stresses in patients with irritable colon and ulcerative colitis. *New England Journal of Medicine*, **282**, 14–17.

Meuret, G., Bitzi, A. & Hammer, B. (1978) Macrophage turnover in Crohn's disease and ulcerative colitis. *Gastroenterology*, **74**, 501–503.

Meuwissen, S. G. M., Nadorp, J. H. S. M. & Tytgat, G. N. J. (1977) Crohn's disease: a review of immunopathological aspects. *Netherlands Journal of Medicine*, **20**, 78–89.

Meuwissen, S. G. M., Schellekens, P. Th. A., Huismans, L. & Tytgat, G. N. (1975) Impaired anamnestic cellular immune response in patients with Crohn's disease. *Gut*, **16**, 854–860.

Meuwissen, S. G. M., Feltkamp-Vroom, Th. M., Brutel de la Riviere, A., von dem Borne, A. E. G. Kr. & Tytgat, G. N. J. (1976) Analysis of the lymphoplasmacytic infiltrate in Crohn's disease, with special reference to identification of lymphocyte-subpopulations. *Gut*, **17**, 770–780.

Meyers, S., Sachar, D. B., Taub, R. N. & Janowitz, H. D. (1976) Anergy to dinitrochlorobenzene and depression of T lymphocytes in Crohn's disease and ulcerative colitis. *Gut*, **17**, 911–915.

Meyers, S., Sachar, D. B., Taub, R. N. & Janowitz, H. D. (1978) Significance of anergy to dinitrochlorobenzene (DNCB) in inflammatory bowel disease: family and postoperative studies. *Gut*, **19**, 249–252.

Mitchell, D. N. & Rees, R. J. (1970) Agent transmissible from Crohn's disease tissue. *Lancet*, **ii**, 168–171.

Mitchell, D. N. & Rees, R. J. W. (1976) Further observations on the transmissibility of Crohn's disease. *Annals of the New York Academy of Sciences*, **278**, 546–558.

Mitchell, D. N., Rees, R. J. & Goswami, K. K. (1976) Transmissible agents from human sarcoid and Crohn's disease tissues. *Lancet*, **ii**, 761–765.

Monk, M., Mendeloff, A. I., Siegel, C. I. & Lilienfeld, A. (1970) An epidemiological study of ulcerative colitis and regional enteritis among adults in Baltimore. III. Psychological and possible stress-precipitating factors. *Journal of Chronic Diseases*, **22**, 565–578.

Monteiro, E., Fossey, J., Shiner, M., Drasar, B. S. & Allison, A. C. (1971) Antibacterial antibodies in rectal and colonic mucosa in ulcerative colitis. *Lancet*, **i**, 249–251.

Morowitz, D. A., Allen, L. W. & Kirsner, J. B. (1968) Thrombocytosis in chronic inflammatory bowel disease. *Annals of Internal Medicine*, **68**, 1013–1021.

Munro, J., Mayberry, J. F., Matthews, N. & Rhodes, J. (1979) Chlamydia and Crohn's disease (letter). *Lancet*, **ii**, 45–46.

Murray, C. B. (1930) Psychogenic factors in the etiology of ulcerative colitis and bloody diarrhea. *American Journal of Medical Science*, **180**, 239–248.

Nairn, R. C., Fothergill, J. E., McEntegart, M. G. & Porteous, I. R. (1962) Gastrointestinal-specific antigen: an immunohistological and serological study. *British Medical Journal*, **i**, 1788–1790.

Nielsen, H., Petersen, P. H. & Svehag, S. E. (1978) Circulating immune complexes in ulcerative colitis. II. Correlation with serum protein concentrations and complement conversion products. *Clinical and Experimental Immunology*, **31**, 81–91.

Nielsen, H., Binder, V., Dougherty, H. & Svehag, S. E. (1978) Circulating immune complexes in ulcerative colitis. I. Correlation to disease activity. *Clinical and Experimental Immunology*, **31**, 72–80.

O'Donoghue, D. P. & Kumar, P. (1979) Rectal IgE cells in inflammatory bowel disease. *Gut*, **20**, 149–153.

Orr, M. M. (1975) Experimental intestinal granulomas. *Proceedings of the Royal Society of Medicine*, **68**, 14.

Parent, K. & Mitchell, P. (1976) Bacterial variants: etiologic agents in Crohn's disease? *Gastroenterology*, **71**, 365–368.

Parent, K. & Mitchell, P. (1978) Cell wall defective variants of pseudomonas-like (Group Va) bacteria in Crohn's disease. *Gastroenterology*, **75**, 368–372.

Parent, K., Mitchell, P. & Krueger, M. (1978) Serological evidence supporting an etiological role for pseudomonas-like bacteria in Crohn's disease (abstract). *Gastroenterology*, **74**, 1074.

Perlmann, P., Lagercrantz, R. & Gustafsson, B. E. (1965) Antigen from colon of germfree rats and antibodies in human ulcerative colitis. *Annals of the New York Academy of Sciences*, **124**, 377–394.

Perlmann, P., Hammarstrom, S., Lagercrantz, R. & Campbell, D. (1967) Auto-antibodies to colon in rats and human ulcerative colitis: cross-reactivity with Escherichia coli 014 antigen. *Proceedings of the Society for Experimental Biology and Medicine*, **125**, 975–980.

Phillpotts, R. J., Weston-Underwood, J., Brooke, B. N. & Hermon-Taylor, J. (1977) Immune-electron microscopy of stool specimens from patients with Crohn's disease. *Lancet*, **i**, 1213.

Rabin, B. S. & Rogers, S. J. (1976) Nonpathogenicity of anti-intestinal antibody in the rabbit. *American Journal of Pathology*, **83**, 269–278.

Ramachandar, K., Sachar, D. B., Janowitz, H. D., Forman, S. P., Douglas, S. D. & Taub, R. N. (1974) B lymphocytes in inflammatory bowel disease. *Lancet*, **ii**, 45–46.

Rao, S. N. (1973) Mast cells as a component of the granulomata in Crohn's disease. *Journal of Pathology*, **109**, 79–82.

Rawcliffe, D. M. & Truelove, S. C. (1978) Breakfast and Crohn's disease – 1. *British Medical Journal*, **ii**, 539–540.

Reichert, F. L. & Mathes, M. E. (1936) Experimental lymphoedema of the intestinal tract and its relation to regional cicatrizing enteritis. *Annals of Surgery*, **104**, 601–616.

Riemann, J. F. (1977) Further electron microscopic evidence of virus-like particles in Crohn's disease. *Acta Hepato-Gastroenterologica*, **24**, 116–118.

Rimpila, J. J., O'Neal, S. T., Drab, I. M., Diab, I. M., Roth, L. J. & Kraft, S. C. (1976) Immunohistochemical studies of inflammatory bowel disease using a freeze-dried tissue technique (abstract). *Gastroenterology*, **70**, 929.

Sachar, D. B. & Auslander, M. O. (1978) Missing pieces in the puzzle of Crohn's disease. *Gastroenterology*, **75**, 745–748.

Sachar, D. B., Taub, R. N., Brown, S. M., Present, D., Korelitz, B. & Janowitz, H. D. (1973) Impaired lymphocyte responsiveness in inflammatory bowel disease. *Gastroenterology*, **64**, 203–209.

Sachar, D. B., Taub, R. N., Ramachandar, K., Meyers, S., Forman, S. P., Douglas, S. D. & Janowitz, H. D. (1976) T and B lymphocytes and cutaneous anergy in inflammatory bowel disease. *Annals of the New York Academy of Sciences*, **278**, 565–573.

Salley, G. O., Winkleman, R. K. & Rovelstad, R. A. (1975) Correlation between regional enterocolitis and cutaneous polyarteritis nodosa. Two case reports and review of the literature. *Gastroenterology*, **69**, 235–239.

Schneierson, S. S., Garlock, J. H., Shore, B., Stuart, W. D., Steinglass, M. & Aronson, B. (1962) Studies on the viral etiology of regional enteritis and ulcerative colitis. A negative report. *American Journal of Digestive Diseases*, **7**, 839–843.

Schuller, J. L., Piket-van Ulsen, J., Veeken, I. V. D., Michel, M. F. & Stolz, E. (1979) Antibodies against chlamydia of lymphogranuloma-venereum type in Crohn's disease. *Lancet*, **i**, 19–20.

Segal, A. W. & Loewi, G. (1976) Neutrophil dysfunction in Crohn's disease. *Lancet*, **ii**, 219–221.

Sharon, P., Ligunsky, M., Rachmilewitz, D. & Zor, U. (1978) Role of prostaglandins in ulcerative colitis. Enhanced production during active disease and inhibition by sulfasalazine. *Gastroenterology*, **75**, 638–640.

Shorter, R. G., Cardoza, M., Huizenga, K. A., ReMine, S. G. & Spencer, R. J. (1969b) Further studies of in vitro cytotoxicity of lymphocytes for colonic epithelial cells. *Gastroenterology*, **57**, 30–35.

Shorter, R. G., Cardoza, M., Spencer, R. J. & Huizenga, K. A. (1969a) Further studies of an in vitro cytotoxicity of lymphocytes from patients with ulcerative and granulomatous colitis for allogeneic colonic epithelial cells, including the effect of colectomy. *Gastroenterology*, **56**, 304–309.

Shorter, R. G., Huizenga, K. A., ReMine, S. G. & Spencer, R. J. (1970b) Effects of preliminary incubation of lymphocytes with serum on their cytotoxicity for colonic epithelial cells. *Gastroenterology*, **58**, 843–850.

Shorter, R. G., Huizenga, K. A. & Spencer, R. J. (1972) A working hypothesis for the etiology and pathogenesis of nonspecific inflammatory bowel disease. *American Journal of Digestive Diseases*, **17**, 1024–1032.

Shorter, R. G., Huizenga, K. A., Spencer, R. J. & Guy, S. K. (1972) Inflammatory bowel disease: the role of lymphotoxin in the cytotoxicity of lymphocytes for colon epithelial cells. *American Journal of Digestive Diseases*, **17**, 689–696.

Shorter, R. G., Spencer, R. J. & Huizenga, K. A. (1968) Inhibition of in vitro cytotoxicity of lymphocytes from patients with ulcerative colitis and granulomatous colitis for allogeneic colonic epithelial cells using horse anti-human thymus serum. *Gastroenterology*, **54**, 227–231.

Shorter, R. G., Cardoza, M. R., ReMine, S. G., Spencer, R. J. & Huizenga, K. A. (1970a) Modification of in vitro cytotoxicity of lymphocytes from patients with chronic ulcerative colitis or granulomatous colitis for allogeneic colonic epithelial cells. *Gastroenterology*, **58**, 692–698.

Shorter, R. G., Huizenga, K. A., Spencer, R. J., Aas, J. & Guy, S. K. (1971) Cytophilic antibody and the cytotoxicity of lymphocytes for colonic cells *in vitro*. *American Journal of Digestive Diseases*, **16**, 673–679.

Shorter, R. G., Huizenga, K. A., Spencer, R. J. & Weedon, D. (1973) Lymphotoxin in nonspecific inflammatory bowel disease lymphocytes. *American Journal of Digestive Diseases*, **18**, 79–83.

Siegelbaum, S. P., Fazio, T. L., Schwartz, S. E., Hubbell, C. & Henry, J. B. (1979) Evidence supporting a genetic pathogenesis for regional enteritis – a prospective familial study (abstract). *Gastroenterology*, **76**, 1247.

Simonowitz, D., Block, G., Riddell, R. H., Kraft, S. C. & Kirsner, J. B. (1977) The production of an unusual tissue reaction in rabbit bowel injected with Crohn's disease homogenates. *Surgery*, **82**, 211–218.

Sinzinger, H., Silberbauer, K. & Seyfried, H. (1979) Rectal mucosa prostacyclin formation in ulcerative colitis (letter). *Lancet*, **i**, 444.

Soltis, R. D., Hasz, D., Morris, M. J. & Wilson, I. D. (1979) Evidence against the presence of circulating immune complexes in chronic inflammatory bowel disease. *Gastroenterology*, **76**, 1380–1385.

Soltoft, J., Petersen, L. & Kruse, P. (1972) Immunoglobulin deficiency and regional enteritis. *Scandinavian Journal of Gastroenterology*, **7**, 233–236.

Sommers, S. C. (1966) Mast cells and Paneth cells in ulcerative colitis. *Gastroenterology*, **51**, 841–851.

Sommers, S. C. & Korelitz, B. I. (1975) Mucosal-cell counts in ulcerative and granulomatous colitis. *American Journal of Clinical Pathology*, **63**, 359–365.

Sorensen, S. F. & Hoj, L. (1977) Lymphocyte subpopulations in Crohn's disease and chronic ulcerative colitis. *Acta Pathologica et Microbiologica Scandinavica*. Section C, **85**, 41–48.

Stanford, J. L., White, S. A., Burnham, W. R., Lennard-Jones, J. E. & Bird, R. G. (1979) Mycobacteria and inflammatory bowel disease (letter). *Lancet*, **i**, 444.

Stobo, J. D., Tomasi, T. B., Huizenga, K. A., Spencer, R. J. & Shorter, R. G. (1976) In vitro studies of inflammatory bowel disease. Surface receptors of the mononuclear cell required to lyse allogenic colon epithelial cells. *Gastroenterology*, **70**, 171–176.

Strickland, R. G. & Sachar, D. B. (1977) The immunology of inflammatory bowel disease. In *Progress in Gastroenterology*, Volume III (Ed.) Jerzy Glass, G.B. pp. 821–838.

Strickland, R. G., Husby, G., Black, W. C. & Williams, R. G. Jr (1975) Peripheral blood and intestinal lymphocyte sub-populations in Crohn's disease. *Gut*, **16**, 847–853.

Strickland, R. G., Volpicelli, N. A., Roninson, J. M., Greenlee, L. S. & McLaren, L. C. (1979) Isolation of infectious agents from patients with inflammatory bowel disease (abstract). *Clinical Research*, **27**, 29.

Sullivan, A. J. (1935) Psychogenic factors in ulcerative colitis. *American Journal of Digestive Diseases and Nutrition*, **2**, 651–656.

Swarbrick, E. T., Kingham, J. G. C., Price, H. L., Blackshaw, A. J., Griffiths, P. D., Darougar, S. & Bucknell, N. A. (1979) Chlamydia, cytomegalovirus, and yersinia in inflammatory bowel disease. *Lancet*, **ii**, 11–12.

Syverton, J. T. (1961) Enteroviruses. *Gastroenterology*, **40**, 331–337.

Taub, R. N., Sachar, D. B., Siltzbach, L. E. & Janowitz, H. D. (1974) Transmission of ileitis and sarcoid granulomas to mice. *Transactions of the Association of American Physicians*, **87**, 219–224.

Taub, R. N., Sachar, D. B., Janowitz, H. D. & Siltzbach, L. E. (1976) Induction of granulomas in mice by inoculation of tissue homogenates from patients with inflammatory bowel disease and sarcoidosis. *Annals of the New York Academy of Sciences*, **278**, 560–564.

Taylor, F. W. (1971) Seat-belt injury resulting in regional enteritis and intestinal obstruction. *Journal of the American Medical Association*, **215**, 1154–1155.

Taylor, K. B. & Truelove, S. C. (1961) Circulating antibodies to milk proteins in ulcerative colitis. *British Medical Journal*, **ii**, 924–929.

Taylor-Robinson, D., O'Morain, C. A., Thomas, B. J. & Levi, A. J. (1979) Low frequency of chlamydial antibodies in patients with Crohn's disease and ulcerative colitis. *Lancet*, **i**, 1162–1163.

Thayer, W. R. Jr (1976) Are the inflammatory bowel diseases immune complex diseases? *Gastroenterology*, **70**, 136–137.

Thayer, W. R., Brown, M., Huyett Sangree, M., Katz, J. & Hersh, T. (1969) Escherichia coli 0:14 and colon hemagglutinating antibodies in inflammatory bowel disease. *Gastroenterology*, **57**, 311–318.

Thomas, B. J., Jarrett, R. J. & Keen, H. (1977) Breakfast and Crohn's disease. *British Medical Journal*, **ii**, 641.

Truelove, S. C. (1961) Ulcerative colitis provoked by milk. *British Medical Journal*, **i**, 154–160.

Wackers, F. J., Tytgat, G. N. & Vreeken, J. (1979) Necrotizing vasculitis and ulcerative colitis. *British Medical Journal*, **iv**, 83–84.

Walker, J. E. G. (1978) Possible diagnostic test for Crohn's disease by use of buccal mucosa. *Lancet*, **ii**, 759–760.

Warren, S. & Sommers, S. C. (1949) Pathogenesis of ulcerative colitis. *American Journal of Pathology*, **25**, 657–674.

Watson, D. & Martucci, R. (1975) Sensitivity to mycobacterial antigens in patients with chronic inflammatory bowel disease. *Clinical Research*, **23**, 100.

Weinstock, H. I. (1962) Successful treatment of ulcerative colitis by psychoanalysis: a survey of 28 cases with follow-up. *Journal of Psychosomatic Diseases*, **6**, 243–249.

Whorwell, P. J., Phillips, C. A., Beeken, W. L., Little, P. K. & Roessner, K. D. (1977) Isolation of reovirus-like agents from patients with Crohn's disease. *Lancet*, **i**, 1169–1170.

Wolf, S. & Goodell, H. (1968) *Harold G. Wolff's Stress and Disease*. Second edition. pp. 66–73, Springfield, Illinois: Charles C. Thomas.

Workshop on Infectious Agents in Inflammatory Bowel Disease; National Foundation for Ileitis and Colitis (1978) Tarrytown, N.Y., November 17–19.

Wright, R. & Truelove, S. C. (1965a) A controlled therapeutic trial of various diets in ulcerative colitis. *British Medical Journal*, **ii**, 138–141.

Wright, R. & Truelove, S. C. (1965b) Circulating antibodies to dietary proteins in ulcerative colitis. *British Medical Journal*, **ii**, 142–144.

Wright, R. & Truelove, S. C. (1966a) Autoimmune reactions in ulcerative colitis. *Gut*, **7**, 32–40.

Wright, R. & Truelove, S. C. (1966b) Serial rectal biopsy in ulcerative colitis during the course of a controlled therapeutic trial of various diets. *American Journal of Digestive Diseases*, **11**, 847–857.

Yassinger, S., Adelman, R., Cantor, D., Halsted, C. H. & Bolt, R. J. (1976) Association of inflammatory bowel disease and large vascular lesions. *Gastroenterology*, **71**, 844–846.

Zeromski, J., Perlmann, P., Lagercrantz, R., Hammarstrom S. & Gustafsson, B. E. (1970) Immunological studies in ulcerative colitis. VII. Anti-colon antibodies of different immunoglobulin classes. *Clinical and Experimental Immunology*, **7**, 469–475.

Section I
Defining targets by understanding aetiopathogenesis of gut inflammation

2
Development of novel drugs for inflammatory bowel disease based on molecular targets

S. SCHREIBER

INTRODUCTION

Inflammatory bowel disease (IBD) now serves as a model for modern drug development. Genetic exploration has defined the first disease gene for a chronic inflammatory, polygenic condition. The clear phenotype, which appears to allow the definition of 'hard' outcome parameters such as mucosal inflammation by endoscopy, has attracted clinical trials with new therapeutic principles. Clinical trials of novel drugs for registration as a treatment for IBD are often pursued on a 'proof-of-principle' basis in the development strategy of companies that aim for larger markets in other chronic inflammatory conditions (e.g. rheumatoid arthritis, psoriasis). Drug companies are attracted by the successful development story of the first anti-tumour necrosis factor (TNF) agent, which has been followed as a paradigm for the development of other experimental drugs. With only two phase II–III multicentre trials, registration needs were satisfied for Crohn's disease. Approval for rheumatoid arthritis could be achieved with one additional large, placebo-controlled trial. With the advent of oral drugs that target inflammatory molecules previously identified as effective targets by biologicals, drug development strategies will return to the traditionally structured schemes of three development phases (phase I, toxicity; phase II, dose ranging and definition of application schedule; phase III, clinical efficacy and side-effects).

PRIMARY DISEASE GENES OR PATHOPHYSIOLOGY – WHERE ARE SUCCESSFUL TARGETS?

It appears unclear whether primary disease genes will be suitable targets for novel drugs. Our current understanding of the genetic aetiology of IBD assumes

33

the existence of several disease genes that have to interact in order to precipitate into a disease risk. A promising approach may be the analysis of disease pathophysiology that is based on primary genetic variants. It is expected that primary pathways will converge and that more generic mechanisms that are secondary to the primary causes may be inhibited with a broader therapeutic success than by targeting disease genes. On the other hand subsegmentation of disease may be no hindrance to therapeutic strategies if predictive molecular markers are identified that could be used to target the appropriate patient subgroups.

AVAILABLE PATHOPHYSIOLOGY-BASED TARGETED THERAPIES: TNF-BINDING AGENTS

The development of TNF-neutralizing drugs may serve as a showcase for the application of pathophysiological insights into actual therapy. It should be pointed out that many other pathophysiology-based therapeutic principles with similar prospects of efficacy are under current development.

Pathophysiological role of TNF

Enhanced secretion of TNF plays an important role in the pathophysiology of IBD[1-3]. TNF induces activation of nuclear factor kappa B (NF-κB) amongst other signalling events. Activation of NF-κB, which is strongly observed in Crohn's disease contributes to many of the destructive cellular and functional events observed in IBD, which are induced or regulated by TNF. Genetic variants in the promoter of the TNF gene, or in the TNF molecule itself, are not involved as primary factors in the aetiology of IBD[4]. However, certain single-nucleotide polymorphisms in the TNF promoter induce an increase in TNF expression[5], which could result in an increased severity factor in Crohn's disease. From its central role in pathophysiology it appears likely that the majority of disease genes that will subsequently be unveiled as important in IBD could be involved in the regulation of TNF or TNF-related processes. For example, the recent discovery of the first major disease for Crohn's disease, NOD 2, suggests that an altered regulation of NF-κB activation (and hence activation of TNF) plays an important role in NOD 2-related pathophysiology[6].

Therapeutic efficacy

The clinical efficacy of the first targeted approach to IBD was exciting news in 1995. The successful design and presumed efficacy of a drug, infliximab, to specifically inhibit an immunological mediator, TNF-α, was quite exciting in the field, when compared to the broad drug discovery strategies employed in the past[7]. Infliximab is an IgG1 molecule of murine descent that is directed against human TNF and which has been chimaerized by replacement of large parts of the antibody's signalling sequence with human DNA sequence. For the first time in IBD therapy, a drug was successfully engineered all the way from the laboratory bench to the bedside. The neutralization of TNF by parenteral administration of infliximab leads to a vast improvement in some but not all patients with Crohn's disease[8-11].

Through repeated administration of infliximab, a subset of patients with Crohn's disease can be maintained in remission[11] and their fistulas apparently remain closed[12] if therapy is continued over a 1-year period. The efficacy of infliximab in ulcerative colitis is unclear; first trials could not generate a positive signal[13].

Potential differences between TNF-binding drugs

Most interestingly, different agents that neutralize TNF through binding appear to convey different clinical efficacies in Crohn's disease. Etanercept (a fusion protein between TNF-receptor II and an immunoglobulin) has not shown any statistically significant clinical efficacy in comparison with placebo in a small trial[15]. The clinical development of humicade (CDP571, a humanized mouse monoclonal against TNF, that is of IgG1 subclass) appears to run into problems, although therapeutic efficacy has been demonstrated in comparison with placebo[16]. Results of the clinical exploration of TBP-1 (recombinant soluble TNF-receptor I) and CDP870 (polyethylene glycol conjugated ('PEGylated') F(ab')2 fragments directed against TNF) are expected from ongoing clinical trials, although positive signals have been observed in small studies. Adalizumab (D2E7, a completely human monoclonal antibody directed against TNF (developed using phage-display technology) is just entering clinical trials in Crohn's disease, but will be approved for therapy of rheumatoid arthritis within the next year.

Anti-TNF compounds may differ in their biological actions, thus resulting in different levels of clinical efficacy. Differentiating factors could include the ability to induce reverse signalling through binding of membrane-expressed TNF[16,17], as well as cytotoxic or pro-apoptotic capabilities[18-20].

Interindividual differences in drug response – pharmacogenetic aspects

There is significant diversity in drug response in the patient population[8,9]. Four weeks after a single infusion of infliximab (5 mg/kg bodyweight) about 30–40% of patients are in complete remission, while in others an incomplete response or no effect is seen. A repeat infusion within 2 weeks induces response (drop of CDAI by at least 70 points) in an additional 13% of patients[11]. It appears that non-responsiveness is not a general phenomenon but rather the result of a differential ability of the TNF-binding antibody to modulate the underlying disease process[9]. While remission rates are very high 1 week after treatment with a single infusion of infliximab this effect declines with time[9], leaving only a few patients (up to 13% 1 year after single infusion) as long-term responders[11]. Immunological studies suggest that the underlying disease process rebounds, with reactivation of TNF expression and NF-κB activation[9].

The variability of response among patients and the stability of the pattern after re-exposure appears to be a good starting point for pharmacogenetic exploration. Genetic markers would be highly useful as part of the therapeutic algorithm if one could select patients who have a particularly high chance for induction of remission, or are at a particular risk for certain side-effects before administration of the

- novel therapeutic principles
- highly selective mechanism of action
- highly effective in patient subgroups
- high therapeutic costs
- potential for severe side effects

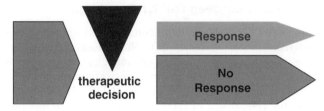

Fig. 1 Therapeutic decisions in biologic therapies in inflammatory bowel disease

drug (Fig. 1). Two cohorts from multicentre, placebo-controlled trials have been investigated. The combination of the two cohorts results in a high specificity and an adequate power to reject negative findings. In a first series of experiments genetic variation in the TNF gene itself and the TNF receptor (I and II) genes could be excluded as pharmacogenetic markers[21]. This is an important finding when one considers previous positive reports that were generated in a retrospective, small series[22,23]. An association between therapeutic outcome and variations in the CARD 15 (NOD 2) gene can also be rejected with the necessary statistical power on the basis of the two-cohort design described above[24]. This is in agreement with a study of an outpatient population in which no association could be found between NOD 2 variations and outcome[25]. The variations in the NOD 2 gene, which were tested (G908R; R702W; 3020insC) are considered primary aetiological factors for the development of Crohn's disease[26–28].

Side-effects

Immunosuppression leading to clinical benefits is accompanied by sometimes severe side-effects, which apparently relate to the very effect of the drug[29]. These side-effects include the occurrence of infectious complications including sepsis and tuberculosis[30,31]. Therefore, the use of immunosuppressive agents should be preceded by adequate screening procedures and – if necessary – the appropriate anti-infective treatment or prophylaxis. An enhanced development of malignant diseases including lymphoma in patients who received treatment with infliximab has been suggested. This has not been evident in larger case series as observed malignancy rates do not statistically differ from those expected in the general population[32].

Immunization against foreign protein is a problem inherent to the application of recombinant proteins. The extent of murine sequence may be one predictor for immunogenicity. However, as even completely 'human' proteins induce neodeterminants (that are not previously known to the immune systems) it is somewhat difficult to predict immunogenicity for new compounds. The main problem is not that of adverse drug reaction at the time of infusion (acute infusion reactions) or in the days thereafter (delayed hypersensitivity, type IV 'serum sickness' reaction), as this can be managed by standard care interventions including glucocorticoids, H1 antagonists and α-adrenergic substances. However, patients who frequently receive recombinant proteins as a last resort are rendered unresponsive to future treatments with that particular drug if they have been immunized.

FUTURE DEVELOPMENTS – PRIMARY DISEASE GENES

Partitioning of Crohn's disease – primary disease genes

With the discovery of the first disease gene in Crohn's disease (NOD 2)[26–28], it has become clear that Crohn's disease itself is a syndrome rather than a single condition, in which several genes in combination determine complex phenotypes and, perhaps, response to some drugs. All three variants in the CARD 15 gene that are associated with Crohn's disease affect the leucine-rich region of the gene, that is a putative interaction site with bacterial and protein antigens. The most important variation, SNP 13, results in a shift of the open reading frame that truncates the protein in this region. Homozygosity or compound heterozygosity for the SNP 13 is associated with a greatly increased susceptibility to develop adult Crohn's disease; it is also associated with an ileal/right colonic phenotype. It is expected that additional disease genes are located on several chromosomes including chromosome 16 with the 'IBD1' susceptibility area[33], chromosome 6 ('IBD3'[4,34–38]), chromosome 12 ('IBD2'[36,37–39]), chromosome 4 ('IBD4'[36,40]) and chromosome 5[41] (Table 1). The next steps in molecular exploration will broaden our understanding of the interplay between different genetic susceptibility factors in this disease, and may identify genetic variations, which may exclusively determine response to specific anti-inflammatory treatments. However, at present it is unclear whether primary disease genes in themselves will be suitable targets for new drugs.

Table 1 Chromosomal locations for suspected disease genes as listed in the OMIM database. The listing includes the first disease gene (CARD 15) that has been identified in Crohn's disease

Name	Chromosome	Sample	Publications
IBD1 (CARD 15)	16q12	F/USA/D	Hugot, Nature 2001; Cho, Nature 2001; Hampe, Lancet 2001
IBD8	16 q/p	D	Hampe, PNAS 2002
IBD2	12p13.2-q24.1	UK	Duerr, AJHG 1998; IBD Consort, AJHG 2001; Satsangi, Nat Gen 1996
IBD3	6p	D	Hampe, AJHG 1999; Dechairo, EJHG 2001
IBD4	14q11/12	USA	Duerr, AJHG 2000; Mah, IBD 1999
IBD5	5q31	Ca	Rioux Nat Gen, 2001; Rioux, AJHG 2000
IBD6	19p13	Ca	Rioux, AJHG 2000
IBD7	1p36	USA	Cho, PNAS 1998; Cho, Hum Mol Gen 2000

ONGOING CLINICAL DEVELOPMENTS BASED ON DISEASE PATHOPHYSIOLOGY

Other targets

Crohn's disease has become a playing field for pharmaceutical developments, which subsequently aim at larger markets such as rheumatoid arthritis and psoriasis. A host of potential drug targets has become available, with animal models having a limited capacity to identify the most promising ones. The tempting advantage of having an efficacy parameter as clear as mucosal inflammation has led to the introduction of appropriate and less appropriate experimental biological therapies at early stages of drug development in patients. However, one should be aware when assessing the risk–benefit ratio that Crohn's disease leads to a sharp reduction in the quality of life during active phases, but does not result in a general decrease in life expectancy in usually young patients.

The past few years have seen the discovery of many immune-relevant drug targets which include immunological mediators (e.g. interleukins IL-1, IL-6, IL-8, IL-12, IL-16, IL-18), transcription factors (e.g. NF-κB, OCT-1, STAT-1, T-bet), adhesion molecules (e.g. ICAM-1, α4–β7 integrin) cell cycle regulating factors (e.g. CD40/CD40-L, OX-40, OX-40L), proliferation-associated enzymes (e.g. various kinases) among many others. In most cases biologicals have been developed to inhibit or modulate these target genes and proteins.

A particularly interesting case is IL-10. IL-10, which was identified in 1989 as 'cytokine synthesis inhibitory factor', profoundly inhibits effector functions of activated macrophages and monocytes *in vitro* (Fig. 2)[42]. IL-10 down-regulates the production of proinflammatory cytokines, interferon-gamma (IFN-γ) and, to a lesser extent, IL-2 production by type 1 T-helper cells[43]. In various *in-vitro* and *in-vivo* models IL-10 shows a strong anti-inflammatory effect[44–46]. This effect may be mediated by inhibition of the activation of NF-κB[47–49], a transcription factor, which initiates or augments the expression of many proinflammatory mediators. Glucocorticoids exert some of their anti-inflammatory actions in a similar manner to IL-10, by inhibition of the activation of NF-κB[50,51].

Inflammation

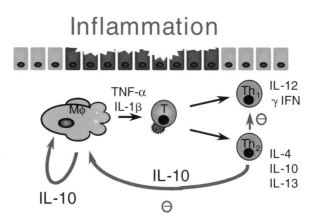

Fig. 2 Anti-inflammatory action of human recombinant IL-10

IL-10 is involved in the maintenance of the normal non-inflammatory state of the intestine[52]. IL-10 inhibits *in vitro* the proinflammatory activities of mononuclear cells which have been isolated from the intestinal lamina propria of patients with IBD[45]. Clinical studies have suggested that IL-10 has some therapeutic activity in mild to moderate, untreated Crohn's disease[53]. In a large trial in chronic active, steroid-refractory Crohn's disease only limited clinical effects were seen[54], and promising data from an earlier pilot study in this condition could not be confirmed[55]. In a blinded subanalysis of the 329 patients included in the trial it appeared that a responder subpopulation with a distinct down-regulation of the NF-κB system was present[54]. Unfortunately, a pharmacogenetic substudy was not part of the development programme.

The clinical response to IL-10 followed a bell-shaped dose–response curve with higher doses of IL-10 leading to reduced clinical efficacy. This appeared mainly due to side-effects including anaemia through the induction of IFN-γ and other immunoregulatory cytokines[56]. While a systemic application of high doses of IL-10 may be not suitable, the topical application[45] is currently being re-studied. Possible genetic approaches, which have generated promising preclinical data, include the use of IL-10-producing lactobacilli[57] or of gut-homing T cells, that are isolated from peripheral blood and transfected with an IL-10 construct *ex vivo* before they are reinfused[58]. Both approaches will generate high mucosal levels of IL-10 and the first clinical results are awaited with great interest.

The most promising new drug developments which approach the approval process are monoclonal antibodies which are directed against the integrin system (e.g. natalizumab directed against α4-integrin) and IFN-β. It also appears important to reassess recombinant IL-1 receptor antagonist (IL-1ra, anakinra) as this molecule apparently failed a small trial for Crohn's disease (results were not published) but has shown strong signs of clinical efficacy in rheumatoid arthritis[59]. Many other novel agents which have either failed or are in the early stages of clinical development have recently been reviewed in detail[60].

The next generation of therapies

While a host of therapeutic trials has been launched, or are currently being prepared, using recombinant proteins to antagonize targets, the first new targeted developments return to orally available small molecules. A particularly interesting concept is the introduction of orally available antisense oligonucleotides which could block the mucosal production of TNF (Orasense by ISIS Pharmaceuticals). However, this compound is still in the early stages of clinical research. Other developments include the refinement of anti-TNF compounds that are based on thalidomide. Thalidomide, approved in many markets for the therapy of lepra[61], has shown some signs of a clinical effect in small trials in Crohn's disease[62,63].

A good example for a targeted development of an oral compound using combinatorial chemistry is the inhibition of MAP-kinase p38, as this molecule has been revealed to be a relevant proximal regulator of TNF expression in Crohn's disease and other autoimmune conditions. Here, a designer drug approach has been adopted to generate a series of small molecule specific inhibitors[64], which are currently making their way into clinical phase II trials in Crohn's disease, rheumatoid arthritis and psoriasis.

OUTLOOK

Crohn's disease therapy is a field that will witness the successful development of biological drugs that will probably result in potent beneficial effects in patient subpopulations. Biological drugs can identify and confirm targets that will be addressed by subsequent developments of orally available small-molecule compounds. The progress in IBD therapy outlines how the findings that have come about from the present genomic revolution can be used. However, the real test of the value of genomic insights that are generated in IBD will be the effect of novel drugs on the long-term quality of life of the patients.

The induction of mucosal healing by infliximab, which cannot be achieved with glucocorticoids, or requires a long period of treatment with azathioprine (if successful at all), results in a slow but steady redefinition of remission as a clinical endpoint in the general approach to the disease. It is therefore anticipated that future clinical developments will have to address remission rather than response as a clinical endpoint. The definition of remission may have to include endoscopic healing (which is not well defined as of yet[65]) in addition to the clinical presentation as mucosal recovery may be associated with a favourable mid-term prognosis[66].

It is our sincere hope that these developments are accompanied by the definition of molecular markers that help to predict the selective response to some of the drugs. The future of Crohn's disease therapy cannot evolve to a trial-and-error scheme using various recombinant, parenteral therapies, but rather has to develop into a rational use to compounds including oral drugs.

Acknowledgements

The work described in this chapter was partially supported by grants from the BMBF (Competence Network Inflammatory Bowel Disease, German National Genome Research Network) and the Deutsche Forschungsgemeinschaft. Parts of the chapter have appeared in similar form in other publications.

References

1. MacDonald TT, Hutchings P, Choy MY, Murch S, Cooke A. Tumour necrosis factor-alpha and interferon-gamma production measured at the single cell level in normal and inflamed human intestine. Clin Exp Immunol. 1990;81:301–5.
2. Reinecker H-C, Steffen M, Witthoeft T et al. Enhanced secretion of tumour necrosis factor-alpha, IL-6, and IL-1 beta by isolated lamina propria mononuclear cells from patients with ulcerative colitis and Crohn's disease. Clin Exp Immunol. 1993;94:174–81.
3. Schreiber S, Nikolaus S, Hampe J et al. Tumor necrosis factor-α and interleukin 1β in relapse of Crohn's disease. Lancet. 1999;353:459–61.
4. Hampe J, Shaw SH, Saiz R et al. Linkage of inflammatory bowel disease to human chromosome 6p. Am J Hum Genet. 1999;65:1647–55.
5. Bouma G, Crusius JB, Oudkerk-Pool M et al. Secretion of tumour necrosis factor alpha and lymphotoxin alpha in relation to polymorphisms in the TNF genes and HLA-DR alleles. Relevance for inflammatory bowel disease. Scand J Immunol. 1996;43:456–63.
6. Beutler B. Autoimmunity and apoptosis: the Crohn's connection. Immunity. 2001;15:5–14.
7. van Dullemen HM, van Deventer SJH, Hommes DW et al. Treatment of Crohn's disease with anti-tumor necrosis factor chimeric antibody (cA2). Gastroenterology. 1995;109:129–35.

8. Targan SR, Hanauer SB, van Deventer SJH *et al*. A short term study of chimeric monoclonal antibody cA2 to tumor necrosis factor-α for Crohn's disease. N Engl J Med. 1997;337:1029–35.
9. Nikolaus S, Raedler A, Sfikas N, Kühbacher T, Fölsch UR, Schreiber S. Mechanisms in failure of infliximab for Crohn's disease. Lancet. 2000;356:1475–9.
10. Schreiber S, Campieri M, Colombel JF *et al*. Use of anti-tumour necrosis factor agents in inflammatory bowel disease. European Guidelines for 2001–2003. Int J Colorectal Dis. 2001;16:1–11.
11. Hanauer SB, Feagan BG, Lichtenstein GR *et al*. Maintenance infliximab for Crohn's disease: the ACCENT I randomized trial. Lancet. 2002;359:1541–9.
12. Sands WJ, van Deventer S, Bernstein C *et al*. Long-term treatment of fistulizing Crohn's disease: response to infliximab in the ACCENT II trial through 54 weeks. Gastroenterology. 2002;122:A81 (abstract).
13. Probert CSJ, Hearing SD, Schreiber S *et al*. Infliximab in glucocorticoid-resistant ulcerative colitis – a randomized controlled trial. (Submitted.)
14. Sandborn WJ, Hanauer SB, Katz S *et al*. Etanercept for active Crohn's disease: a randomized, double-blind, placebo-controlled trial. Gastroenterology. 2001;121:1088–94.
15. Stack WA, Mann SD, Roy AJ *et al*. Randomised controlled trial of CDP571 antibody to tumour necrosis factor-alpha in Crohn's disease. Lancet. 1997;22:521–4.
16. Kriegler M, Perez C, DeFay K, Albert I, Lu SD. A novel form of TNF/cachectin is a cell surface cytotoxic transmembrane protein: ramifications for the complex physiology of TNF. Cell. 1988; 53:45–53.
17. Waetzig G, Seegert D, Rosenstiel P, Nikolaus N, Schreiber S. p38 mitogen-activated protein kinase is activated and linked to TNF-alpha signaling in inflammatory bowel disease. J Immunol. 2002;168:5342–51.
18. Scallon BJ, Moore MA, Trinh DM, Ghrayeb J. Chimeric anti-TNF – α monoclonal antibody, cA2, binds recombinant transmembrane TNF-α and activates immune effector functions. Cytokine. 1995;7:251–9.
19. ten Hove T, van Montfrans C, Peppelenbosch MP, van Deventer SJ. Infliximab treatment induces apoptosis of lamina propria T lymphocytes in Crohn's disease. Gut. 2002;50:206–11.
20. Lugering A, Schmidt M, Lugering N, Pauels HG, Domschke W, Kucharzik T. Infliximab induces apoptosis in monocytes from patients with chronic active Crohn's disease by using a caspase-dependent pathway. Gastroenterology. 2001;121:1145–57.
21. Mascheretti S, Hampe J, Kühbacher T *et al*. Pharmacogenetic investigation of the TNF/TNF-receptor system in patients with chronic active Crohn's disease treated with infliximab. Pharmacogenomics J. 2002;2:127–36.
22. Taylor KD, Plevy SE, Yang H *et al*. ANCA pattern and LTA haplotype relationships to clinical responses to anti-TNF antibody treatment in Crohn's disease. Gastroenterology. 2001;120:1347–55.
23. Vermeire S, Monsuur F, Groenen P, Peeters M, Vlietinck R, Rutgeerts P. Response to anti-TNFa treatment is associated with the TNFa-308*1 allele. Gastroenterology. 2000;118:A654.
24. Mascheretti S, Hampe J, Croucher PJP *et al*. Response to infliximab treatment in Crohn's disease is not associated with mutations in the CARD15 (NOD2) gene. Pharmacogenetics. 2002; 12: 509–15.
25. Vermeire S, Louis E, Rutgeerts P and the Belgian Group of Infliximab Expanded Access Program and Fondation Jean Dausset CEPH, Paris, France. NOD2/CARD15 does not influence response to infliximab in Crohn's disease. Gastroenterology. 2002;123:106–11.
26. Hugot JP, Chamaillard M, Zouali H *et al*. Association of NOD2 leucine-rich repeat variants with susceptibility to Crohn's disease. Nature. 2001;411:599–603.
27. Ogura Y, Bonen DK, Inohara N *et al*. A frameshift mutation in NOD2 associated with susceptibility to Crohn's disease. Nature. 2001;411:603–6.
28. Hampe J, Cuthbert A, Croucher PJ *et al*. Association between insertion mutation in NOD2 gene and Crohn's disease in German and British populations. Lancet. 2001;357:1925–8.
29. Aithal GP, Mansfield JC. Review article: The risk of lymphoma associated with inflammatory bowel disease and immunosuppressive treatment. Aliment Pharmacol Ther. 2001;15:1101–8.
30. Nunez Martinez O, Ripoll Noiseux C, Carneros Martin JA, Gonzalez Lara V, Gregorio Maranon HG. Reactivation tuberculosis in a patient with anti-TNF-alpha treatment. Am J Gastroenterol. 2001;96:1665–6.
31. Keane J, Gershon S, Wise RP *et al*. Tuberculosis associated with infliximab, a tumor necrosis factor alpha-neutralizing agent. N Engl J Med. 2001;345:1098–104.
32. Bickston SJ, Lichtenstein GR, Arseneau KO, Cohen RB, Cominelli F. The relationship between infliximab treatment and lymphoma in Crohn's disease. Gastroenterology. 1999;117:1433–7.

33. Hampe J, Frenzel H, Mirza MM et al. Evidence for a NOD2 independent susceptibility locus for inflammatory bowel disease on chromosome 16p. Proc Natl Acad Sci USA. 2002;99:321–6.

34. Rioux JD, Silverberg MS, Daly MJ et al. Genomewide search in Canadian families with inflammatory bowel disease reveals two novel susceptibility loci. Am J Hum Genet. 2000;66:1863–70.

35. Satsangi J, Welsh KI, Bunce M et al. Contribution of genes of the major histocompatibility complex to susceptibility and disease phenotype in inflammatory bowel disease. Lancet. 1996;347:1212–17.

36. Hampe J, Schreiber S, Shaw S et al. A genomewide analysis provides evidence for novel linkages in inflammatory bowel disease in a large European cohort. Am J Hum Genet. 1999;64:808–16.

37. Satsangi J, Parkes M, Louis E et al. Two stage genome-wide search in inflammatory bowel disease provides evidence for susceptibility loci on chromosomes 3, 7 and 12. Nat Genet. 1996;14:199–202.

38. Duerr RH, Barnada M, Zhang L et al. Linkage and association between inflammatory bowel disease and a locus on chromosome 12. Am J Hum Genet. 1998;63:95–100.

39. Yang H, Ohmen JD, Ma Y et al. Additional evidence of linkage between Crohn's disease and a putative locus on chromosome 12. Genet Med. 1999;1:194–8.

40. Cho JH, Nicolae DL, Gold LH et al. Identification of novel susceptibility loci for inflammatory bowel disease on chromosomes 1p, 3q, and 4q: evidence for epistasis between 1p and IBD1. Proc Natl Acad Sci USA. 1998;95:7502–7.

41. Rioux JD, Daly MJ, Silverberg MS et al. Genetic variation in the 5q31 cytokine gene cluster confers susceptibility to Crohn disease. Nat Genet. 2001;29:223–8.

42. de Waal Malefyt R, Yssel H, Roncarolo M-G, Spits H, de Vries JE. Interleukin 10. Curr Opin Immunol. 1992;4:314–22.

43. Fiorentino DF, Bond MW, Mosmann TR. Two types of mouse T helper cells. IV. Th2 clones secrete a factor that inhibits cytokine production by Th1 clones. J Exp Med. 1989;170:2081–95.

44. Pajkrt D, Camoglio L, Tiel-van Buul MC et al. Attenuation of proinflammatory response by recombinant human IL-10 in human endotoxemia: effect of timing of recombinant human IL-10 administration. J Immunol. 1997;158:3971–7.

45. Schreiber S, Heinig T, Thiele HG, Raedler A. Immunoregulatory role of interleukin 10 in patients with inflammatory bowel disease. Gastroenterology. 1995;108:1434–44.

46. Asadullah K, Sterry W, Stephanek K et al. IL-10 is a key cytokine in psoriasis. Proof of principle by IL-10 therapy: a new therapeutic approach. J Clin Invest. 1998;101:783–94.

47. Wang P, Wu P, Siegel MI, Egan RW, Billah MM. Interleukin (IL)-10 inhibits nuclear factor kappa B (NF kappa B) activation in human monocytes. IL-10 and IL-4 suppress cytokine synthesis by different mechanisms. J Biol Chem. 1995;270:9558–63.

48. Schreiber S, Nikolaus S, Hampe J. Activation of nuclear factor kappa B in inflammatory bowel disease. Gut. 1998;42:477–85.

49. Schottelius AJ, Mayo MW, Sartor RB, Baldwin AS Jr. Interleukin-10 signaling blocks inhibitor of kappaB kinase activity and nuclear factor kappaB DNA binding. J Biol Chem. 1999;274:31868–74.

50. Scheinman RI, Cogswell PC, Lofquist AK, Baldwin Jr. AS. Role of transcriptional activation by IkB in mediation of immunosuppression by glucocorticoids. Science. 1995;270:283–6.

51. Auphan N, DiDonato JA, Rosette C, Helmberg A, Karin M. Immunosuppression by glucocorticoids: inhibition of NFκB activity through induction of IkB synthesis. Science. 1995;270:286–90.

52. Kühn R, Löhler J, Rennick D, Rajewsky K, Müller W. Interleukin-10-deficient mice develop chronic enterocolitis. Cell. 1993;75:263–74.

53. Fedorak RN, Gangl A, Elson CO et al. Recombinant human interleukin-10 in the treatment of patients with mild to moderately active Crohn's disease. Gastroenterology. 2000;119:1473–82.

54. Schreiber S, Fedorak RN, Nielsen OH et al. Recombinant human interleukin-10 in active Crohn's disease. Gastroenterology. 2000;119:1461–72.

55. Van Deventer SJ, Elson CO, Fedorak RN. Multiple doses of intravenous interleukin 10 in patients with inflammatory bowel disease. Gastroenterology. 1997;1113:383–9.

56. Tilg H, van Montfrans C, van Den Ende A et al. Treatment of Crohn's disease with recombinant human interleukin 10 induces the proinflammatory cytokine interferon gamma. Gut. 2002;50:191–5.

57. Steidler L, Hans W, Schotte L et al. Treatment of murine colitis by Lactococcus lactis secreting interleukin-10. Science. 2000;289:1352–5.

58. Van Deventer SJ. The future of inflammatory bowel disease therapy. Inflamm Bowel Dis. 2002;8:301–5.
59. Jiang Y, Genant HK, Watt I et al. A multicenter, double-blind, dose-ranging, randomized, placebo-controlled study of recombinant human interleukin-1 receptor antagonist in patients with rheumatoid arthritis: radiologic progression and correlation of Genant and Larsen scores. Arthritis Rheum. 2000;43:1001–9.
60. Sandborn WJ, Targan SR. Biologic therapy of inflammatory bowel disease. Gastroenterology. 2002;122:1592–608.
61. Iyer CG, Languillon J, Ramanujam K et al. WHO co-ordinated short-term double-blind trial with thalidomide in the treatment of acute lepra reactions in male lepromatous patients. Bull World Health Org. 1971;45:719–32.
62. Vasiliauskas EA, Kam LY, Abreu-Martin MT et al. An open-label pilot study of low-dose thalidomide in chronically active, steroid-dependent Crohn's disease. Gastroenterology. 1999;117:1278–87.
63. Ehrenpreis ED, Kane SV, Cohen LB, Cohen RD, Hanauer SB. Thalidomide therapy for patients with refractory Crohn's disease: an open-label trial. Gastroenterology. 1999;117:1271–7.
64. Pargellis C, Tong L, Churchill L et al. Inhibition of p38 MAP kinase by utilizing a novel allosteric binding site. Nat Struct Biol. 2002;9:268–72.
65. Cellier C, Sahmoud T, Froguel E et al. Correlations between clinical activity, endoscopic severity, and biological parameters in colonic or ileocolonic Crohn's disease. A prospective multicentre study of 121 cases. Groupe d'Études Thérapeutiques des Affections Inflammatoires Digestives. Gut. 1994;35:231–5.
66. Allez M, Lemann M, Bonnet J, Cattan P, Jian R, Modigliani R. Long term outcome of patients with active Crohn's disease exhibiting extensive and deep ulcerations at colonoscopy. Am J Gastroenterol. 2002;97:947–53.

3
On the role of innate immunity during mucosal defence and intestinal infections: are there new therapeutic targets for intervention?

S. BAUER

INTRODUCTION

In vertebrates the immune system can be broadly categorized as an adaptive and innate system. Adaptive immunity relies on clonally distributed T and B cells which confer a specific and memory response against pathogens. The innate immune system has developed germ-line encoded pattern recognition receptors (PRR) that promote rapid responses to microbial pathogens during the invading phase. Cueing on conserved pathogen-associated molecular patterns (PAMP) which are not present in the host, cells of the innate immune system activate and direct the emanating response against pathogens[1]. Two classes of PRR on antigen-presenting cells (APC) have been identified: one class of receptors facilitate uptake of pathogens such as the membrane anchored mannose-binding receptor. These receptors lead to internalization of pathogens with subsequent presentation of antigen via major histocompatibility complex (MHC) molecules but do not activate these cells. In contrast, Toll-like receptors, as members of the second class of PRR, activate APC after engagement of their cognate PAMP to express costimulatory molecules and to secrete proinflammatory (tumor-necrosis factor (TNF)-α, interleukin (IL)-6) and regulatory cytokines (IL-12, IL-18)[2]. Overall the innate immune system is central in sensing an infection and directing the adaptive immune response[3].

MUCOSA, TOLL-LIKE RECEPTORS AND INNATE IMMUNITY

The mucosal surface of the gastrointestinal tract is challenged with a large quantity of microbes and, in the colon for example, up to 10^9 microorganisms are present per millilitre of luminal content. A single layer of polarized intestinal epithelial

44

cells (IEC) separates the lumen of the gastrointestinal tract from the underlying gut-associated lymphoid tissue. Over the past decade it has been shown that IECs not only provide a barrier for luminal microorgansims but are also capable of modulating the mucosal immune response. For example, IECs secrete cytokines and chemokines, and interact with cells of myeloid origin, e.g. T cells, dendritic cells and polymorphonuclear lymphocytes[4]. Furthermore, IECs express immunologically relevant molecules on their cell surface such as Toll-like receptors which are implicated in innate immune responses[5].

Toll receptors are transmembranal proteins which are conserved in evolution between insects and vertebrates[6]. In *Drosophila*, toll was first identified as an essential molecule for dorsal–ventral patterning of the embryo, and subsequently as a key molecule for the antifungal immune response in the adult animal[7]. A homologous family of toll receptors, termed toll-like receptors (TLR), exists in vertebrates[6]. In humans 10 members (TLR1–10) have been reported which are fundamental in recognition of PAMP[6,8,9]. TLR2 and TLR4 recognize different cell wall components of Gram-positive and Gram-negative bacteria as well as heat-shock proteins[10]. TLR3 and TLR5 are fundamental for the recognition of double-stranded RNA[11] and flagellin[12], respectively. TLR9 recognizes bacterial CpG-DNA[13]. TLR1 and TLR6 form heterodimers with TLR2 and broaden the spectrum of ligand recognition[14,15]. Recently we identified a synthetic antiviral compound, the imidazoquinoline resiquimod (R-848), as activator for TLR7[16] and for TLR8[17]. The natural ligands for TLR7, TLR8 and TLR10 have not yet been identified (Fig. 1).

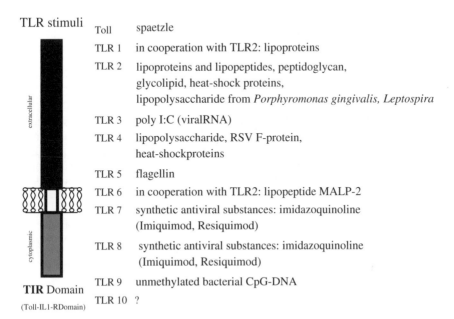

TLR stimuli	Toll	spaetzle
	TLR 1	in cooperation with TLR2: lipoproteins
	TLR 2	lipoproteins and lipopeptides, peptidoglycan, glycolipid, heat-shock proteins, lipopolysaccharide from *Porphyromonas gingivalis, Leptospira*
	TLR 3	poly I:C (viralRNA)
	TLR 4	lipopolysaccharide, RSV F-protein, heat-shockproteins
	TLR 5	flagellin
	TLR 6	in cooperation with TLR2: lipopeptide MALP-2
	TLR 7	synthetic antiviral substances: imidazoquinoline (Imiquimod, Resiquimod)
	TLR 8	synthetic antiviral substances: imidazoquinoline (Imiquimod, Resiquimod)
	TLR 9	unmethylated bacterial CpG-DNA
	TLR 10	?

TIR Domain
(Toll-IL1-RDomain)

Fig. 1 TLRs and their ligands

TLRs sense PAMPs and activate immune cells via the MyD88-dependent TLR/IL-1R signalling pathway which involves downstream mediators such as myeloid differentiation primary response gene 88 (MyD88), IL-1 receptor-associated kinase (IRAK), and TNF receptor-associated factor 6 (TRAF-6). Oligomerization of TRAF-6 leads to the activation of mitogen-activated protein kinases (MAPK), stress-activated protein kinase c-Jun N-terminal kinase (JNK), p38 and the transcription factors activating protein-1 (AP-1) and nuclear factor-κB (NF-κB)[18,19].

TOLL-LIKE RECEPTORS ON IECs IN INFLAMMATORY BOWL DISEASE (IBD)

Inflammatory bowel disease is thought to result from sustained and inappropriate activation of the mucosal immune system driven by the luminal flora. Defects in the barrier function of IECs and the mucosal immune system may facilitate this aberrant response[20]. Genetic factors contribute to susceptibility to inflammatory bowel diseases such as Crohn's disease and ulcerative colitis. Mapping of chromosome 16 has recently resulted in the identification of NOD2 which, at least in part, is linked to susceptibility to Crohn's disease[21,22]. NOD2 is expressed in macrophages and may serve as a PRR for bacterial lipopolysaccharide. Surprisingly, NOD2 variants are responsible for reduced macrophage activation of NF-κB in response to lipopolysaccharide[23]. The immune response and inflammatory pathways involved in the mucosa from patients with Crohn's disease or ulcerative colitis is different. The mucosa of patients with established Crohn's disease is dominated by CD4$^+$ T cells with a type 1 helper T cell phenotype. These cells produce interferon-γ (IFN-γ) and interleukin-2 (IL-2). In contrast, the mucosa of ulcerative colitis patients is dominated by CD4$^+$ T cells with an atypical type 2 helper T cell (Th2) phenotype which is characterized by the production of transforming growth factor-β (TGF-β) and IL-5[20].

The expression of TLRs in healthy humans and patients with Crohn's disease or ulcerative colitis has recently been analysed by polymerase chain reaction or antibodies against TLRs. IECs of healthy donors strongly express TLR3 and TLR5[5,24]. Interestingly, TLR5 is highly expressed on the basolateral surface of intestinal epithelial cells, giving an explanation of how IECs regulate their ability to direct their response to bacterial products, e.g. the TLR5 ligand flagellin[24]. Since flagellin should be present at high doses in the gut lumen, apical expression of TLR5 and constant signalling of non- and pathogenic bacteria would not be favourable. Basolateral expression detects only infiltrating bacteria which need to be controlled by an appropriate immune response initiated by TLR5 signalling. The polarized and functional expression of TLR2 and TLR4 is less clear. Lipopolysaccharide (LPS) recognition by TLR4 requires two more proteins, namely MD-2 and CD14, which are not highly expressed in IECs[25,26]. Nevertheless functional responses to LPS have been reported in IECs, and recent data show that TLR4 expression is detected in the Golgi apparatus and colocalizes with internalized LPS[5,27].

Interestingly, TLR expression in IECs of Crohn's disease patients and patients with ulcerative colitis is different compared to control samples. Whereas control

IECs show strong expression of TLR3 and TLR5, and weak expression of TLR2 and TLR4, IECs from Crohn's disease patients up-regulate TLR4 expression. In contrast, IECs from patients with ulcerative colitis also up-regulate TLR4, but strongly down-regulate TLR3. Taken together these data imply that IBD may be associated with distinctive changes in selective TLR expression in the intestinal epithelium[28].

Considering the different Th1 and Th2 phenotype of Crohn's disease and ulcerative colitis, one could speculate that stimulation with TLR ligands or antagonist may be beneficial for the treatment of the diseases.

References

1. Medzhitov R, Janeway Jr CA. Innate immunity: impact on the adaptive immune response. Curr Opin Immunol. 1997;9:4–9.
2. Medzhitov R, Janeway Jr C. Innate immunity. N Engl J Med. 2000;343:338–44.
3. Janeway CA Jr, Medzhitov R. Introduction: the role of innate immunity in the adaptive immune response. Semin Immunol. 1998;10:349–50.
4. Eckmann L, Kagnoff MF. Cytokines in host defense against *Salmonella*. Microbes Infect. 2001; 3:1191–200.
5. Cario E, Rosenberg IM, Brandwein SL, Beck PL, Reinecker HC, Podolsky DK. Lipopolysaccharide activates distinct signaling pathways in intestinal epithelial cell lines expressing Toll-like receptors. J Immunol. 2000;164:966–72.
6. Rock FL, Hardiman G, Timans JC, Kastelein RA, Bazan JF. A family of human receptors structurally related to *Drosophila* Toll. Proc Natl Acad Sci USA. 1998;95:588–93.
7. Lemaitre B, Nicolas E, Michaut L, Reichhart JM, Hoffmann JA. The dorsoventral regulatory gene cassette spatzle/Toll/cactus controls the potent antifungal response in *Drosophila* adults. Cell. 1996;86:973–83.
8. Du X, Poltorak A, Wei Y, Beutler B. Three novel mammalian toll-like receptors: gene structure, expression, and evolution. Eur Cytokine Netw. 2000;11:362–71.
9. Chuang T, Ulevitch RJ. Identification of hTLR10: a novel human Toll-like receptor preferentially expressed in immune cells. Biochim Biophys Acta. 2001;1518:157–61.
10. Medzhitov R. Toll-like receptors and innate immunity. Nature Rev Immunol. 2001;1:135–45.
11. Alexopoulou L, Holt AC, Medzhitov R, Flavell RA. Recognition of double-stranded RNA and activation of NF-kappaB by Toll-like receptor 3. Nature. 2001;413:732–8.
12. Hayashi F, Smith KD, Ozinsky A *et al.* The innate immune response to bacterial flagellin is mediated by Toll-like receptor 5. Nature. 2001;410:1099–103.
13. Hemmi H, Takeuchi O, Kawai T *et al.* A Toll-like receptor recognizes bacterial DNA. Nature. 2000;408:740–5.
14. Hajjar AM, O'Mahony DS, Ozinsky A *et al.* Cutting edge: functional interactions between toll-like receptor (TLR) 2 and TLR1 or TLR6 in response to phenol-soluble modulin. J Immunol. 2001; 166:15–19.
15. Takeuchi O, Kawai T, Muhlradt PF *et al.* Discrimination of bacterial lipoproteins by Toll-like receptor 6. Int Immunol. 2001;13:933–40.
16. Hemmi H, Kaisho T, Takeuchi O *et al.* Small anti-viral compounds activate immune cells via the TLR7 MyD88-dependent signaling pathway. Nat Immunol. 2002;3:196–200.
17. Jurk M, Heil F, Vollmer J *et al.* Human TLR7 or TLR8 independently confer responsiveness to the antiviral compound R-848. Nat Immunol. 2002;3:499.
18. Medzhitov R, Preston-Hurlburt P, Kopp E *et al.* MyD88 is an adaptor protein in the hToll/IL-1 receptor family signaling pathways. Mol Cell. 1998;2:253–8.
19. Baud V, Liu ZG, Bennett B, Suzuki N, Xia Y, Karin M. Signaling by proinflammatory cytokines: oligomerization of TRAF2 and TRAF6 is sufficient for JNK and IKK activation and target gene induction via an amino-terminal effector domain. Genes Dev. 1999;13:1297–308.
20. Podolsky DK. Inflammatory bowel disease. N Engl J Med. 2002;347:417–29.
21. Ogura Y, Bonen DK, Inohara N *et al.* A frameshift mutation in NOD2 associated with susceptibility to Crohn's disease. Nature. 2001;411:603–6.

22. Hugot JP, Chamaillard M, Zouali H *et al.* Association of NOD2 leucine-rich repeat variants with susceptibility to Crohn's disease. Nature. 2001;411:599–603.
23. Ogura Y, Inohara N, Benito A, Chen FF, Yamaoka S, Nunez G. Nod2, a Nod1/Apaf-1 family member that is restricted to monocytes and activates NF-kappaB. J Biol Chem. 2001;276:4812–18.
24. Gewirtz AT, Navas TA, Lyons S, Godowski PJ, Madara JL. Cutting edge: bacterial flagellin activates basolaterally expressed TLR5 to induce epithelial proinflammatory gene expression. J Immunol. 2001;167:1882–5.
25. Shimazu R, Akashi S, Ogata H *et al.* MD-2, a molecule that confers lipopolysaccharide responsiveness on Toll-like receptor 4. J Exp Med. 1999;189:1777–82.
26. Akashi S, Ogata H, Kirikae F *et al.* Regulatory roles for CD14 and phosphatidylinositol in the signaling via toll-like receptor 4-MD-2. Biochem Biophys Res Commun. 2000;268:172–7.
27. Hornef MW, Frisan T, Vandewalle A, Normark S, Richter-Dahlfors A. Toll-like receptor 4 resides in the Golgi apparatus and colocalizes with internalized lipopolysaccharide in intestinal epithelial cells. J Exp Med. 2002;195:559–70.
28. Cario E, Podolsky DK. Differential alteration in intestinal epithelial cell expression of toll-like receptor 3 (TLR3) and TLR4 in inflammatory bowel disease. Infect Immun. 2000;68:7010–17.

4
Enteric bacteria: innocent bystanders, therapeutic targets or vehicles for mucosal delivery of therapeutic molecules?

R. B. SARTOR

Bacteria are involved in each of the four aetiological hypotheses for inflammatory bowel disease (IBD) (Table 1)[1,2]. Persistent infection with a specific pathogen is an attractive theory with obvious therapeutic ramifications, but no single agent has been validated to date. *Mycobacterium paratuberculosis*, which causes a chronic granulomatous ileocaecal inflammation (Johne's disease) in ruminants has been found in increased frequency by polymerase chain reaction and *in-situ* hybridization in Crohn's disease tissues, particularly those with granulomas, relative to inflammatory controls and normals[3-5], but there is no convincing evidence for this agent as an aetiological cause for inflammation. It is likely that this organism is present in contaminated milk and possibly meat products, with preferential absorption across the ulcerated mucosa of Crohn's disease. A similar explanation can be provided for immunohistochemical evidence of *Listeria monocytogenes* in Crohn's disease[6]. There has been a notable lack of evidence for cell-mediated immune responses to either organism in Crohn's disease patients. An ongoing trial of triple antibiotic therapy in Australia and the United States may help settle the mycobacterial issue, although the investigated broad-spectrum antibiotics (clarithromycin, ethambutol and rifabutin) will also suppress commensal enteric bacteria. There is no convincing evidence to date that measles infection or immunization causes Crohn's disease[7,8]. However, the Lille group have convincingly demonstrated enteroadherent/invasive *Escherichia coli* in mucosal biopsies of patients with early recurrence of Crohn's disease after segmental resection[9]. This is an example of subtle alterations in the virulence factors of commensal bacteria that can have profound implications for the pathogenesis of chronic inflammation.

Evidence from both clinical studies and experimental models indicates that the balance of injurious vs. protective commensal enteric bacteria is altered in

Table 1 Aetiological hypotheses for the pathogenesis of inflammatory bowel diseases

---

1. Persistent infection with a pathogen:
   Mycobacterium paratuberculosis, measles, *Listeria monocytogenes, Helicobacter* species

2. Dysbiosis:
   Aggressive commensals: *Bacteroides vulgatus, Enterococcus faecalis, E. coli*
   Protective commensals (probiotics): *Lactobacillus* species, *Bifidobacterium* species

3. Defective mucosal protection or healing:
   Mucus, intestinal trefoil factor, growth factors, tight junctions, bacterial killing

4. Dysregulated immune responses:
   Defective tolerance (IL-10, TGF-β, prostaglandins)
   Aggressive effector cells (TNF, IL-1, IL-12, IFN-γ, IL-18)
   Defective apoptosis of effector lymphocytes and macrophages

---

chronic inflammation and that therapeutic manipulation can prevent and treat intestinal disease[1]. Results from animal models suggest that *Bacteroides vulgatus, Enterococcus faecalis*, and *E. coli* are involved in intestinal inflammation/injury[10–12] while the probiotic species *Lactobacillus* and *Bifidobacterium* provide protective responses[13–15]. In human studies *E. coli* and *Bacteroides* species are selectively expanded[16] and enteroadherent/invasive *E. coli* are associated with the mucosa of ulcerative colitis and Crohn's disease patients[9,16]. Similarly, probiotic agents effective in humans include *Lactobacillus* species, *Bifidobacterium* species, and a protective *E. coli* species (*E. coli Nissle*)[17,18].

In the past several years there have been excellent examples from clinical and experimental model studies that indicate that defective mucosal barrier function can lead to chronic inflammation[16,19,20]. The epithelial barrier is composed of a mucus layer which traps bacteria, thereby preventing epithelial adherence. Mucus viscosity is increased by intestinal trefoil factor. Secreted defensins provide local bactericidal activity, while secretory IgA complexes bacterial antigens to prevent mucosal uptake. Epithelial injury is promptly repaired by epithelial restitution, which is mediated by secreted intestinal trefoil factor and local production of growth factors such as transforming growth factor beta (TGF-β) and members of the fibroblast growth factor family[21]. Elegant evidence of increased mucosal adherence of bacteria with epithelial invasion is provided by Swidsinski *et al*[16]. In these studies epithelial adherence by bacteria was increased 1000-fold with selective increases in *E. coli* and *Bacteroides* species. As-yet-unidentified intracellular bacteria were detected within epithelial cells by electron microscopy.

A number of knockout and transgenic mouse and rat studies demonstrate that dysregulated immune responses can lead to loss of tolerance to enteric bacterial species. The mechanisms of this loss of tolerance include defective immunosuppressive molecules (TGF-β, interleukin 10 (IL-10) and prostaglandins), overly aggressive cellular immune responses (tumour necrosis factor (TNF), IL-1, IL-12, IL-18, etc.) and defective apoptosis.

Recently the molecular mechanisms of signalling by the bacterial adjuvants lipopolysaccharide (LPS, endotoxin), peptidoglycan and bacterial DNA (CpG) have been elucidated[22–24]. LPS binds to toll-like receptor (TLR) 4 while peptidoglycan and CpG motifs bind to TLR 2 and TLR 9, respectively. When bound by bacterial products, these activated receptors signal a common central pathway of NF-κB which transduces signals leading to transcriptional activation of a number of proinflammatory cytokines, adhesion molecules, costimulatory molecules and MHC class II molecules. Very recently Nunez and colleagues have demonstrated homologous intracellular NOD 1 and 2 molecules which bind LPS and peptido-glycan to stimulate the NF-κB pathway in a similar fashion[25]. Direct evidence that defective bacterial signalling contributes to the pathogenesis of IBD is provided by detection of polymorphisms in NOD 2 in 25–30% of Crohn's dis-ease patients[26,27]. The three most common single nucleotide polymorphisms in Crohn's disease are within the leucine-rich region (LLR) of NOD 2 which is the portion of this molecule that binds LPS and peptidoglycan. NOD 2 is expressed in monocytes, macrophages, dendritic cells and activated epithelial cells in the intestine[28].

We propose the *hypothesis* that chronic intestinal and extraintestinal inflam-mation in susceptible hosts is due to an overly aggressive cell-mediated immune response to a subset of luminal enteric bacteria. Susceptibility is determined by genes encoding immune responses and barrier function, while onset/reactivation of inflammation is triggered by environmental stimuli. In the normal state the host exists in homeostasis with the enteric bacteria, with immigration of activated macrophages and T cells to the lamina propria but no inflammation (controlled inflammation) (Fig. 1). However, exposure to environment triggers, i.e. self-limited enteric infections or non-steroidal anti-inflammatory drugs, leads to acute injury in all hosts. The normal host rapidly heals with no residual inflammation due to the net down-regulatory profile of intestinal cytokines and T cells. However, the genetically susceptible host develops chronic inflammation driven by the constant antigenic stimulation of luminal bacterial antigens. This

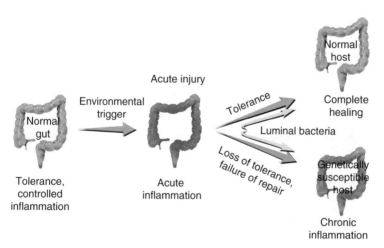

Fig. 1 Proposed pathogenesis of IBD. Variable outcomes of non-specific inflammation dependent on the genetic susceptibility of the host. Normal (resistant) hosts down-regulate immune responses to commensal bacterial antigens and adjuvants, while genetically susceptible hosts mount aggressive immune responses leading to chronic, spontaneously relapsing intestinal inflammation. (Used with permission of the American Gastroenterologic Association)

genetic susceptibility is governed by a loss of tolerance due to defective immunoregulation, a failure of epithelial repair, or lack of effective clearance of invading bacteria.

The consequences of increased uptake of the adjuvants and antigens produced by the predominantly anaerobic microflora of the distal ileum and colon are activation of resident lamina propria macrophages and T lymphocytes (Fig. 2).

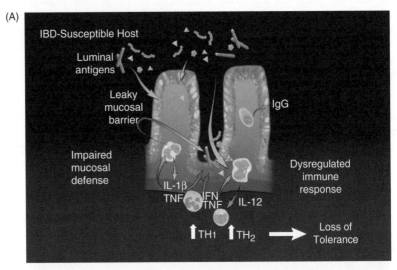

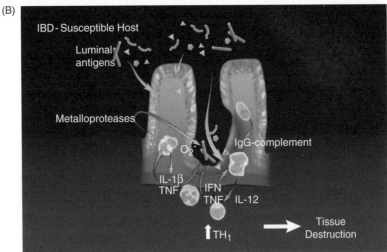

Fig. 2 Response to commensal enteric bacteria in genetically susceptible hosts. **A**: Increased uptake of bacterial antigens, adjuvants and viable bacteria activates lamina propria macrophages and lymphocytes, which secrete proinflammatory products. **B**: These proinflammatory cytokines induce release of metalloproteases and reactive oxygen metabolites that cause tissue damage, leading to the invasion of viable bacteria to perpetuate the inflammatory response. (Used with permission from the American Gastroenterologic Association)

These activated cells produce proinflammatory cytokines and chemokines that recruit additional effector cells to the inflammatory focus. These recently recruited effector cells secrete TNF, IL-1β and interferon gamma (IFN-γ), reactive oxygen metabolites and metalloproteases, which injure epithelial cells and destroy matrix proteins, leading to ulceration. This ulceration potentiates the uptake of luminal adjuvants and antigens, dietary components and secondary invasion of viable bacteria which perpetuates the inflammatory response.

Thus, luminal bacteria could be considered to be either secondary invaders or primary stimulants of intestinal inflammation. Evidence for a primary role is provided by clinical observations with intestinal bypass. Following ileocecal resection with primary anastomosis, clinical recurrence is 85% and endoscopic recurrence is almost universal[29]. However, with a diversion of faecal contents with a proximal ostomy, no inflammation occurs in the bypassed ileum[30]. However, following a take-down of the proximal ostomy, recurrence occurs within 1 month by endoscopic criteria. D'Haens et al. demonstrated that infusion of ileostomy contents into the bypass distal ileum induced histological and immunological evidence of inflammation within 1 week[31]. Similar studies have been performed with colonic inflammation with a diverting split ileostomy[32]. These studies clearly implicate luminal contents in the pathogenesis of recurrent Crohn's disease[33].

Studies in gnotobiotic rodents indicate a conclusive role for enteric bacteria in the induction of intestinal inflammation in genetically susceptible hosts[1]. In at least 11 different models of spontaneous inflammation in genetically engineered rats and mice or in induced models of inflammation in rodents, there is no immune activation and no colitis in the absence of bacteria (sterile or germ-free rodents). However, as early as 1 week after colonization of genetically susceptible hosts with normal commensal bacteria devoid of detectable pathogens, there is clear evidence of macrophage and Th1 lymphocyte activation with histological evidence of colitis[34]. We have demonstrated bacterial antigen-specific CD4+ immune responses in an Enterococcus faecalis-monoassociated IL-10 knockout murine model[11]. CD4+ MLN T cells secrete IFN-γ in response to lysed E. faecalis, but show almost undetectable responses to E. coli and Bacteroides vulgatus[35]. A primary effect of these immune responses is suggested by the onset of Th1-mediated immune activation prior to the onset of clinical and histological evidence of intestinal inflammation. In this monoassociated model, histological inflammation is not present until 10–12 weeks after E. faecalis colonization; however, mucosal secretion of IL-12 and IFN-γ responses to E. faecalis by purified CD4+ mesenteric lymph node lymphocytes is apparent by 5 weeks[35].

Studies in animal models demonstrate bacterial species specificity in various host genetic backgrounds and, very importantly, that different bacterial species in the same host lead to inflammation in different regions of the intestine. For example, germ-free HLA B27 transgenic rats do not display any colitis, but colonization with unfractionated caecal pathogen free bacteria leads to aggressive colitis[10]. Selective colonization of B. vulgatus induces moderate colitis, but B27 transgenic rats monoassociated with E. coli have no inflammation or immune activation[36]. Moreover Lactobacillus GG decreases colitis following caecal bacterial colonization[15]. However, IL-10 knockout mice selectively colonized with B. vulgatus do not develop colitis[34] but a murine E. coli strain induces a vigorous colonic inflammation and bacterial specific T cell response (Kim SC, Sartor RB, unpublished observations). Of considerable interest, *E. faecalis*-monoassociated IL-10 knockout mice develop a slow onset of colitis preferentially located in the distal colon[11] while selective colonization with *E. coli* induces an aggressive early onset of inflammation targeting the caecum and proximal colon.

These experimental observations indicate that different host genetic backgrounds selectively respond to different enteric bacterial species and that different commensal bacterial species can cause inflammation in different regions of the intestine in a single host. In clinical studies it is apparent that heterogeneous groups of patients display variable responses to antibiotics and bacterial diagnostic markers. These observations support the *hypothesis* that each genetically and phenotypically distinct subset of patients will have a *unique* dominant bacterial species and will *selectively* respond to a defined therapeutic intervention. The clear clinical implications of this hypothesis are that clinical trials of antibiotics, probiotics and prebiotics should be designed with adequate power to substratify for different clinical phenotypes and genotypes.

Clinical trials support this hypothesis and indicate the clinical usefulness of altering the composition of the enteric bacterial milieu[37]. In a North American multicentre trial, Sutherland *et al.* demonstrated that metronidazole significantly decreased the Crohn's disease activity index (CDAI) in an unfractionated Crohn's disease population, although no differences in clinical remission rates were detected[38]. However, subgroup analysis clearly indicated that patients with isolated ileal disease did not reproducibly respond to metronidazole treatment, whereas significantly enhanced responses over placebo values were demonstrated for those patients with ileocolitis or isolated colonic inflammation. This selective response of Crohn's disease patients with colonic involvement has been recapitulated in every antibiotic trial to date in which disease location has been evaluated[39–43].

Other antibiotic and probiotic trials in IBD patients suggest that therapeutic manipulation of the luminal flora can be effective[42,44,45]. Rutgeerts *et al.* demonstrated that postoperative administration of metronidazole significantly decreased endoscopic evidence of recurrent Crohn's disease 12 weeks after surgery and decreased clinical recurrence rates at 1 year relative to placebo values[46]. The protective role of metronidazole was evident up to 3 years after metronidazole administration, although treatment was continued for only 3 months after surgery. Similar preventive responses were seen with nitroimidizol antibiotics[47]. Madden *et al.* demonstrated a clear role for metronidazole treatment of pouchitis[48], which appears to respond to a wide spectrum of antibiotic treatments. Clinical trials of antibiotics in Crohn's disease indicate that metronidazole, ciprofloxacin, the combination of these two agents, and possibly clarithromycin have a role in Crohn's colitis and ileal colitis, but toxicity of metronidazole is high, and ciprofloxacin and clarithromycin are quite expensive. Although highly suggestive, more convincing studies are needed to firmly establish a role for antibiotics in the therapy of Crohn's disease. Studies of antibiotics in ulcerative colitis suggest a possible adjunctive role for ciprofloxacin[49], but results with other agents are not promising. The efficacy of non-absorbable agents such as rifaximin needs to be investigated. In contrast, antibiotics have a clear role in the primary treatment of pouchitis with metronidazole, ciprofloxacin and rifaximin having documented therapeutic roles[48,50,51].

Studies with probiotics, which are commensal bacteria with beneficial physiological or therapeutic activities, are provocative but so far non-definitive[44,45,52]. Probiotic bacteria, which most commonly include *Lactobacillus* and *Bifidobacterium* species along with *E. coli Nissle*, have several potential mechanisms of action. These agents have been documented to inhibit the growth of pathogenic bacteria (colonization resistance) by decreasing luminal pH and liberating bactericidal proteins. In addition, these agents can improve epithelial function by secreting short-chain fatty acids, particularly butyrate, which promote epithelial differentiation and barrier function as well as stimulate mucus secretion[53]. An immunoregulatory effect is suggested by enhanced production of IL-10 and secretory IgA with decreased TNF production by isolated immune cells and mucosa of treated rats, mice and humans[54]. In human clinical trials *E. coli 1917 Nissle* is equal to low-dose 5-amino salicylic acid (5-ASA) in ulcerative colitis[18,55] and superior to placebo in Crohn's disease[56]. In uncontrolled studies the VSL3 combination of eight probiotic bacteria induced a 75% remission rate in a 12-month trial of ulcerative colitis (Fedorak F, Gionchetti P, unpublished results). However, a single *Lactobacillus* species (*Lactobacillus GG*) had no effect on prevention of postoperative relapse of Crohn's disease[57]. Strong evidence of the potential for probiotics to have an effect in IBD is provided by the impressive result of VSL3 in prevention of relapse of refractory pouchitis. Gionchetti and colleagues demonstrated that 85% of patients who received daily administration of VSL3 (6 g/day) for 9 months maintained a remission of their refractory pouchitis after induction of remission with antibiotics compared with 0% of the placebo control population[17]. In preliminary studies, prophylactic administration of VSL3 beginning immediately after pouch closure decreased the onset of clinically detectable pouchitis[58]. These combined studies suggest that probiotics have potential for treating IBD but there is still limited support for their efficacy in ulcerative colitis and Crohn's disease. However, probiotics appear very promising for maintenance of remission of refractory pouchitis. Clearly we need large multicentre double-blind placebo-controlled trials for the primary and adjunctive treatment of active ulcerative colitis and Crohn's disease, prevention of relapse of steroid-treated ulcerative colitis and Crohn's and prevention of postoperative recurrence of Crohn's disease and pouchitis with and without antibiotics.

The exciting possibility of mucosal delivery of therapeutic molecules by recombinant bacteria has been raised by recent studies. Steidler and colleagues engineered *Lactococcus lactis* to secrete IL-10 and suggested potential therapeutic use of this agent by demonstrating that colonization of mice with this engineered bacterium could decrease colitis in two separate murine models[59]. These results raise the possibility for potential application of other therapeutic molecules, including immunosuppressive cytokines (IL-10, TGF-β) and agents inducing epithelial restitution (i.e. intestinal trefoil factor). Advantages of these genetically engineered luminal bacteria include selective local therapy with increased efficacy, decreased toxicity and a cost-effective approach, particularly if chronic colonization could be accomplished following a single administration. However, there are a number of unresolved environmental consequences which prevent widespread use of these agents in the near future. For example, how will faecal material from treated patients be disposed of, and what are the long-term implications of chronic secretion of immunosuppressive cytokines or growth factors of the intestine of either IBD patients or normal hosts? Could the engineered gene be transmitted to normal commensal bacteria by plasmid transfer? Environmental consequences of genetically engineered bacteria would be minimized if these agents could be created with an inducible promoter (other than tetracycline, which can have activity and side-effects) so that there is no constitutive expression of the therapeutic gene.

Additional novel approaches to prevent the detrimental effects of commensal enteric bacteria in intestinal inflammation which extend past the traditional antibiotic and probiotic approaches include blockade of lipopolysaccharide, peptidoglycan and bacterial DNA receptors (TLR 4, TLR 2, and TLR 9 respectively) on the membrane of innate immune cells, as well as intracellular receptors such as NOD 1 or NOD 2. Activation of innate immune cells by bacterial adjuvants could also be prevented by blocking the signal transduction pathways of NF-κB, AP1 and MAP kinases.

There is little doubt that commensal luminal bacteria have both primary and secondary effects on intestinal inflammation. Indeed, perpetuation of initial non-specific inflammation triggered by environmental transient infections and non-steroidal anti-inflammatory drugs may be a critical mechanism in the pathogenesis of IBD. Secondary uptake of bacterial adjuvants and antigens with translocation of viable bacteria across the ulcerated mucosa will potentiate the inflammatory response and expand T cell activation in a polyclonal fashion. This more complex and expanded activation of innate and acquired immune responses will lead not only to more extensive tissue damage but also to more refractory disease, which could become unresponsive to selective blockade of specific targets.

In conclusion, it is my firm contention that luminal commensal bacteria in IBD represent key therapeutic targets rather than merely being innocent bystanders. Therapeutic options to block the ability of selected components of the commensal flora to induce disease include antibiotics, probiotics, prebiotics (dietary substances which foster the growth and activation state of endogenous probiotic bacterial species) as well as blockade of bacterial receptors and signal transduction pathways of these receptors. However, to optimize treatment of IBD, I believe that we should adopt a comprehensive approach in which we not only eliminate the antigenic drive and inhibit Th1 and innate immune responses but we should promote regulatory T cells (Th1 and Th3 lymphocytes that secrete IL-10 and TGF-β, respectively) while restoring the mucosal barrier with proper nutrition, intestinal trefoil factor and metabolic fuels (i.e. butyrate). It is likely that only such a comprehensive approach will reproducibly heal the mucosa and change the natural history of these spontaneously relapsing chronic conditions. Recent advances in our understanding of genetic subsets of Crohn's disease and ulcerative colitis offer the possibility to match selective therapy with genetically determined defects in pathophysiology to increase efficacy and eliminate the random sequential approach to treatment of IBD. Selective targeting of the pathogenic members of the commensal bacteria in genetically defined subsets offer great promise for modulating the balance of proinflammatory and anti-inflammatory bacteria.

Acknowledgements

Original work by the author was supported by NIH grants RO1 DK 40249, RO1 DK 53347 and P30 DK 34987. The author thanks Susie May for excellent secretarial support, and the many postdoctoral fellows, graduate students and technicians who contributed to this work.

References

1. Sartor RB. Microbial factors in the pathogenesis of Crohn's disease, ulcerative colitis and experimental intestinal inflammation. In: Kirsner JB, editor. Inflammatory Bowel Diseases, 5th edn. Philadelphia: Saunders, 1999:153–78.
2. Sartor RB. Intestinal microflora in human and experimental inflammatory bowel disease. Curr Opin Gastroenterol. 2001;17:324–30.
3. Fidler HM, Thurrel W, Johnson NM, Rook GA, McFadden JJ. Specific detection of *Mycobacterium paratuberculosis* DNA associated with granulomatous tissue in Crohn's disease. Gut. 1994;35:506–10.
4. Hulten K, El-Zimaity HM, Karttunen TJ *et al.* Detection of *Mycobacterium avium* subspecies paratuberculosis in Crohn's diseased tissues by *in situ* hybridization. Am J Gastroenterol. 2001;96:1529–35.
5. Hermon-Taylor J. Protagonist. *Mycobacterium avium* subspecies paratuberculosis is a cause of Crohn's disease. Gut. 2001;49:755–6.
6. Liu Y, Van Kruiningen HJ, West AB, Cartun RW, Cortot A, Colombel JF. Immunocytochemical evidence of *Listeria, Escherichia coli*, and *Streptococcus* antigens in Crohn's disease. Gastroenterology. 1995;108:1396–404.
7. Robertson DJ, Sandler RS. Measles virus and Crohn's disease: a critical appraisal of the current literature. Inflamm Bowel Dis. 2001;7:51–7.
8. Ghosh S, Armitage E, Wilson D, Minor PD, Afzal MA. Detection of persistent measles virus infection in Crohn's disease: current status of experimental work. Gut. 2001;48:748–52.
9. Darfeuille-Michaud A, Neut C, Barnich N *et al.* Presence of adherent *Escherichia coli* strains in ileal mucosa of patients with Crohn's disease. Gastroenterology. 1998;115:1405–13.
10. Rath HC, Herfarth HH, Ikeda JS *et al.* Normal luminal bacteria, especially *Bacteroides* species, mediate chronic colitis, gastritis, and arthritis in HLA-B27/human beta2 microglobulin transgenic rats. J Clin Invest. 1996;98:945–53.
11. Kim SC, Tonkonogy SL, Balish E, Brackett DR, Warner T, Sartor RB. IL-10 deficient mice monoassociated with nonpathogenic *Enterococcus faecalis* develop chronic colitis. Gastroenterology. 2001;120:A82(abstract).
12. Balish E, Warner T. *Enterococcus faecalis* induces inflammatory bowel disease in interleukin-10 knockout mice. Am J Pathol. 2002;160:2253–7.
13. Madsen KL, Tavernini MM, Mosmann TR, Fedorak RN. Interleukin 10 modulates ion transport in rat small intestine. Gastroenterology. 1996;111:936–44.
14. Madsen KL, Doyle JS, Jewell LD, Tavernini MM, Fedorak RN. *Lactobacillus* species prevents colitis in interleukin 10 gene-deficient mice. Gastroenterology. 1999;116:1107–14.
15. Dieleman LA, Goerres M, Arends A *et al.* *Lactobacillus GG* prevents recurrence of colitis in HLA-B27 transgenic rats after antibiotic treatment. Gut. 2002(In press).
16. Swidsinski A, Ladhoff A, Pernthaler A *et al.* Mucosal flora in inflammatory bowel disease. Gastroenterology. 2002;122:44–54.
17. Gionchetti P, Rizzello F, Venturi A *et al.* Oral bacteriotherapy as maintenance treatment in patients with chronic pouchitis: a double-blind, placebo-controlled trial. Gastroenterology. 2000;119:305–9.
18. Kruis W, Schutz E, Fric P, Fixa B, Judmaier G, Stolte M. Double-blind comparison of an oral *Escherichia coli* preparation and mesalazine in maintaining remission of ulcerative colitis. Aliment Pharmacol Ther. 1997;11:853–8.
19. Mashimo H, Wu DC, Podolsky DK, Fishman MC. Impaired defense of intestinal mucosa in mice lacking intestinal trefoil factor. Science. 1996;274:262–5.
20. Hermiston ML, Gordon JI. Inflammatory bowel disease and adenomas in mice expressing a dominant negative N-cadherin. Science. 1995;270:1203–7.

21. Dignass AU, Podolsky DK. Cytokine modulation of intestinal epithelial cell restitution: central role of transforming growth factor beta. Gastroenterology. 1993;105:1323–32.
22. Beutler B. Toll-like receptors: how they work and what they do. Curr Opin Hematol. 2002;9:2–10.
23. Inohara N, Ogura Y, Nunez G. Nods: a family of cytosolic proteins that regulate the host response to pathogens. Curr Opin Microbiol. 2002;5:76–80.
24. Kimbrell DA, Beutler B. The evolution and genetics of innate immunity. Nature Rev Genet. 2001;2:256–67.
25. Ogura Y, Inohara N, Benito A, Chen FF, Yamaoka S, Nunez G. Nod2, a Nod1/Apaf-1 family member that is restricted to monocytes and activates NF-kappaB. J Biol Chem. 2001;276:4812–18.
26. Ogura Y, Bonen DK, Inohara N et al. A frameshift mutation in NOD2 associated with suscepti-bility to Crohn's disease. Nature. 2001;411:603–6.
27. Hugot JP, Laurent-Puig P, Gower-Rousseau C et al. Mapping of a susceptibility locus for Crohn's disease on chromosome 16. Nature. 1996;379:821–3.
28. Gutierrez O, Pipaon C, Inohara N et al. Induction of Nod2 in myelomonocytic and intestinal epithelial cells via nuclear factor-κB activation. J Biol Chem. 2002(In press).
29. Rutgeerts P, Geboes K, Vantrappen G, Beyls J, Kerremans R, Hiele M. Predictability of the postoperative course of Crohn's disease. Gastroenterology. 1990;99:956–63.
30. Rutgeerts P, Geboes K, Peeters M et al. Effect of faecal stream diversion on recurrence of Crohn's disease in the neoterminal ileum. Lancet. 1991;338:771–4.
31. D'Haens GR, Geboes K, Peeters M, Baert F, Penninckx F, Rutgeerts P. Early lesions of recurrent Crohn's disease caused by infusion of intestinal contents in excluded ileum. Gastroenterology. 1998;114:262–7.
32. Harper PH, Lee EC, Kettlewell MG, Bennett MK, Jewell DP. Role of the faecal stream in the maintenance of Crohn's colitis. Gut. 1985;26:279–84.
33. Sartor RB. Postoperative recurrence of Crohn's disease: the enemy is within the fecal stream. Gastroenterology. 1998;114:398–400.
34. Sellon RK, Tonkonogy S, Schultz M et al. Resident enteric bacteria are necessary for develop-ment of spontaneous colitis and immune system activation in interleukin-10-deficient mice. Infect Immun. 1998;66:5224–31.
35. Kim SC, Tonkonogy SL, Balish E, Sartor RB. Bacterial antigen specific T cell activation precedes intestinal inflammation in E. faecalis monoassociated IL-10 deficient mice. Gastroenterology. 2002;122:A85(abstract).
36. Rath HC, Wilson KH, Sartor RB. Differential induction of colitis and gastritis in HLA-B27 transgenic rats selectively colonized with Bacteroides vulgatus and Escherichia coli. Infect Immun. 1999;67:2969–74.
37. Sartor RB. Intestinal microflora in human and experimental inflammatory bowel disease. Curr Opin Gastroenterol. 2001;17:555–61.
38. Sutherland L, Singleton J, Sessions J et al. Double blind, placebo controlled trial of metronidazole in Crohn's disease. Gut. 1991;32:1071–5.
39. Greenbloom SL, Steinhart AH, Greenberg GR. Combination ciprofloxacin and metronidazole for active Crohn's disease. Can J Gastroenterol. 1998;12:53–6.
40. Ursing B, Alm T, Barany F et al. A comparative study of metronidazole and sulfasalazine for active Crohn's disease: the cooperative Crohn's disease study in Sweden. II. Result. Gastroenterology. 1982;83:550–62.
41. Colombel JF, Lemann M, Cassagnou M et al. A controlled trial comparing ciprofloxacin with mesalazine for the treatment of active Crohn's disease. Groupe d'Etudes Therapeutiques des Affections Inflammatoires Digestives (GETAID). Am J Gastroenterol. 1999;94:674–8.
42. Colombel JF, Cortot A, Van Kruiningen HJ. Antibiotics in Crohn's disease. Gut. 2001;48:647.
43. Steinhart AH, Feagan BG, Wong CJ et al. Combined budesonide and antibiotic therapy for active Crohn's disease: a randomized controlled trial. Gastroenterology. 2002;123:33–40.
44. Shanahan F. Probiotics and inflammatory bowel disease: is there a scientific rationale? Inflamm Bowel Dis. 2000;6:107–15.
45. Gionchetti P, Rizzello F, Campieri M. Probiotics and antibiotics in inflammatory bowel diseases. Curr Opin Gastroenterol. 2001;17:331–5.
46. Rutgeerts P, Hiele M, Geboes K et al. Controlled trial of metronidazole treatment for prevention of Crohn's recurrence after ileal resection. Gastroenterology. 1995;108:1617–21.
47. Rutgeerts PJ, D'Haens G, Baert F et al. Nitroimidazole antibiotics are efficacious for prophylaxis of postoperative recurrence of Crohn's disease: a placebo controlled trial. Gastroenterology. 1999;116:G3506(abstract).

48. Madden MV, McIntyre AS, Nicholls RJ. Double-blind crossover trial of metronidazole versus placebo in chronic unremitting pouchitis. Dig Dis Sci. 1994;39:1193–6.
49. Turunen UM, Farkkila MA, Hakala K et al. Long-term treatment of ulcerative colitis with ciprofloxacin: a prospective, double-blind, placebo-controlled study. Gastroenterology. 1998; 115:1072–8.
50. Gionchetti P, Rizzello F, Venturi A et al. Antibiotic combination therapy in patients with chronic, treatment-resistant pouchitis. Aliment Pharmacol Ther. 1999;13:713–18.
51. Mimura T, Rizzello F, Helwig U et al. Four-week open-label trial of metronidazole and ciprofloxacin for the treatment of recurrent or refractory pouchitis. Aliment Pharmacol Ther. 2002;16:909–17.
52. Schultz M, Sartor RB. Probiotics and inflammatory bowel diseases. Am J Gastroenterol. 2000;95:S19–21.
53. Mack DR, Michail S, Wei S, McDougall L, Hollingsworth MA. Probiotics inhibit enteropathogenic *E. coli* adherence *in vitro* by inducing intestinal mucin gene expression. Am J Physiol. 1999;276:G941–50.
54. Ulisse S, Gionchetti P, D'Alo S et al. Expression of cytokines, inducible nitric oxide synthase, and matrix metalloproteinases in pouchitis: effects of probiotic treatment. Am J Gastroenterol. 2001;96:2691–9.
55. Kruis W, Kalk EK, Fric P, Stolte M. Maintenance of remission in ulcerative colitis is equally effective with *Escherichia coli Nissle* 1917 and with standard mesalamine. Gastroenterology. 2001;120:A127(abstract).
56. Malchow HA. Crohn's disease and *Escherichia coli*. A new approach in therapy to maintain remission of colonic Crohn's disease? J Clin Gastroenterol. 1997;25:653–8.
57. Prantera C, Scribano ML, Falasco G, Andreoli A, Luzi C. Ineffectiveness of probiotics in preventing recurrence after curative resection for Crohn's disease: a randomised controlled trial with *Lactobacillus GG*. Gut. 2002;51:405–9.
58. Gionchetti P, Rizzello F, Venturi A et al. Prophylaxis of pouchitis onset with probiotic therapy: a double-blind placebo controlled trial. Gastroenterology. 2000;118:A190(abstract).
59. Steidler L, Hans W, Schotte L et al. Treatment of murine colitis by *Lactococcus lactis* secreting interleukin-10. Science. 2000;289:1352–5.

Section II
Tools for therapeutic development

5
Do animal models always give the right direction for therapy?

C. O. ELSON, Y. CONG, N. IQBAL and C. T. WEAVER

INTRODUCTION

The development in the past decade of many new experimental models of inflammatory bowel disease (IBD) has added tremendously to our understanding of the basic cellular and molecular mechanisms involved in IBD. Experimental models have been and continue to be used to study many phases and aspects of IBD, including genetic predisposition, mechanisms involved in initiation or triggering of disease, factors involved in progression or perpetuation of inflammation, immune regulation, and healing. Insights have been achieved in all of these areas[1]. In this chapter the question posed in the title will be subdivided into two aspects. First, have animal models provided new targets for therapy? Second, are animal models always predictive of efficacy in humans of a potential therapeutic agent?

Before addressing these questions the design of experiments used to test potential therapeutic agents in experimental models needs to be considered (Fig. 1). In many models the timing of disease onset can be precisely controlled, for instance by the feeding of an agent such as dextran sulphate sodium (DSS) or by transfer of pathogenic T cells. One experimental design is to administer the potential therapeutic agent simultaneously with the induction of colitis. This design thus studies whether a given agent can prevent the induction of inflammation. The second common experimental design is to induce inflammation and let it become established prior to the administration of a potential therapeutic agent. This design tests whether the agent can treat pre-existing, active inflammation. The first design is more analogous to maintenance of remission and the second more analogous to treatment of active flares of disease.

HAVE ANIMAL MODELS PROVIDED NEW TARGETS FOR THERAPY?

Experimental models have identified a number of factors that are important in the perpetuation or progression of chronic intestinal inflammation. The first of

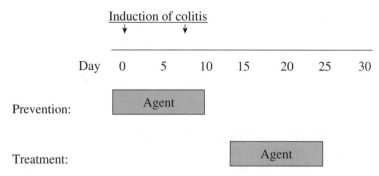

Fig. 1 Comparison of prevention vs treatment protocols commonly used in experimental models

these is a prolonged increase in inflammatory cytokines such as tumour necrosis factor alpha (TNF-α), interferon gamma (IFN-γ), and interleukins IL-1α, IL-12 and IL-18. In regard to pathogenic Th1 responses a sustained increase of IL-12 over weeks or months is required[2,3]. IL-12 is produced by antigen-presenting cells and acts on Th1 cells via a specific heterodimeric IL-12 receptor. This signals Th1 cells to produce more IFN-γ, as well as other cytokines. IFN-γ then feeds back on the antigen-presenting cell to stimulate the production of more IL-12, creating a self-sustaining loop. Co-stimulatory interactions between the surface molecule CD40 on antigen-presenting cells (APCs) and CD40L (CD40 ligand) on Th1 cells is required for IL-12 production[4] and blockade of this interaction with monoclonal antibodies can ameliorate colitis[3,5]. This IL-12–IFN-γ loop also stimulates the production of large amounts of TNF-α. Inhibitors of TNF-α are already in use in the clinic and have shown efficacy in the treatment of at least a subset of patients with Crohn's disease[6]. A human monoclonal antibody to IL-12 is in clinical trials in patients with Crohn's disease and clinical trials are planned for inhibitors of CD40L. Neutralization of IL-12 has been efficacious as a prevention and treatment for trinitrobenzene sulphonic acid (TNBS)-ethanol-induced colitis and in mice deficient in IL-10[2,7]. Anti-IL-12 has also worked as a prevention of colitis in IL-2-deficient mice[8]. Interestingly, in IL-10-deficient mice the age of the mice at the time of administration of anti-IL-12 was an important factor in response. Anti-IL-12 administered to 10-day-old mice had a very significant amelioration of disease; however, anti-IL-12 given to 3-month-old IL-10 mice with established disease showed substantially less efficacy[7]. This may be due to a shift from predominant Th1-mediated inflammation and to more of a Th2, IL-4-dependent inflammation later in the disease course[9]. Most of the inflammatory cytokines are under the control of the NF-κB signal transduction pathway. Blockade of the NF-κB pathway with an anti-sense oligonucleotide was shown to be effective in two different experimental animal models when given either topically or systemically[10]. Studies with this same inhibitor of NF-κB, namely an anti-sense phosphorothioate nucleotide to the p65 component of NF-κB, are under way in humans. The preliminary report indicates that a single enema in steroid-refractory or -dependent patients with distal colitis or proctitis resulted in a 71% improvement rate vs 25% in the placebo group. Two patients who received this agent apparently went into prolonged remission[11].

A second factor required for perpetuation or progression of IBD is continued recruitment of effector cells into the lesions. Activated effector cells are short-lived and undergo apoptosis. Thus they must be renewed constantly for an inflammatory lesion to continue. Inflammatory cells traffic into tissues and into inflammatory sites in a multistep process that is reasonably well understood[12]. Such trafficking requires a series of interactions among surface molecules on lymphoid cells with ligands on endothelial cells. With regard to cells trafficking into the intestine, interactions between $\alpha 4\beta 7$ integrin on leucocytes and MAdCAM-1 on endothelial cells is required. A blockade of the interaction between these molecules by monoclonal antibodies has shown efficacy in the treatment of experimental colitis[13,14]. This success has led to two clinical trials of a recombinant humanized monoclonal antibody specific for $\alpha 4$ integrin (Natalizumab, Antegren). This agent given once to patients at 3 mg/kg resulted in 39% remission 2 weeks later vs 8% in the placebo group[15]. A subsequent phase 2 trial of two doses of Natalizumab given at 0 and 4 weeks found a 46% remission rate at 6 weeks in the treatment group vs 27% in placebo[16]. Other strategies being pursued in this arena that have shown some benefit in experimental models include an antibody to $\alpha 4\beta 7$ integrin, an antibody to MAdCAM-1[14], and a lymphotoxin β–Ig fusion protein which interrupts lymphoid architecture and thus indirectly affects cell trafficking[17].

A third factor found in experimental models that is required for perpetuation, and that may have therapeutic benefit, is continuous bacterial stimulation. This has been demonstrated best in the transgenic $\varepsilon 26$ adoptive transfer model of colitis[18]. Pathogenic effector CD4$^+$ T cells from colitic Tg$\varepsilon 26$ mice, when transferred into conventional immunodeficient RAG$^{-/-}$ mice, result in colitis. However, when the same pathogenic CD4$^+$ effector T cells were transferred into germ-free RAG$^{-/-}$ mice no colitis ensued, even though in both instances activated memory T cells were present in the colon. This result implies that interruption of the antigenic drive to pathogenic T cells might be an effective prevention or therapy. This result might help explain the benefit of bypass surgery in Crohn's disease in which the faecal stream is diverted. It also provides some rationale for delivery of probiotic organisms to patients or, alternatively, genetically altered bacteria producing inhibitory cytokines such as IL-10[19]. These are but a few examples that can be cited of new targets identified from experimental models. Thus, the answer to the first question posed is that experimental models have certainly provided many new targets of therapy.

DO RESULTS IN ANIMALS ALWAYS PREDICT EFFICACY IN HUMANS?

The answer to that question is 'not necessarily'. In at least two instances promising results in experimental models did not translate to efficacy in human trials.

IL-10 is an inhibitory cytokine which down-regulates most inflammatory cytokines including IL-12 and TNF-α. Absence of IL-10 results in enterocolitis in mice, and exogenous IL-10 was effective in preventing colitis in IL-10-deficient mice, in the CD45RB transfer model[20], and in experimental granulomatous colitis in the rat[21]. Thus, its use as a potential therapeutic agent has an excellent rationale. On the other hand, IL-10 was relatively ineffective in treating established inflammation; e.g. there was only a partial benefit of IL-10 therapy in IL-10-deficient mice already ill at the time of administration[22] and no effect of IL-10 as a treatment in either the CD45RB transfer model[20] or in the HLA-B27 rat[23]. The initial trial of IL-10 given intravenously to patients with refractory Crohn's disease showed some beneficial effect. However, five subsequent studies of IL-10 in moderately active Crohn's disease, in chronic active Crohn's disease and steroid-dependent Crohn's disease, in maintenance of remission after surgery in Crohn's disease, and in moderately active ulcerative colitis, all failed[24]. IL-10 seems to be a key cytokine produced by regulatory cells, which have been shown to be able to suppress active inflammation in a number of models. Thus, the failure of these trials in humans may relate more to the systemic route of administration rather than a lack of efficacy if it could be delivered directly to the intestinal lesions. Support of this notion comes from work reported recently in which *Lactococcus lactis* bacteria were genetically engineered to produce IL-10 in the colon itself. This local administration resulted in a therapeutic benefit in two different animal models of colitis[19].

A second model in which promising results in experimental models failed to translate to the clinic is keratinocyte growth factor-1 (KGF-1) or Repafirmin. KGF-1 is a growth factor for epithelial cells, including intestinal epithelial cells. The rationale for its use in IBD is to speed epithelial restitution and repair. KGF-1 had beneficial effects as a preventive in two different animal models, DSS colitis and the $CD4^+,CD45RB^{high}$ transfer model. However, a phase 2 trial of KGF-1 in patients with ulcerative colitis failed to show any benefit[24]. In these two instances the beneficial effect in experimental animals was more for prevention of induction rather than treatment of active disease, and perhaps that is a lesson to be learned and applied to considerations for future agents. These two instances illustrate the point that the results in experimental animal models do not always translate into beneficial effects in humans. However, this should not be surprising, in that only a small percentage of agents that get to clinical trials end up as a new therapeutic in the clinic.

SUGGESTED GUIDELINES

With regard to the choice of an appropriate model for preclinical assessment, some guidelines can be suggested. First, the model should be coherent with the presumed mechanism of action of the therapeutic agent. Second, treatment of established disease is perhaps a better predictor of success than an agent that is able simply to prevent the disease. Third, models with chronic intestinal inflammation are probably better tests of potential therapy than models of acute injury or inflammation such as DSS-induced colitis, although these simpler models might be useful for screening compounds and for establishing a dose range to use in more complex models.

References

1. Elson CO. Experimental models of intestinal inflammation. New insights into mechanisms of mucosal homeostasis. In: Ogra PL, Mestecky J, Lamm ME, Strober W, McGhee JR, Bienenstock J, editors. Mucosal Immunology, 2nd edn. San Diego: Academic Press, 1999:1007–24.
2. Neurath MF, Fuss I, Kelsall B, Meyer zum Buschenfelde KH, Strober W. Effect of IL-12 and anti-bodies to IL-12 on established granulomatous colitis in mice. Ann NY Acad Sci. 1996;795:368–70.
3. Cong Y, Weaver CT, Lazenby A, Elson CO. Colitis induced by enteric bacterial antigen-specific CD4⁺ T cells requires CD40–CD40 ligand interactions for a sustained increase in mucosal IL-12. J Immunol. 2000;165:2173–82.
4. Kelsall BL, Stuber E, Neurath M, Strober W. Interleukin-12 production by dendritic cells. The role of CD40-CD40L interactions in Th1 T-cell responses. Ann NY Acad Sci. 1996;795:116–26.
5. De Jong YP, Comiskey M, Kalled SL et al. Chronic murine colitis is dependent on the CD154/CD40 pathway and can be attenuated by anti-CD154 administration. Gastroenterology. 2000;119:715–23.
6. Targan SR, Hanauer SB, van Deventer SJ et al. A short-term study of chimeric monoclonal antibody cA2 to tumor necrosis factor alpha for Crohn's disease. Crohn's Disease cA2 Study Group. N Engl J Med. 1997;337:1029–35.
7. Davidson NJ, Hudak SA, Lesley RE, Menon S, Leach MW, Rennick DM. IL-12, but not IFN-gamma, plays a major role in sustaining the chronic phase of colitis in IL-10-deficient mice. J Immunol. 1998;161:3143–9.
8. Ludviksson BR, Gray B, Strober W, Ehrhardt RO. Dysregulated intrathymic development in the IL-2-deficient mouse leads to colitis-inducing thymocytes. J Immunol. 1997;158:104–11.
9. Spencer DM, Veldman GM, Banerjee S, Willis J, Levine AD. Distinct inflammatory mechanisms mediate early versus late colitis in mice. Gastroenterology. 2002;122:94–105.
10. Neurath MF, Pettersson S, Meyer zum Buschenfelde KH, Strober W. Local administration of antisense phosphorothioate oligonucleotides to the p65 subunit of NF-kappa B abrogates estab-lished experimental colitis in mice. Nature Med. 1996;2:998–1004.
11. Lofberg R, Neurath M, Ost A, Pettersson S. Topical NF-κB p65 antisense oligonucleotides in patients with active distal colonic IBD. A randomized controlled pilot trial. Gastroenterology. 2002;122(suppl. 1):A60.
12. Butcher EC, Picker LJ. Lymphocyte homing and homeostasis. Science. 1996;272:60–6.
13. Podolsky DK, Lobb R, King N et al. Attenuation of colitis in the cotton-top tamarin by anti-alpha 4 integrin monoclonal antibody. J Clin Invest. 1993;92:372–80.
14. Picarella D, Hurlbut P, Rottman J, Shi X, Butcher E, Ringler DJ. Monoclonal antibodies specific for beta 7 integrin and mucosal addressin cell adhesion molecule-1 (MAdCAM-1) reduce inflam-mation in the colon of scid mice reconstituted with CD45RBhigh CD4+ T cells. J Immunol. 1997;158:2099–106.
15. Gordon FH, Lai CW, Hamilton MI et al. A randomized placebo-controlled trial of a humanized monoclonal antibody to alpha 4 integrin in active Crohn's disease. Gastroenterology. 2001;121:268–74.
16. Ghosh S, Goldin E, Malchow H et al. A randomized, double-blind, placebo-controlled, pan-European study of a recombinant humanized antibody to alpha 4 integrin (Antegren) in moder-ate to severely active Crohn's disease. Gastroenterology. 2001;120:A127–8.
17. Mackay F, Browning JL, Lawton P et al. Both the lymphotoxin and tumor necrosis factor path-ways are involved in experimental murine models of colitis. Gastroenterology. 1998;115:1464–75.
18. Velkamp C, Tonkonogy SL, De long YP et al. Continuous stimulation by normal luminal bacte-ria is essential for the development and perpetuation of colitis in Tg epsilon 26 mice. Gastroenterology. 2001;120:900–13.
19. Steidler L, Hans W, Schotte L et al. Treatment of murine colitis by Lactococcus lactis secreting interleukin-10. Science. 2000;289:1352–5.
20. Powrie F, Leach MW, Mauze S, Menon S, Caddle LB, Coffman RL. Inhibition of Th1 responses prevents inflammatory bowel disease in scid mice reconstituted with CD45RBhi CD4+ T cells. Immunity. 1994;1:553–62.
21. Herfarth HH, Mohanty SP, Rath HC, Tonkonogy S, Sartor RB. Interleukin 10 suppresses experi-mental chronic, granulomatous inflammation induced by bacterial cell wall polymers. Gut. 1996;39:836–45.

22. Rennick DM, Fort MM. Lessons from genetically engineered animal models. XII. IL-10-deficient (IL-10(−/−)) mice and intestinal inflammation. Am J Physiol – Gastrointest Liver Physiol. 2000;278:G829–33.
23. Bertrand V, Quere S, Guimbaud R et al. Effects of murine recombinant interleukin-10 on the inflammatory disease of rats transgenic for HLA-B27 and human beta 2-microglobulin. Eur Cytokine Netw. 1998;9:161–70.
24. Sandborn WJ, Targan SR. Biologic therapy of inflammatory bowel disease. Gastroenterology. 2002;122:1592–608.

6
Are cell lines and cultures a good way to develop therapeutic approaches?

G. ROGLER

INTRODUCTION

Cell lines have brought incredible advances in the understanding of mucosal physiology and cell–cell interactions during the past 30 years. They have been used to study cytokine and chemokine secretion, regulation of gene transcription, cell activation by proinflammatory mediators and more recently for array technology to compare cellular responses. However, typical cell lines are derived from tumours and have an uncontrolled number of mutations and functional alterations. HT-29 cells, which are frequently used as a model for intestinal epithelial cells (IEC), were derived from colonic cancer and, for example, have mutations in the interleukin-15 (IL-15) gene as well as a complete lack of bcl-2 expression. RAW cells used as a model for monocytes form tumours when injected into mice. These are just a few of the limitations of cell lines and *in-vitro* results.

Animal models have brought much progress to the field of drug development and drug testing. They reflect better the complex interactions of cells which take place during mucosal inflammation *in vivo*. However, researchers had to learn that a large number of completely different approaches cause intestinal inflammation in mice, and that therapeutic strategies highly effective in animal models can frequently fail in patients with inflammatory bowel diseases (IBD).

Cell culture models of primary human cells avoid two disadvantages. The scientist does not need to work with transformed cell lines, and species differences do not play a role in the interpretation of the results. Primary human cells from the intestinal mucosa have been difficult to isolate or culture in the past, but recent years have brought some progress. We can now isolate and culture primary human IEC. We can isolate and culture intestinal macrophages and dendritic cells, as well as primary human intestinal fibroblasts or mast cells. This is an approach to make complex systems simple. After studying isolated functions of single components of an immunological network we are now able to move from the simple systems to more complex ones such as three-dimensional co-culture systems. For drug development in dermatology three-dimensional 'skin reconstructs' have become important, and are widely used. Similar three-dimensional 'mucosa reconstructs' are needed in the future. We are on the way to developing these three-dimensional 'mucosa reconstructs', but will they really be a good way to develop therapeutic approaches?

The final proof of a therapeutic approach can be obtained only from clinical studies, from the 'human experiment'. However, at present, strategies are tested in patients that have previously not been evaluated sufficiently in test systems. If a recombinant protein is mainly anti-apoptotic but not anti-inflammatory in mucosal cells expressing the receptor it is not reasonable to test this protein in a mainly anti-inflammatory-focused therapeutic setting.

Before testing new therapeutic approaches in patients the new cell culture systems, as well as animal models and cell lines, should be used to gain as much information as is available.

PROBLEMS WITH THE INTERPRETATION OF RESULTS FROM ANIMAL MODELS

During the past two decades animal models have received more and more interest in IBD research. Results from animal models were the basis for a number of clinical trials indicating that new therapeutic strategies were derived from those models. In fact, positive results in animal studies have become the most important argument for the start of clinical studies with IBD patients. We have to ask whether that is justified.

A large number of animal models have been described; Table 1 gives a few examples. We have animals spontaneously developing bowel inflammation such as the cottontop tamarin, a monkey, which frequently contracts chronic diarrhoea if kept in cages, but not in its normal habitat[1-12]. A mouse strain (C3H/HeJ) spontaneously showing symptoms of chronic colitis has also been described[13-18]. Unfortunately, in this case outbreeding has occurred, and this model is no longer available. There may be more species developing chronic bowel inflammation. Veterinarians report chronic gut inflammation in dogs or cats, which can be

Table 1 Some examples for animal models of colonic inflammation or inflammatory bowel disease. Which one to choose for a particular study?

Spontaneous	*Transfer models*
Cottontop tamarin	CD45RB^{high} transfer
C3H/HeJ	
	Knockouts and transgenics
Induced colitis	IL-10$^{-/-}$
TNBS colitis	IL-2$^{-/-}$
DSS colitis (acute and chronic)	HLA-B27 transgenic rats
Indomethacin colitis	Mdr-1$^{-/-}$
PG-PS colitis	N-cadherin dominant negative

successfully treated by steroids, but this has never been scientifically compared with features of human IBD (perhaps we should do that in the future).

Several models of induced colitis are known. One of the most frequently used models for acute and chronic colitis is the dextran–sodium sulphate (DSS) model[14,19–44]. Other chemicals have been used to induce colitis, such as trinitrobenzene sulphonic acid (TNBS)[8,36,45–57], Indomethacin[58–63] or a preparation of bacterial wall products, the PG-PS model[64–71]. Besides induction of colitis by administration of chemicals, colitis can be induced by the transfer of CD45RB[high] T cells[72–82].

Finally chronic bowel inflammation is found in a number of knockout models or transgenic rodents such as the IL-2$^{-/-}$ model[83–94], the IL-10$^{-/-}$ model[93,95–109], mdr-1$^{-/-}$ mice[110], or the HLA-B27 transgenic rats[111–122].

The problem with this large number of different models is to choose the right one. No-one can tell which model is more appropriate to resemble features of human IBD. It is not surprising that IL-10-deficient mice with chronic gut inflammation can be successfully treated with IL-10; this is exactly what those mice are lacking. More and more investigators recommend that a new therapeutic approach must be successful in more than one animal model before the start of a clinical trial with IBD patients. There is still major discussion as to which model might be favourable, and we will have to live with this problem for the next few years.

Besides the question of which animal could be the right model, there are other problems that limit the interpretation of animal studies. No model resembles typical IBD courses that are usually characterized by acute flares and times of remission. Usually we either have inflammation or we do not. In fact the lifespan of rodents is too short to observe something like 'remission' or 'flare'. The definitions of chronic inflammation reflect that. In TNBS colitis inflammation is regarded as chronic after 10 days; in DSS colitis after 3 months.

Another problem that cannot be avoided if working with rodent models is the fundamental difference in the mucosal immune system between those animals and humans. There is no clear Th1/Th2 dichotomy in humans as is found in mice. In addition dendritic cells can be specifically identified in mice with the CD11b surface antigen, which is much less specific in humans and also expressed on monocytes and macrophages, and other cells.

Unfortunately we also do not have an animal model developing strictures and fistulas, typical features of human Crohn's disease. Mice do not show signs of fibrosis, possibly due to their short lifespan. However, as we are able to treat the inflammation in IBD more and more effectively, but not the strictures and fistulas, those models are urgently needed.

During recent years a number of new therapeutic strategies have proved to be very successful in animal models, such as experimental therapies with IL-10 or IL-11[68,69,117,123–126], but the clinical trials in patients were disappointing[127–135]. This has led to some frustration among IBD researchers, and some loss of confidence in the results from animal models.

Taken together we have to admit that animal models have a number of important limitations. They are still used as the main tool to test and develop new therapeutic approaches by most investigators. However, due to the limitations of animal models mentioned above, human primary cell culture models and cell lines will probably gain more attention in the upcoming years.

ADVANTAGES AND DISADVANTAGES OF
CELL CULTURES AND CELL LINES

Clearly cell cultures and cell lines are *not* an easy and straightforward way to develop new therapeutic strategies. They have certain disadvantages. As cell culture models are used in an attempt to make complex systems more simple by isolating certain functions, they of course do not resemble and mimic the complex interactions that are found in the intestinal mucosa. A functional change in cell culture or a cell–cell interaction model cannot tell us whether there will be a reduction of inflammation *in vivo*. The whole is more than its parts, and the mucosal immune system is not really reflected by a careful analysis of its components.

Nevertheless we can gain important information from cell culture experiments. It is not just a disadvantage, but also a great advantage, that the analysis of cell culture models and cell lines allows us to isolate specific cellular functions and investigate them in detail. A better understanding of specific cellular functions may allow us to modulate those functions using drugs that finally can be tested further for their therapeutic potential. MAP-kinase inhibitors were developed in cell culture and cell line studies before their potential for IBD therapy was studied further[136–138].

If more complex cell culture models are used, such as the co-culture of two cell types, cell–cell interactions can be studied. Direct cell–cell interactions and the modulation of those interactions cannot be investigated *in vivo*. Methods to evaluate the success of a new approach *in vivo* in a rodent model are limited (usually histology and cytokine secretion), whereas specific functions of the human mucosal immune system can be simulated in cell culture experiments (e.g. antigen presentation, mucus production, oxidative burst reaction, clonal T-cell proliferation).

On the other hand cell cultures and cell lines allow us to investigate specific effects of potential therapeutic interventions. One example is given here: a tissue-protective effect of IL-11 for the intestinal mucosa had been postulated from animal models of IBD, as mentioned above[117]. However, IL-11 responsiveness is clearly restricted to cells that express the IL-11 receptor alpha-chain (IL-11Rα) and an additional signal transducing subunit (gp130). In one of our studies we identified the target cells for IL-11 within the human colon with a new IL-11Rα monoclonal antibody and investigated the effects of IL-11-induced signalling. Mucosal IL-11Rα expression was examined by immunohistochemistry. IL-11-induced cytoprotective effects were investigated by flow cytometry and Western blotting in HT-29 cells and primary human colonic epithelial cells (CEC). Immunohistochemistry revealed expression of the IL-11Rα selectively on CEC. HT-29 and CEC constitutively expressed IL-11Rα mRNA and protein. IL-11 induced signalling through triggering activation of the Jak-STAT pathway, without inducing anti-inflammatory or proliferative effects in CEC. However, IL-11 stimulation resulted in a dose-dependent tyrosine phosphorylation of Akt and a reduced induction of apoptosis in cultured CEC. Therefore, the known beneficial effects of IL-11 therapy are likely to be mediated by epithelial cells via activation of the Akt-survival pathway, mediating anti-apoptotic effects to ensure mucosal integrity. Knowledge of these data might have changed the approach by which IL-11 was tested in the clinical trial. If it acts mainly via reduction of apoptosis it might play a role in mucosal restitution, but not during a phase when reduction of inflammation is very crucial.

CELL CULTURE MODELS FOR THE STUDY OF THE INTESTINAL IMMUNE SYSTEM

During the past 8 years our group have developed a number of new cell culture models for the study of the intestinal immune system.

Culture of primary human intestinal epithelial cells

The classical functions of epithelial cells have mainly been studied in transformed human or rat cell lines. These classical functions are absorption and secretion of fluids, electrolytes, and nutrients as well as the formation of the primary physiological barrier against the multitude of antigens in the gut lumen. In recent years it has also been shown that epithelial cells play an active role in the intestinal immune system. IEC lines express HLA-DR after stimulation with interferon gamma (IFN-γ)[139–161]. After stimulation with IFN or IL-1 they show enhanced expression of adhesion molecules and lymphocyte function-associated antigens (CD58)[162–166]. ICAM-1 could be enhanced in HT-29 and Caco-2 cells by incubation with proinflammatory cytokines; however, the responsiveness to either IFN-α, tumour necrosis factor alpha (TNF-α), or IL-1 treatment was different between those cell lines[165].

In the cell line studies evidence was found that epithelial cells are able to respond to damage or bacterial invasion by secreting cytokines[167–174]. Cytokine production had mainly been studied in human and rat epithelial cell lines such as Caco-2, HT-29, T84 and IEC-6[169–173,175]. However, metabolic events and physiological regulation are clearly different in tumour or murine cell lines compared to primary human cells. Tumour cell lines undergo a number of consecutive mutations after transformation, and it is not possible to characterize all of them as new mutations may occur with every passage.

To allow the investigation of not-transformed primary human IEC we established a new method for the culture of primary human IEC (Fig. 1A,B)[176]. Cells are kept on translucent, permeable filter membranes at the medium/air interface (Fig. 1B) and are viable for about 5 days.

We found that, in contrast to data derived from studies with tumour cell lines, the primary cells did not produce IL-1β or IL-6. As mentioned above, animal models are an important tool to study the function of epithelial cells during an inflammatory event. However, the study of single-cell function is complicated by the complexity of the tissue structure in a living animal. In several animal models a Th1-cell-driven pathogenesis of intestinal inflammation has been proposed[54,177–182]. However, the effects of IFN-γ on IEC physiology and cytokine secretion are still a matter of discussion. Kolios and co-workers showed that IFN-γ did not influence IL-8 secretion in the HT-29 cell line[183]. On the other hand, Eckmann and Kagnoff demonstrated that IFN-γ was effective in up-regulating IL-8 secretion in HT-29, SW620, Caco-2 and T-84 cells[171]. Targan

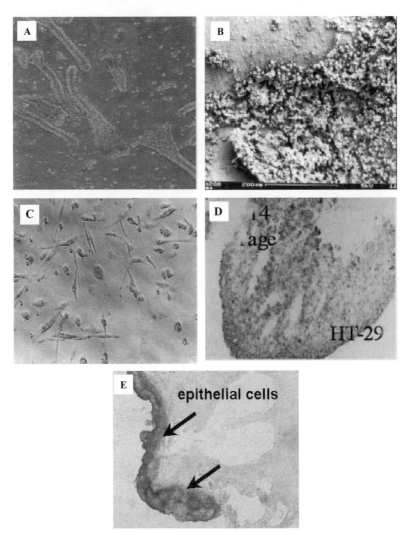

Fig. 1 Examples of cell culture models for the study of the mucosal immune system. **A**: Isolated crypts from human mucosa. **B**: Cultured primary human colonic epithelial cells on filter supports. **C**: Isolated and purified primary colonic macrophages. **D**: MCS of HT-29 cells and monocytes after 7 days of co-culture. **E**: 'organotypic colonic reconstructs'. Staining of EP-4 surface antigens to visualize epithelial cells (HT-29)

and co-workers demonstrated that IFN-γ pre-incubation is necessary for TNF-α or anti-Fas-induced apoptosis in the HT-29 line, but they could not observe co-operative effects of IFN-γ or TNF-α on IL-8 production[184]. To clarify these conflicting data we investigated the influence of IFN-γ on IL-8 secretion in the primary human IEC model.

We found that IFN-γ down-regulated IL-8 secretion and expression in primary human colonic IEC whereas it induced IL-8 secretion in HT-29 cells (Fig. 2).

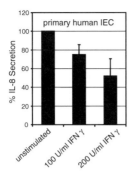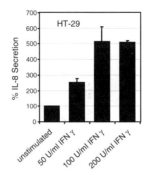

Fig. 2   IL-8 secretion of primary human colonic IEC and HT-29 cells after incubation with IFN-γ. Cells were cultured for 24 h in the presence of IFN-γ. Secretion of IL-8 into the culture medium was measured by ELISA. Whereas there was a reduction of IL-8 secretion in primary human colonic epithelial cells (left panel) in HT-29 cells IL-8 secretion was induced (right panel)

This effect was not due to induction or priming of susceptibility to apoptosis. The data demonstrate that there may be important differences in the response of cell lines and primary cells to stimulation, and that data derived from transformed cell lines may lead to misinterpretation of IEC function.

Isolation and culture of primary human macrophages

Mucosal macrophages (MAC) are central players in the local immune reactions. They originate in the bone marrow from pluripotent stem cells, differentiate via promonocytes into mature monocytes (MO) and enter the circulation within 24 h. After emigration from the circulation into the different tissues of the body the MO differentiate into resident tissue MAC. Intestinal MAC represent one of the largest compartments of the mononuclear phagocyte system in the body. They are localized preferentially at the sites of antigen entry, e.g. in the subepithelial region of the intestinal lamina propria and domes of Peyer's patches[185–188]. Resident MAC constitute 10–20% of the mononuclear cells in the lamina propria, as determined by immunohistochemistry and tissue-disaggregating experiments[189–191].

Intestinal macrophages are able to secrete a large number of different mediators, and these molecules may pass the basement membrane of the epithelium and influence epithelial cells of the intestinal mucosa. The investigation of direct interactions between intestinal macrophages and epithelial cells has been hampered by a lack of methods for the purification and culture of both cell types in the past. Recently we could establish a technique for the purification and short-time culture of human intestinal macrophages[188]. Lamina propria mononuclear cells (LPMNC) were isolated from normal and Crohn's disease mucosa specimens. Macrophages were labelled with immunomagnetic MicroBeads armed with CD33 antibody and purified twice with the help of type AS separation columns (Miltenyi Biotec)[188]. LPMNC with magnetically labelled macrophages were passed through an AS separation column which was placed in the permanent magnet SuperMACS. The magnetically labelled cells were retained in the column and separated from the unlabelled cells, which passed through. After removal of the column from the magnetic field the retained fraction could be eluted. Eluted cells were passed through a second AS separation column to increase purification of macrophages to a final purity of >95%. The purified intestinal macrophages could be seeded on FALCON Primaria® plates and kept in culture for several days (Fig. 1C).

Three-dimensional spheroids for the differentiation of mucosal macrophages

Several models have been established for the *in-vitro* differentiation of MAC[192–202]. A well-established model system is the culture of isolated monocytes (MO) in plastic dishes or Teflon® bags with 2% human AB serum for 7 days[197–199]. Under these conditions differentiation of MAC is associated with high surface expression of CD14[199]. MAC induced in serum free cultures with large amounts of albumin, immunoglobulin or with M-CSF also showed expression of CD14.

The differentiation/maturation of MAC has been studied in three-dimensional culture systems (multicellular spheroids, MCS)[203,204]. In these three-dimensional aggregates different conditions, for example O_2-gradient, pH, extracellular matrix production and cell proliferation, are similar to the *in-vivo* situation[205–210]. We used the MCS technique to induce close contact of MO with IEC in a three-dimensional environment. In the MCS cells form cell–cell and cell–matrix contacts (Fig. 1D)[211–213].

The typical phenotype of intestinal MAC from normal mucosa with a lack of CD14, CD16 and CD11b expression, as well as a lack of expression of co-stimulatory molecules, had not so far been induced *in vitro*. IEC are separated only by the basement high expression membrane from these MAC. We therefore assumed that IEC could possibly influence the differentiation of intestinal MAC. To investigate this possibility we used the MCS technique to allow close association of monocytes with IEC in a three-dimensional environment similar to the lamina propria.

During the 7 days of co-culture a significant change in the surface antigen expression of the MAC could be observed. CD14 and CD11b, which had been detected after 24 h of co-culture, had disappeared after 7 days but were still present in the spheroids of non-intestinal origin[214]. Flow cytometry showed a reduction of cells positive for both CD14 and CD68 from 81% of total CD68-positive cells at the 24 h time point to 7.6% after 7 days. This was not observed with carcinoma cell lines from non-intestinal origin[214].

These results indicate that, in the three-dimensional model of MCS, IEC induce an intestinal-like phenotype in the invading MAC. Therefore, IEC play an important role in the differentiation process of intestinal MAC.

An interesting question arises from these findings: could there be a disturbed differentiation of intestinal MAC during IBD? Could the inability of epithelial cells to induce the non-reactive normal intestinal MAC phenotype be responsible for the presence of permanently activated MAC in IBD? More complex models such as 'organotypic reconstructs' (Fig. 1E) will hopefully help to answer these questions.

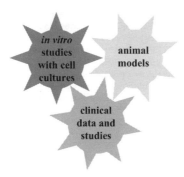

Fig. 3 Data derived from *in-vitro* studies with cell culture models, from animal models and clinical data must be combined for the evaluation of new therapeutic strategies

HOW CAN WE DEVELOP NEW THERAPEUTIC STRATEGIES WITH THESE MODELS?

To come back to the question raised in the title of this chapter: are cell lines and cultures a good way to develop therapeutic approaches? The answer is simple: despite all the advances demonstrated here they are not. These models may provide flexible tools that can be set together to understand basic functions of human mucosal immunology, but they are not complex enough to really represent the network of the human mucosal immune system. Therefore all these models cannot predict responses in humans. However, we also had to learn that animal models do not allow these predictions, as the differences between rodents and humans are significant.

We should therefore request a combined effort before the start of new clinical trials. Studies from cell culture models must be provided, as well as studies on animal models and trials with healthy volunteers, before a trial with patients can be performed (Fig. 3). Experts should review these data from cell culture models and animal models, as well as volunteers, to decide whether the time is ripe for new clinical trials. Too many trials have been performed based on only one of these three fundamentals, leading to frustrating results for the participating patients and the clinical researcher.

References

1. Wood JD, Peck OC, Tefend KS *et al*. Evidence that colitis is initiated by environmental stress and sustained by fecal factors in the cotton-top tamarin (*Saguinus oedipus*). Dig Dis Sci. 2000;45:385–93.
2. Wood JD, Peck OC, Tefend KS *et al*. Colitis and colon cancer in cotton-top tamarins (*Saguinus oedipus oedipus*) living wild in their natural habitat. Dig Dis Sci. 1998;43:1443–53.
3. Bertone ER, Giovannucci EL, King NW, Jr, Petto AJ, Johnson LD. Family history as a risk factor for ulcerative colitis-associated colon cancer in cotton-top tamarin. Gastroenterology. 1998;114:669–74.
4. Hesterberg PE, Winsor-Hines D, Briskin MJ *et al*. Rapid resolution of chronic colitis in the cotton-top tamarin with an antibody to a gut-homing integrin alpha 4 beta 7. Gastroenterology. 1996;111:1373–80.

5. Johnson LD, Ausman LM, Sehgal PK, King NW, Jr. A prospective study of the epidemiology of colitis and colon cancer in cotton-top tamarins (*Saguinus oedipus*). Gastroenterology. 1996;110:102–15.
6. Podolsky DK, Lobb R, King N *et al*. Attenuation of colitis in the cotton-top tamarin by anti-alpha 4 integrin monoclonal antibody. J Clin Invest. 1993;92:372–80.
7. Clapp N, Henke M, Hansard R, Carson R, Fretland D. Anti-colitic efficacy of SC-41930 in colitic cotton-top tamarins. Agents Actions. 1993;39:C36–8.
8. Kim HS, Berstad A. Experimental colitis in animal models. Scand J Gastroenterol. 1992;27:529–37.
9. Targan SR, Landers CJ, King NW, Podolsky DJ, Shanahan F. Ulcerative colitis-linked antineutrophil cytoplasmic antibody in the cotton-top tamarin model of colitis. Gastroenterology. 1992;102:1493–8.
10. Clapp NK, Henke MA, Hansard RM *et al*. Inflammatory mediators in cotton-top tamarins (CTT) with acute and chronic colitis. Agents Actions. 1991;34:178–80.
11. Podolsky DK, Madara JL, King N, Sehgal P, Moore R, Winter HS. Colonic mucin composition in primates. Selective alterations associated with spontaneous colitis in the cotton-top tamarin. Gastroenterology. 1985;88:20–5.
12. Madara JL, Podolsky DK, King NW, Sehgal PK, Moore R, Winter HS. Characterization of spontaneous colitis in cotton-top tamarins (*Saguinus oedipus*) and its response to sulfasalazine. Gastroenterology. 1985;88:13–19.
13. Elson CO, Cong Y, Sundberg J. The C3H/HeJBir mouse model: a high susceptibility phenotype for colitis. Int Rev Immunol. 2000;19:63–75.
14. Stevceva L, Pavli P, Buffinton G, Wozniak A, Doe WF. Dextran sodium sulphate-induced colitis activity varies with mouse strain but develops in lipopolysaccharide-unresponsive mice. J Gastroenterol Hepatol. 1999;14:54–60.
15. Mahler M, Bristol IJ, Sundberg JP *et al*. Genetic analysis of susceptibility to dextran sulfate sodium-induced colitis in mice. Genomics. 1999;55:147–56.
16. Cong Y, Brandwein SL, McCabe RP *et al*. CD4+ T cells reactive to enteric bacterial antigens in spontaneously colitic C3H/HeJBir mice: increased T helper cell type 1 response and ability to transfer disease. J Exp Med. 1998;187:855–64.
17. Brandwein SL, McCabe RP, Cong Y *et al*. Spontaneously colitic C3H/HeJBir mice demonstrate selective antibody reactivity to antigens of the enteric bacterial flora. J Immunol. 1997;159:44–52.
18. Sundberg JP, Elson CO, Bedigian H, Birkenmeier EH. Spontaneous, heritable colitis in a new substrain of C3H/HeJ mice. Gastroenterology. 1994;107:1726–35.
19. Wang QY, Chen CL, Wang JD, Lai ZS, Liu R, Zhang YL. Establishment of dextran sulfate sodium-induced ulcerative colitis model in mice. Di Yi Jun Yi Da Xue Xue Bao. 2002;22:608–10.
20. ten Hove T, Drillenburg P, Wijnholds J, Te Velde AA, van Deventer SJ. Differential susceptibility of multidrug resistance protein-1 deficient mice to DSS and TNBS-induced colitis. Dig Dis Sci. 2002;47:2056–63.
21. Obermeier F, Dunger N, Deml L, Herfarth H, Scholmerich J, Falk W. CpG motifs of bacterial DNA exacerbate colitis of dextran sulfate sodium-treated mice. Eur J Immunol. 2002;32:2084–92.
22. Seril DN, Liao J, Ho KL, Warsi A, Yang CS, Yang GY. Dietary iron supplementation enhances DSS-induced colitis and associated colorectal carcinoma development in mice. Dig Dis Sci. 2002;47:1266–78.
23. Kitajima S, Morimoto M, Sagara E. A model for dextran sodium sulfate (DSS)-induced mouse colitis: bacterial degradation of DSS does not occur after incubation with mouse cecal contents. Exp Anim. 2002;51:203–6.
24. Sivakumar PV, Westrich GM, Kanaly S *et al*. Interleukin 18 is a primary mediator of the inflammation associated with dextran sulphate sodium induced colitis: blocking interleukin 18 attenuates intestinal damage. Gut. 2002;50:812–20.
25. Sayer B, Lu J, Green C, Soderholm JD, Akhtar M, McKay DM. Dextran sodium sulphate-induced colitis perturbs muscarinic cholinergic control of colonic epithelial ion transport. Br J Pharmacol. 2002;135:1794–800.
26. Kitajima S, Morimoto M, Sagara E, Shimizu C, Ikeda Y. Dextran sodium sulfate-induced colitis in germ-free IQI/Jic mice. Exp Anim. 2001;50:387–95.
27. Farkas S, Herfarth H, Rossle M *et al*. Quantification of mucosal leucocyte endothelial cell interaction by *in vivo* fluorescence microscopy in experimental colitis in mice. Clin Exp Immunol. 2001;126:250–8.

28. Egger B, Bajaj-Elliott M, MacDonald TT, Inglin R, Eysselein VE, Buchler MW. Characterisation of acute murine dextran sodium sulphate colitis: cytokine profile and dose dependency. Digestion. 2000;62:240–8.

29. Diaz-Granados N, Howe K, Lu J, McKay DM. Dextran sulfate sodium-induced colonic histopathology, but not altered epithelial ion transport, is reduced by inhibition of phosphodiesterase activity. Am J Pathol. 2000;156:2169–77.

30. Marrero JA, Matkowskyj KA, Yung K, Hecht G, Benya RV. Dextran sulfate sodium-induced murine colitis activates NF-kappaB and increases galanin-1 receptor expression. Am J Physiol Gastrointest Liver Physiol. 2000;278:G797–804.

31. Herfarth H, Brand K, Rath HC, Rogler G, Scholmerich J, Falk W. Nuclear factor-kappa B activity and intestinal inflammation in dextran sulphate sodium (DSS)-induced colitis in mice is suppressed by gliotoxin. Clin Exp Immunol. 2000;120:59–65.

32. Kitajima S, Takuma S, Morimoto M. Changes in colonic mucosal permeability in mouse colitis induced with dextran sulfate sodium. Exp Anim. 1999;48:137–43.

33. Hamamoto N, Maemura K, Hirata I, Murano M, Sasaki S, Katsu K. Inhibition of dextran sulphate sodium (DSS)-induced colitis in mice by intracolonically administered antibodies against adhesion molecules (endothelial leucocyte adhesion molecule-1 (ELAM-1) or intercellular adhesion molecule-1 (ICAM-1)). Clin Exp Immunol. 1999;117:462–8.

34. Kitajima S, Takuma S, Morimoto M. Tissue distribution of dextran sulfate sodium (DSS) in the acute phase of murine DSS-induced colitis. J Vet Med Sci. 1999;61:67–70.

35. Dieleman LA, Palmen MJ, Akol H et al. Chronic experimental colitis induced by dextran sulphate sodium (DSS) is characterized by Th1 and Th2 cytokines. Clin Exp Immunol. 1998;114:385–91.

36. Rogler G, Andus T. Cytokines in inflammatory bowel disease. World J Surg. 1998;22:382–9.

37. Mahler M, Bristol IJ, Leiter EH et al. Differential susceptibility of inbred mouse strains to dextran sulfate sodium-induced colitis. Am J Physiol. 1998;274:G544–51.

38. van Meeteren ME, van Bergeijk JD, van Dijk AP, Tak CJ, Meijssen MA, Zijlstra FJ. Intestinal permeability and contractility in murine colitis. Mediators Inflamm. 1998;7:163–8.

39. Kojouharoff G, Hans W, Obermeier F et al. Neutralization of tumour necrosis factor (TNF) but not of IL-1 reduces inflammation in chronic dextran sulphate sodium-induced colitis in mice. Clin Exp Immunol. 1997;107:353–8.

40. Dieleman LA, Ridwan BU, Tennyson GS, Beagley KW, Bucy RP, Elson CO. Dextran sulfate sodium-induced colitis occurs in severe combined immunodeficient mice. Gastroenterology. 1994;107:1643–52.

41. Axelsson LG, Landstrom E, Goldschmidt TJ, Gronberg A, Bylund-Fellenius AC. Dextran sulfate sodium (DSS) induced experimental colitis in immunodeficient mice: effects in CD4(+)-cell depleted, athymic and NK-cell depleted SCID mice. Inflamm Res. 1996;45:181–91.

42. Zijlstra FJ, Garrelds IM, van Dijk AP, Wilson JH. Experimental colitis in mice: effects of olsalazine on eicosanoid production in colonic tissue. Agents Actions. 1992; Special issue, C76–8.

43. Hans W, Scholmerich J, Gross V, Falk W. The role of the resident intestinal flora in acute and chronic dextran sulfate sodium-induced colitis in mice. Eur J Gastroenterol Hepatol. 2000;12:267–73.

44. Hans W, Scholmerich J, Gross V, Falk W. Interleukin-12 induced interferon-gamma increases inflammation in acute dextran sulfate sodium induced colitis in mice. Eur Cytokine Netw. 2000;11:67–74.

45. Camoglio L, Juffermans NP, Peppelenbosch M et al. Contrasting roles of IL-12p40 and IL-12p35 in the development of hapten-induced colitis. Eur J Immunol. 2002;32:261–9.

46. Ten Hove T, Corbaz A, Amitai H et al. Blockade of endogenous IL-18 ameliorates TNBS-induced colitis by decreasing local TNF-alpha production in mice. Gastroenterology. 2001;121:1372–9.

47. Camoglio L, te Velde AA, de Boer A, ten Kate FJ, Kopf M, van Deventer SJ. Hapten-induced colitis associated with maintained Th1 and inflammatory responses in IFN-gamma receptor-deficient mice. Eur J Immunol. 2000;30:1486–95.

48. McCafferty DM, Miampamba M, Sihota E, Sharkey KA, Kubes P. Role of inducible nitric oxide synthase in trinitrobenzene sulphonic acid induced colitis in mice. Gut. 1999;45:864–73.

49. Stallmach A, Wittig B, Giese T et al. Protection of trinitrobenzene sulfonic acid-induced colitis by an interleukin 2-IgG2b fusion protein in mice. Gastroenterology. 1999;117:866–76.

50. Dohi T, Fujihashi K, Rennert PD, Iwatani K, Kiyono H, McGhee JR. Hapten-induced colitis is associated with colonic patch hypertrophy and T helper cell 2-type responses. J Exp Med. 1999;189:1169–80.
51. Wittig B, Schwarzler C, Fohr N, Gunthert U, Zoller M. Curative treatment of an experimentally induced colitis by a CD44 variant V7-specific antibody. J Immunol. 1998;161:1069–73.
52. Neurath MF, Fuss I, Pasparakis M et al. Predominant pathogenic role of tumor necrosis factor in experimental colitis in mice. Eur J Immunol. 1997;27:1743–50.
53. Neurath MF, Pettersson S, Meyer zum Buschenfelde KH, Strober W. Local administration of antisense phosphorothioate oligonucleotides to the p65 subunit of NF-kappa B abrogates established experimental colitis in mice. Nat Med. 1996;2:998–1004.
54. Neurath MF, Fuss I, Kelsall BL, Stuber E, Strober W. Antibodies to interleukin 12 abrogate established experimental colitis in mice. J Exp Med. 1995;182:P1281–90.
55. Duchmann R, Schmitt E, Knolle P, Meyer zum Buschenfelde KH, Neurath M. Tolerance towards resident intestinal flora in mice is abrogated in experimental colitis and restored by treatment with interleukin-10 or antibodies to interleukin-12. Eur J Immunol. 1996;26:934–8.
56. Neurath MF, Fuss I, Kelsall BL, Presky DH, Waegell W, Strober W. Experimental granulomatous colitis in mice is abrogated by induction of TGF-beta-mediated oral tolerance. J Exp Med. 1996;183:2605–16.
57. Elson CO, Beagley KW, Sharmanov AT et al. Hapten-induced model of murine inflammatory bowel disease: mucosa immune responses and protection by tolerance. J Immunol. 1996;157:2174–85.
58. Karmeli F, Cohen P, Rachmilewitz D. Cyclo-oxygenase-2 inhibitors ameliorate the severity of experimental colitis in rats. Eur J Gastroenterol Hepatol. 2000;12:223–31.
59. Banerjee A. Thromboxanes, indomethacin, and experimental colitis. Gastroenterology. 1993;104:1891–2.
60. Gurbindo C, Russo P, Sabbah S, Lohoues MJ, Seidman E. Interleukin-2 activity of colonic lamina propria mononuclear cells in a rat model of experimental colitis. Gastroenterology. 1993;104:964–72.
61. Empey LR, Walker K, Fedorak RN. Indomethacin worsens and a leukotriene biosynthesis inhibitor accelerates mucosal healing in rat colitis. Can J Physiol Pharmacol. 1992;70:660–8.
62. Topalian SL, Ziegler MM. Necrotizing enterocolitis: a review of animal models. J Surg Res. 1984;37:320–36.
63. Mann NS, Demers LM. Experimental colitis studied by colonoscopy in the rat: effect of indomethacin. Gastrointest Endosc. 1983;29:77–82.
64. Yamada T, Sartor RB, Marshall S, Specian RD, Grisham MB. Mucosal injury and inflammation in a model of chronic granulomatous colitis in rats. Gastroenterology. 1993;104:759–71.
65. Fitzpatrick LR, Wang J, Le T. Gliotoxin, an inhibitor of nuclear factor-kappa B, attenuates peptidoglycan-polysaccharide-induced colitis in rats. Inflamm Bowel Dis. 2002;8:159–67.
66. Kandil HM, Argenzio RA, Sartor RB. Low endogenous prostaglandin E2 predisposes to relapsing inflammation in experimental rat enterocolitis. Dig Dis Sci. 1999;44:2110–18.
67. van Tol EA, Holt L, Li FL et al. Bacterial cell wall polymers promote intestinal fibrosis by direct stimulation of myofibroblasts. Am J Physiol. 1999;277:G245–55.
68. Herfarth HH, Bocker U, Janardhanam R, Sartor RB. Subtherapeutic corticosteroids potentiate the ability of interleukin 10 to prevent chronic inflammation in rats. Gastroenterology. 1998;115:856–65.
69. Herfarth HH, Mohanty SP, Rath HC, Tonkonogy S, Sartor RB. Interleukin 10 suppresses experimental chronic, granulomatous inflammation induced by bacterial cell wall polymers. Gut. 1996;39:836–45.
70. Sartor RB, Rath HC, Lichtman SN, van Tol EA. Animal models of intestinal and joint inflammation. Baillières Clin Rheumatol. 1996;10:55–76.
71. Sartor RB, Bond TM, Schwab JH. Systemic uptake and intestinal inflammatory effects of luminal bacterial cell wall polymers in rats with acute colonic injury. Infect Immun. 1988;56:2101–8.
72. Scheerens H, Hessel E, de Waal-Malefyt R, Leach MW, Rennick D. Characterization of chemokines and chemokine receptors in two murine models of inflammatory bowel disease: IL-10$^{-/-}$ mice and Rag-2$^{-/-}$ mice reconstituted with CD4$^+$CD45RBhigh T cells. Eur J Immunol. 2001;31:1465–74.

73. Liu Z, Geboes K, Colpaert S *et al.* Prevention of experimental colitis in SCID mice reconstituted with CD45RBhigh CD4+ T cells by blocking the CD40–CD154 interactions. J Immunol. 2000;164:6005–14.

74. Kawachi S, Morise Z, Jennings SR *et al.* Cytokine and adhesion molecule expression in SCID mice reconstituted with CD4+ T cells. Inflamm Bowel Dis. 2000;6:171–80.

75. Chu A, Hong K, Berg EL, Ehrhardt RO. Tissue specificity of E- and P-selectin ligands in Th1-mediated chronic inflammation. J Immunol. 1999;163:5086–93.

76. De Winter H, Cheroutre H, Kronenberg M. Mucosal immunity and inflammation. II. The yin and yang of T cells in intestinal inflammation: pathogenic and protective roles in a mouse colitis model. Am J Physiol. 1999;276:G1317–21.

77. Claesson MH, Bregenholt S, Bonhagen K *et al.* Colitis-inducing potency of CD4+ T cells in immunodeficient, adoptive hosts depends on their state of activation, IL-12 responsiveness, and CD45RB surface phenotype. J Immunol. 1999;162:3702–10.

78. Ito H, Fathman CG. CD45RBhigh CD4+ T cells from IFN-gamma knockout mice do not induce wasting disease. J Autoimmun. 1997;10:455–9.

79. Aranda R, Sydora BC, McAllister PL *et al.* Analysis of intestinal lymphocytes in mouse colitis mediated by transfer of CD4+, CD45RBhigh T cells to SCID recipients. J Immunol. 1997;158:3464–73.

80. Leach MW, Bean AG, Mauze S, Coffman RL, Powrie F. Inflammatory bowel disease in C.B-17 scid mice reconstituted with the CD45RBhigh subset of CD4+ T cells. Am J Pathol. 1996;148: 1503–15.

81. Powrie F, Correa-Oliveira R, Mauze S, Coffman RL. Regulatory interactions between CD45RBhigh and CD45RBlow CD4+ T cells are important for the balance between protective and pathogenic cell-mediated immunity. J Exp Med. 1994;179:589–600.

82. Powrie F, Leach MW, Mauze S, Caddle LB, Coffman RL. Phenotypically distinct subsets of CD4+ T cells induce or protect from chronic intestinal inflammation in C. B-17 scid mice. Int Immunol. 1993;5:1461–71.

83. Johansson AC, Hansson AS, Nandakumar KS, Backlund J, Holmdahl R. IL-10-deficient B10.Q mice develop more severe collagen-induced arthritis, but are protected from arthritis induced with anti-type II collagen antibodies. J Immunol. 2001;167:3505–12.

84. Garrelds IM, van Meeteren ME, Meijssen MA, Zijlstra FJ. Interleukin-2-deficient mice: effect on cytokines and inflammatory cells in chronic colonic disease. Dig Dis Sci. 2002;47:503–10.

85. Boone DL, Dassopoulos T, Lodolce JP, Chai S, Chien M, Ma A. Interleukin-2-deficient mice develop colitis in the absence of CD28 costimulation. Inflamm Bowel Dis. 2002;8: 35–42.

86. Schultz M, Tonkonogy SL, Sellon RK *et al.* IL-2-deficient mice raised under germfree conditions develop delayed mild focal intestinal inflammation. Am J Physiol. 1999;276:G1461–72.

87. Yang F, de Villiers WJ, Lee EY, McClain CJ, Varilek GW. Increased nuclear factor-kappaB activation in colitis of interleukin-2- deficient mice. J Lab Clin Med. 1999;134:378–85.

88. Ehrhardt RO, Ludviksson B. Induction of colitis in IL2-deficient-mice: the role of thymic and peripheral dysregulation in the generation of autoreactive T cells. Res Immunol. 1997;148:582–8.

89. Baumgart DC, Olivier WA, Reya T, Peritt D, Rombeau JL, Carding SR. Mechanisms of intestinal epithelial cell injury and colitis in interleukin 2 (IL2)-deficient mice. Cell Immunol. 1998;187:52–66.

90. Davidson NJ, Hudak SA, Lesley RE, Menon S, Leach MW, Rennick DM. IL-12, but not IFN-gamma, plays a major role in sustaining the chronic phase of colitis in IL-10-deficient mice. J Immunol. 1998;161:3143–9.

91. Sadlack B, Merz H, Schorle H, Schimpl A, Feller AC, Horak I. Ulcerative colitis-like disease in mice with a disrupted interleukin-2 gene. Cell. 1993;75:253–61.

92. Ehrhardt RO, Ludviksson BR, Gray B, Neurath M, Strober W. Induction and prevention of colonic inflammation in IL-2-deficient mice. J Immunol. 1997;158:566–73.

93. Podolsky DK. Lessons from genetic models of inflammatory bowel disease. Acta Gastroenterol Belg. 1997;60:163–5.

94. Autenrieth IB, Bucheler N, Bohn E, Heinze G, Horak I. Cytokine mRNA expression in intestinal tissue of interleukin-2 deficient mice with bowel inflammation. Gut. 1997;41:793–800.

95. Berg DJ, Zhang J, Weinstock JV *et al.* Rapid development of colitis in NSAID-treated IL-10-deficient mice. Gastroenterology. 2002;123:1527–42.

96. Mahler M, Most C, Schmidtke S et al. Genetics of colitis susceptibility in IL-10-deficient mice: backcross versus F2 results contrasted by principal component analysis. Genomics. 2002;80:274.

97. Madsen KL. Inflammatory bowel disease: lessons from the IL-10 gene-deficient mouse. Clin Invest Med. 2001;24:250–7.

98. Sturlan S, Oberhuber G, Beinhauer BG et al. Interleukin-10-deficient mice and inflammatory bowel disease associated cancer development. Carcinogenesis. 2001;22:665–71.

99. Bristol IJ, Farmer MA, Cong Y et al. Heritable susceptibility for colitis in mice induced by IL-10 deficiency. Inflamm Bowel Dis. 2000;6:290–302.

100. Kennedy RJ, Hoper M, Deodhar K, Erwin PJ, Kirk SJ, Gardiner KR. Interleukin 10-deficient colitis: new similarities to human inflammatory bowel disease. Br J Surg. 2000;87: 1346–51.

101. McCafferty DM, Sihota E, Muscara M, Wallace JL, Sharkey KA, Kubes P. Spontaneously developing chronic colitis in IL-10/iNOS double-deficient mice. Am J Physiol Gastrointest Liver Physiol. 2000;279:G90–9.

102. Davidson NJ, Fort MM, Muller W, Leach MW, Rennick DM. Chronic colitis in IL-10$^{-/-}$ mice: insufficient counter regulation of a Th1 response. Int Rev Immunol. 2000;19:91–121.

103. Madsen KL, Doyle JS, Tavernini MM, Jewell LD, Rennie RP, Fedorak RN. Antibiotic therapy attenuates colitis in interleukin 10 gene-deficient mice. Gastroenterology. 2000; 118:1094–105.

104. Madsen KL, Doyle JS, Jewell LD, Tavernini MM, Fedorak RN. Lactobacillus species prevents colitis in interleukin 10 gene-deficient mice. Gastroenterology. 1999;116:1107–14.

105. Leach MW, Davidson NJ, Fort MM, Powrie F, Rennick DM. The role of IL-10 in inflammatory bowel disease: 'of mice and men'. Toxicol Pathol. 1999;27:123–33.

106. Sellon RK, Tonkonogy S, Schultz M et al. Resident enteric bacteria are necessary for development of spontaneous colitis and immune system activation in interleukin-10-deficient mice. Infect Immun. 1998;66:5224–31.

107. Rennick DM, Fort MM, Davidson NJ. Studies with IL-10$^{-/-}$ mice: an overview. J Leukoc Biol. 1997;61:389–96.

108. Kuhn R, Lohler J, Rennick D, Rajewsky K, Muller W. Interleukin-10-deficient mice develop chronic enterocolitis. Cell. 1993;75:263–74.

109. Berg DJ, Davidson N, Kuhn R et al. Enterocolitis and colon cancer in interleukin-10-deficient mice are associated with aberrant cytokine production and CD4(+) TH1-like responses. J Clin Invest. 1996;98:1010–20.

110. Panwala CM, Jones JC, Viney JL. A novel model of inflammatory bowel disease: mice deficient for the multiple drug resistance gene, mdr1a, spontaneously develop colitis. J Immunol. 1998;161:5733–44.

111. Rath HC, Schultz M, Freitag R et al. Different subsets of enteric bacteria induce and perpetuate experimental colitis in rats and mice. Infect Immun. 2001;69:2277–85.

112. Greenwood-Van Meerveld B, Tyler K, Keith JC, Jr. Recombinant human interleukin-11 modulates ion transport and mucosal inflammation in the small intestine and colon. Lab Invest. 2000;80:1269–80.

113. Sartor RB. Colitis in HLA-B27/beta 2 microglobulin transgenic rats. Int Rev Immunol. 2000;19:39–50.

114. Taurog JD, Maika SD, Satumtira N et al. Inflammatory disease in HLA-B27 transgenic rats. Immunol Rev. 1999;169:209–23.

115. Rath HC, Wilson KH, Sartor RB. Differential induction of colitis and gastritis in HLA-B27 transgenic rats selectively colonized with Bacteroides vulgatus or Escherichia coli. Infect Immun. 1999;67:2969–74.

116. Rath HC, Ikeda JS, Linde HJ, Scholmerich J, Wilson KH, Sartor RB. Varying cecal bacterial loads influences colitis and gastritis in HLA- B27 transgenic rats. Gastroenterology. 1999;116: 310–19.

117. Peterson RL, Wang L, Albert L, Keith JC, Jr, Dorner AJ. Molecular effects of recombinant human interleukin-11 in the HLA-B27 rat model of inflammatory bowel disease. Lab Invest. 1998;78:1503–12.

118. Bertrand V, Quere S, Guimbaud R et al. Effects of murine recombinant interleukin-10 on the inflammatory disease of rats transgenic for HLA-B27 and human beta 2-microglobulin. Eur Cytokine Netw. 1998;9:161–70.

119. Lundin PD, Ekstrom G, Erlansson M, Lundin S, Westrom BR. Intestinal inflammation and barrier function in HLA-B27/beta 2-microglobulin transgenic rats. Scand J Gastroenterol. 1997;32:700–5.

120. Rath HC, Herfarth HH, Ikeda JS et al. Normal luminal bacteria, especially Bacteroides species, mediate chronic colitis, gastritis, and arthritis in HLA-B27/human beta2 microglobulin transgenic rats. J Clin Invest. 1996;98:945–53.

121. Aiko S, Grisham MB. Spontaneous intestinal inflammation and nitric oxide metabolism in HLA-B27 transgenic rats. Gastroenterology. 1995;109:142–50.

122. Gough AW, Mosley RL, Stubbs CJ. Immunopathologic characterization of typhlitis and colitis in juvenile HLA-B27 transgenic rats. Pathobiology. 1994;62:221–31.

123. Steidler L. In situ delivery of cytokines by genetically engineered Lactococcus lactis. Antonie Van Leeuwenhoek. 2002;82:323–31.

124. De Winter H, Elewaut D, Turovskaya O et al. Regulation of mucosal immune responses by recombinant interleukin 10 produced by intestinal epithelial cells in mice. Gastroenterology. 2002;122:1829–41.

125. Barbara G, Xing Z, Hogaboam CM, Gauldie J, Collins SM. Interleukin 10 gene transfer prevents experimental colitis in rats. Gut. 2000;46:344–9.

126. Grool TA, van Dullemen H, Meenan J et al. Anti-inflammatory effect of interleukin-10 in rabbit immune complex-induced colitis. Scand J Gastroenterol. 1998;33:754–8.

127. Schmit A, Carol M, Robert F et al. Dose-effect of interleukin-10 and its immunoregulatory role in Crohn's disease. Eur Cytokine Netw. 2002;13:298–305.

128. Tilg H, van Montfrans C, van den Ende A et al. Treatment of Crohn's disease with recombinant human interleukin 10 induces the proinflammatory cytokine interferon gamma. Gut. 2002; 50:191–5.

129. Herfarth H, Scholmerich J. IL-10 therapy in Crohn's disease: at the crossroads. Treatment of Crohn's disease with the anti-inflammatory cytokine interleukin 10. Gut. 2002;50:146–7.

130. Lindsay JO, Hodgson HJ. Review article: The immunoregulatory cytokine interleukin-10 – a therapy for Crohn's disease? Aliment Pharmacol Ther. 2001;15:1709–16.

131. Colombel JF, Rutgeerts P, Malchow H et al. Interleukin 10 (Tenovil) in the prevention of post-operative recurrence of Crohn's disease. Gut. 2001;49:42–6.

132. Fedorak RN, Gangl A, Elson CO et al. Recombinant human interleukin 10 in the treatment of patients with mild to moderately active Crohn's disease. The Interleukin 10 Inflammatory Bowel Disease Cooperative Study Group. Gastroenterology. 2000;119:1473–82.

133. Schreiber S, Fedorak RN, Nielsen OH et al. Safety and efficacy of recombinant human interleukin 10 in chronic active Crohn's disease. Crohn's Disease IL-10 Cooperative Study Group. Gastroenterology. 2000;119:1461–72.

134. Sands BE, Winston BD, Salzberg B et al. Randomized, controlled trial of recombinant human interleukin-11 in patients with active Crohn's disease. Aliment Pharmacol Ther. 2002;16: 399–406.

135. Sands BE, Bank S, Sninsky CA et al. Preliminary evaluation of safety and activity of recombinant human interleukin 11 in patients with active Crohn's disease. Gastroenterology. 1999;117:58–64.

136. Wong CK, Zhang JP, Ip WK, Lam CW. Activation of p38 mitogen-activated protein kinase and nuclear factor-kappaB in tumour necrosis factor-induced eotaxin release of human eosinophils. Clin Exp Immunol. 2002;128:483–9.

137. Laufer SA, Wagner GK. From imidazoles to pyrimidines: new inhibitors of cytokine release. J Med Chem. 2002;45:2733–40.

138. Xiao YQ, Malcolm K, Worthen GS et al. Cross-talk between ERK and p38 MAPK mediates selective suppression of pro-inflammatory cytokines by transforming growth factor-beta. J Biol Chem. 2002;277:14884–93.

139. Zimmer KP, Buning J, Weber P, Kaiserlian D, Strobel S. Modulation of antigen trafficking to MHC class II-positive late endosomes of enterocytes. Gastroenterology. 2000;118: 128–37.

140. Ruemmele FM, Gurbindo C, Mansour AM, Marchand R, Levy E, Seidman EG. Effects of interferon gamma on growth, apoptosis, and MHC class II expression of immature rat intestinal crypt (IEC-6) cells. J Cell Physiol. 1998;176:120–6.

141. Christ AD, Blumberg RS. The intestinal epithelial cell: immunological aspects. Springer Semin Immunopathol. 1997;18:449–61.

142. Donnet-Hughes A, Borel Y, Schiffrin EJ. The modulation of class I and class II MHC molecules on intestinal epithelial cells at different stages of differentiation. Adv Exp Med Biol. 1995; 371A:247–9.

143. Schiffrin EJ, Borel Y, Donnet-Hughes A. Modulation of the MHC class I and II molecules by bacterial products on intestinal epithelial cells. Adv Exp Med Biol. 1995; 371A:195–6.

144. Brandeis JM, Sayegh MH, Gallon L, Blumberg RS, Carpenter CB. Rat intestinal epithelial cells present major histocompatibility complex allopeptides to primed T cells. Gastroenterology. 1994;107:1537–42.

145. Matsumoto S, Setoyama H, Umesaki Y. Differential induction of major histocompatibility complex molecules on mouse intestine by bacterial colonization. Gastroenterology. 1992;103: 1777–82.

146. Keren DF. Antigen processing in the mucosal immune system. Semin Immunol. 1992;4:217–26.

147. Fais S, Capobianchi MR, Marcheggiano A, Iannoni C, Pallone F. MHC class II antigens on the epithelial cells of the human gastrointestinal tract. Gastroenterology. 1992;102:377–8.

148. Blumberg RS, Terhorst C, Bleicher P et al. Expression of a nonpolymorphic MHC class I-like molecule, CD1D, by human intestinal epithelial cells. J Immunol. 1991;147:2518–24.

149. Salomon P, Pizzimenti A, Panja A, Reisman A, Mayer L. The expression and regulation of class II antigens in normal and inflammatory bowel disease peripheral blood monocytes and intestinal epithelium. Autoimmunity. 1991;9:141–9.

150. Geboes K, Rutgeerts P, Penninckx F, Desmet V, Vantrappen G. Changes in small intestinal epithelial expression of MHC class II antigen after terminal ileal resection for Crohn's disease. Int J Colorectal Dis. 1988;3:102–8.

151. Shao L, Serrano D, Mayer L. The role of epithelial cells in immune regulation in the gut. Semin Immunol. 2001;13:163–76.

152. Laiping So A, Pelton-Henrion K, Small G et al. Antigen uptake and trafficking in human intestinal epithelial cells. Dig Dis Sci. 2000;45:1451–61.

153. So AL, Small G, Sperber K et al. Factors affecting antigen uptake by human intestinal epithelial cell lines. Dig Dis Sci. 2000;45:1130–37.

154. Hershberg RM, Mayer LF. Antigen processing and presentation by intestinal epithelial cells – polarity and complexity. Immunol Today. 2000;21:123–8.

155. Mayer L. Review article: Local and systemic regulation of mucosal immunity. Aliment Pharmacol Ther. 1997;11 (Suppl. 3):81–5; discussion 85–8.

156. Mayer L. Current concepts in mucosal immunity. I. Antigen presentation in the intestine: new rules and regulations. Am J Physiol. 1998;274:G7–9.

157. Fitzpatrick JL, Mayer SJ, Vilela C, Bland PW, Stokes CR. Cytokine-induced major histocompatibility complex class II antigens on cultured bovine mammary gland epithelial cells. J Dairy Sci. 1994;77:2940–8.

158. Mayer L. The role of the epithelial cell in immunoregulation: pathogenetic and therapeutic implications. Mt Sinai J Med. 1990;57:279–82.

159. Mayer L, Eisenhardt D, Salomon P, Bauer W, Plous R, Piccinini L. Expression of class II molecules on intestinal epithelial cells in humans. Differences between normal and inflammatory bowel disease. Gastroenterology. 1991;100:3–12.

160. Mayer L, Shlien R. Evidence for function of Ia molecules on gut epithelial cells in man. J Exp Med. 1987;166:1471–83.

161. Mayer L. The role of epithelial cells as accessory cells. Adv Exp Med Biol. 1987;216A:209–18.

162. Kaiserlian D, Rigal D, Abello J, Revillard JP. Expression, function and regulation of the inter-cellular adhesion molecule-1 (ICAM-1) on human intestinal epithelial cell lines. Eur J Immunol. 1991;21:2415–21.

163. Kvale D, Krajci P, Brandtzaeg P. Expression and regulation of adhesion molecules ICAM-1 (CD54) and LFA-3 (CD58) in human intestinal epithelial cell lines. Scand J Immunol. 1992;35:669–76.

164. Smart CJ, Calabrese A, Oakes DJ, Howdle PD, Trejdosiewicz LK. Expression of the LFA-1 beta 2 integrin (CD11a/CD18) and ICAM-1 (CD54) in normal and coeliac small bowel mucosa. Scand J Immunol. 1991;34:299–305.

165. Dippold W, Wittig B, Schwaeble W, Mayet W, Meyer zum Buschenfelde KH. Expression of intercellular adhesion molecule 1 (ICAM-1, CD54) in colonic epithelial cells. Gut. 1993;34: 1593–7.

166. Bloom S, Simmons D, Jewell DP. Adhesion molecules intercellular adhesion molecule-1 (ICAM-1), ICAM-3 and B7 are not expressed by epithelium in normal or inflamed colon. Clin Exp Immunol. 1995;101:157–63.

167. Gibson P, Rosella O. Interleukin 8 secretion by colonic crypt cells *in vitro*: response to injury suppressed by butyrate and enhanced in inflammatory bowel disease. Gut. 1995;37: 536–43.

168. McGee DW, Beagley KW, Aicher WK, McGhee JR. The regulation of IL-6 secretion from IEC-6 intestinal epithelial cells by cytokines and mucosally important antigens. Adv Exp Med Biol. 1995;371A:229–32.

169. Kelly CP, Keates S, Siegenberg D, Linevsky JK, Pothoulakis C, Brady HR. IL-8 secretion and neutrophil activation by HT-29 colonic epithelial cells. Am J Physiol. 1994;267:G991–7.

170. Schuerer-Maly CC, Eckmann L, Kagnoff MF, Falco MT, Maly FE. Colonic epithelial cell lines as a source of interleukin-8: stimulation by inflammatory cytokines and bacterial lipopolysaccharide. Immunology. 1994;81:85–91.

171. Eckmann L, Jung HC, Schurer-Maly C, Panja A, Morzycka-Wroblewska E, Kagnoff MF. Differential cytokine expression by human intestinal epithelial cell lines: regulated expression of interleukin 8. Gastroenterology. 1993;105:1689–97.

172. Eckmann L, Kagnoff MF, Fierer J. Epithelial cells secrete the chemokine interleukin-8 in response to bacterial entry. Infect Immun. 1993;61:4569–74.

173. Grimm MC, Elsbury SK, Pavli P, Doe WF. Interleukin 8: cells of origin in inflammatory bowel disease. Gut. 1996;38:90–8.

174. Mascarenhas JO, Goodrich ME, Eichelberger H, McGee DW. Polarized secretion of IL-6 by IEC-6 intestinal epithelial cells: differential effects of IL-1 beta and TNF-alpha. Immunol Invest. 1996;25:333–40.

175. Gross V, Andus T, Daig R, Aschenbrenner E, Scholmerich J, Falk W. Regulation of interleukin-8 production in a human colon epithelial cell line (HT-29). Gastroenterology. 1995;108: 653–61.

176. Rogler G, Daig R, Aschenbrenner E *et al.* Establishment of long-term primary cultures of human small and large intestinal epithelial cells. Lab Invest. 1998;78:889–90.

177. Powrie F, Leach MW, Mauze S, Menon S, Caddle LB, Coffman RL. Inhibition of Th1 responses prevents inflammatory bowel disease in scid mice reconstituted with CD45RBhi CD4+ T cells. Immunity. 1994;1:553–62.

178. Davidson NJ, Leach MW, Fort MM *et al.* T helper cell 1-type CD4+ T cells, but not B cells, mediate colitis in interleukin 10-deficient mice. J Exp Med. 1996;184:241–51.

179. Simpson SJ, Shah S, Comiskey M *et al.* T cell-mediated pathology in two models of experimental colitis depends predominantly on the interleukin 12/Signal transducer and activator of transcription (Stat)-4 pathway, but is not conditional on interferon gamma expression by T cells. J Exp Med. 1998;187:1225–34.

180. Williams AM, Whiting CV, Bonhagen K *et al.* Tumour necrosis factor-alpha (TNF-alpha) transcription and translation in the CD4+ T cell-transplanted scid mouse model of colitis. Clin Exp Immunol. 1999;116:415–24.

181. Yamamoto M, Yoshizaki K, Kishimoto T, Ito H. IL-6 is required for the development of Th1 cell-mediated murine colitis. J Immunol. 2000;164:4878–82.

182. Cottrez F, Hurst SD, Coffman RL, Groux H. T regulatory cells 1 inhibit a Th2-specific response *in vivo*. J Immunol. 2000;165:4848–53.

183. Kolios G, Robertson DA, Jordan NJ *et al.* Interleukin-8 production by the human colon epithelial cell line HT-29: modulation by interleukin-13. Br J Pharmacol. 1996;119:351–9.

184. Abreu-Martin MT, Vidrich A, Lynch DH, Targan SR. Divergent induction of apoptosis and IL-8 secretion in HT-29 cells in response to TNF-alpha and ligation of Fas antigen. J Immunol. 1995;155:4147–54.

185. Pavli P, Maxwell L, van de Pol E, Doe WF. Distribution of human colonic dendritic cells and macrophages – functional implications. Adv Exp Med Biol. 1995;378:121–3.

186. Pavli P, Maxwell L, Van de Pol E, Doe F. Distribution of human colonic dendritic cells and macrophages. Clin Exp Immunol. 1996;104:124–32.

187. Oshitani N, Kitano A, Kakazu T *et al.* Functional diversity of infiltrating macrophages in inflamed human colonic mucosa ulcerative colitis. Clin Exp Pharmacol Physiol. 1998;25:50–3.

188. Rogler G, Hausmann M, Vogl D *et al.* Isolation and phenotypic characterization of colonic macrophages. Clin Exp Immunol. 1998;112:205–15.

189. Hall PA, Coates PJ, Ansari B, Hopwood D. Regulation of cell number in the mammalian gastrointestinal tract: the importance of apoptosis. J Cell Sci. 1994;107:3569–77.
190. Lou TY, Teplitz C, Thayer WR, Jr. Ultrastructural morphogenesis of colonic PAS-positive macrophages ('colonic histiocytosis'). Hum Pathol. 1971;2:421–39.
191. Dance DR, Nash AG, McCready VR. The uptake of gallium 67 in colonic macrophages. Eur J Nucl Med. 1976;1:27–9.
192. Yokochi T, Nakashima I, Kato N. Effect of capsular polysaccharide of *Klebsiella pneumoniae* on the differentiation and functional capacity of macrophages cultured *in vitro*. Microbiol Immunol. 1977;21:601–10.
193. Hammerstrom J. Human macrophage differentiation *in vivo* and *in vitro*. A comparison of human peritoneal macrophages and monocytes. Acta Pathol Microbiol Scand [C]. 1979;87C: 113–20.
194. D'Onofrio C, Paradisi F. *In-vitro* differentiation of human monocytes into mature macrophages during long-term cultures. Immunobiology. 1983;164:13–22.
195. Schook LB, Gutmann DH, Marlin LE, Niederhuber JE. *In-vitro*-derived bone marrow macrophages. Expression of Ia antigens during macrophage differentiation. Transplantation. 1984;37:585–90.
196. Eppell BA, Newell AM, Brown EJ. Adenosine receptors are expressed during differentiation of monocytes to macrophages *in vitro*. Implications for regulation of phagocytosis. J Immunol. 1989;143:4141–5.
197. Brugger W, Kreutz M, Andreesen R. Macrophage colony-stimulating factor is required for human monocyte survival and acts as a cofactor for their terminal differentiation to macrophages *in vitro*. J Leukoc Biol. 1991;49:483–8.
198. Brugger W, Reinhardt D, Galanos C, Andreesen R. Inhibition of *in vitro* differentiation of human monocytes to macrophages by lipopolysaccharides (LPS): phenotypic and functional analysis. Int Immunol. 1991;3:221–7.
199. Kreutz M, Krause SW, Hennemann B, Rehm A, Andreesen R. Macrophage heterogeneity and differentiation: defined serum-free culture conditions induce different types of macrophages *in vitro*. Res Immunol. 1992;143:107–15.
200. Vincent F, Eischen A, Bergerat JP, Faradji A, Bohbot A, Oberling F. Human blood-derived macrophages: differentiation *in vitro* of a large quantity of cells in serum-free medium. Exp Hematol. 1992;20:17–23.
201. Jungi TW, Miserez R, Brcic M, Pfister H. Change in sensitivity to lipopolysaccharide during the differentiation of human monocytes to macrophages *in vitro*. Experientia. 1994; 50:110–14.
202. Gantner F, Kupferschmidt R, Schudt C, Wendel A, Hatzelmann A. *In vitro* differentiation of human monocytes to macrophages: change of PDE profile and its relationship to suppression of tumour necrosis factor-alpha release by PDE inhibitors. Br J Pharmacol. 1997;121:221–31.
203. Konur A, Kreutz M, Knuchel R, Krause SW, Andreesen R. Cytokine repertoire during maturation of monocytes to macrophages within spheroids of malignant and non-malignant urothelial cell lines. Int J Cancer. 1998;78:648–53.
204. Konur A, Kreutz M, Knuchel R, Krause SW, Andreesen R. Three-dimensional co-culture of human monocytes and macrophages with tumor cells: analysis of macrophage differentiation and activation. Int J Cancer. 1996;66:645–52.
205. Gorlach A, Acker H. pO_2- and pH-gradients in multicellular spheroids and their relationship to cellular metabolism and radiation sensitivity of malignant human tumor cells. Biochim Biophys Acta. 1994;1227:105–12.
206. Casciari JJ, Sotirchos SV, Sutherland RM. Variations in tumor cell growth rates and metabolism with oxygen concentration, glucose concentration, and extracellular pH. J Cell Physiol. 1992; 151:386–94.
207. Kwok TT, Twentyman PR. Effects of changes in oxygen tension, pH, and glucose concentration on the response to CCNU of EMT6 mouse tumor monolayer cells and multicellular spheroids. Int J Radiat Oncol Biol Phys. 1988;14:1221–9.
208. Santini MT, Rainaldi G, Indovina PL. Apoptosis, cell adhesion and the extracellular matrix in the three-dimensional growth of multicellular tumor spheroids. Crit Rev Oncol Hematol. 2000;36:75–87.
209. Bjerkvig R, Laerum OD, Rucklidge GJ. Immunocytochemical characterization of extracellular matrix proteins expressed by cultured glioma cells. Cancer Res. 1989;49:5424–8.

210. Nederman T, Norling B, Glimelius B, Carlsson J, Brunk U. Demonstration of an extracellular matrix in multicellular tumor spheroids. Cancer Res. 1984;44:3090–7.
211. Korff T, Augustin HG. Integration of endothelial cells in multicellular spheroids prevents apoptosis and induces differentiation. J Cell Biol. 1998;143:1341–52.
212. Hohn HP, Grummer R, Bosserhoff S et al. The role of matrix contact and of cell–cell interactions in choriocarcinoma cell differentiation. Eur J Cell Biol. 1996;69:76–85.
213. Boxberger HJ, Meyer TF. A new method for the 3-D in vitro growth of human RT112 bladder carcinoma cells using the alginate culture technique. Biol Cell. 1994;82:109–19.
214. Spottl T, Hausmann M, Kreutz M et al. Monocyte differentiation in intestine-like macrophage phenotype induced by epithelial cells. J Leukoc Biol. 2001;70:241–51.

7
Characterization of intestinal barrier function: a putative target for therapeutic modification

M. GEHRING and J.-D. SCHULZKE

INTRODUCTION

Intestinal inflammation, including chronic inflammatory bowel disease (IBD), is mostly associated with altered barrier function. This impairment of the mucosal barrier has two main consequences. First, small solutes and water can flow into the lumen and cause *leak flux diarrhoea*. In general all types of diarrhoea are driven by osmotic forces, i.e. fluid follows an impaired solute transport. This includes: (a) the malabsorptive diarrhoea due to reduced absorptive area, to defective transporters or to enzymatic maldigestion of luminal macromolecules; (b) secretory diarrhoea due to an excessive active (an)ion secretion; (c) *leak flux diarrhoea* due to an impaired epithelial barrier and a passive back-leak of ions and water into the intestinal lumen. The second consequence concerns larger molecules, which are under normal conditions almost perfectly prevented from being taken up. If the barrier is disturbed, uptake of even small amounts of antigens may aggravate or even initiate inflammation. Besides altered tight junctions, other structural changes in the epithelium such as epithelial cell apoptoses, erosion/ulcer-type lesions and transcytosis also play a role and should be considered. Thus this chapter gives an overview of: (a) intestinal barrier function and its regulation during inflammation; (b) the changes observed in barrier properties in ulcerative colitis and collagenous colitis and (c) therapeutics targeting epithelial dysfunction in IBD.

EPITHELIAL PROPERTIES WHICH DETERMINE INTESTINAL BARRIER FUNCTION

Tight junction down-regulation by proinflammatory cytokines

Many inflammatory diseases of the intestine are associated with enhanced subepithelial cytokine release. It has been shown, in several cell lines and

Table 1 Cytokine effects on epithelial barrier function

Cytokine	Concentration	Duration (h)	Resistance as percentage of initial value	n
control (no cytokine)		24	98 ± 5	12
IFN-γ	1 U/ml	24	$86 \pm 5^{n.s.}$	6
IFN-γ	10 U/ml	24	$86 \pm 5^{n.s.}$	6
IFN-γ	100 U/ml	24	$83 \pm 7^{n.s.}$	15
IFN-γ	1000 U/ml	24	$79 \pm 5^{**}$	15
TNF-α	5 ng/ml	24	$69 \pm 9^{**}$	6
TNF-α + IFN-γ	5 ng/ml + 10 U/ml	24	$23 \pm 4^{***}$	6

In HT-29/B6 cell monolayers the influence of cytokines on electrical resistance was determined. N.s. = not significantly different from control, $^{**}p < 0.01$; $^{***}p < 0.001$.

cytokine knockout models, that proinflammatory cytokines, especially tumour necrosis factor alpha and interferon gamma (TNF-α and IFN-γ), can impair the epithelial barrier. TNF-α is produced by mononuclear cells and TNF-α expression is up-regulated in intestinal diseases including IBD. Serosal addition of TNF-α (5 ng/ml) decreased R^t function by 31% in the colonic epithelial cell line HT-29/B6 (Table 1). This effect was dose-dependent, not reversible as long as TNF-α was present, and could be mimicked by serosal addition of antibodies against the p55 TNF-α receptor[1]. No cytotoxic effects were observed in lactate dehydrogenase (LDH) assays and immunofluorescence localization with anti-ZO-1 antibodies revealed no evidence for disruption of the monolayer after TNF-α treatment. In freeze–fracture electron microscopy, tight junction complexity was decreased by TNF-α as indicated by a decrease in the number of strands from 4.7 to 3.4. A combination of TNF-α with IFN-γ acted synergistically on the epithelial barrier (Table 1).

Regulation of occludin expression in response to proinflammatory cytokines

The 65 kDa protein occludin was the first of a number of proteins identified to be a membrane-spanning part of the epithelial tight junction. Using genome walking cloning of occluding-specific human genomic DNA sequences, a 1853 bp DNA fragment containing the transcription start point of occludin cDNA sequences was amplified and sequenced[2]. In close proximity to the transcription start point for occludin messenger RNA, a number of transcription factor-binding sites, e.g. for nuclear factor interleukin-6 (NF-IL-6), were identified. Subcloning of this fragment in front of the luciferase reporter gene revealed strong expression of enzymatic activity after transfection of the human intestinal cell line HT-29/B6. The decrease in resistance in HT-29/B6 cells induced by TNF-α and IFN-γ was preceded by a decrease in occludin mRNA expression[2]. TNF-α and IFN-γ diminished occludin promoter activity alone, even synergistically suggesting genomic regulation[2].

Preserved barrier properties in occludin-deficient mice

In the occludin knockout mouse model, however, epithelial barrier function was surprisingly not significantly impaired[3], either in small or in large intestine

Table 2 Epithelial barrier function in occludin-deficient mice

	Small intestine	Large intestine
Wild-type	$22 \pm 6\,\Omega/cm^2$ (6)	$70 \pm 5\,\Omega\cdot cm^2$ (7)
Occludin$^{-/-}$	$18 \pm 2\,\Omega/cm^2$ (10)	$65 \pm 5\,\Omega\cdot cm^2$ (10)
p	n.s.	n.s.

In small and large intestine of occludin-deficient mice and respective littermate controls, epithelial resistance was measured by alternating-current impedance analysis. All values are means $\pm$ SEM; numbers of animals are given in parentheses. N.s. = not significantly different from control.

(Table 2). This held true not only for results of alternating-current impedance analysis but also for mannitol tracer flux measurements. The most likely explanation for this phenomenon is that barrier function of *occludin* can be substituted for by other TJ proteins (so-called substitutional redundancy in the tight junction heteropolymer) and that TNF-α not only down-regulates occludin but also prevents its substitution by other tight junction molecules. Potential candidates for such a substitution are members of the claudin protein family. Claudin-1[4] and claudin-4[5] have especially been characterized by stable transfection into MDCK cells to possess barrier properties for the paracellular pathway, while claudin-2 represents a (cation-selective) pore molecule when inserted into the tight junction heteropolymer[6].

Epithelial apoptoses contribute to epithelial barrier dysfunction

Besides tight junctions other epithelial features are also important for barrier function. This is especially the case for apoptotic cells within the epithelium which represent a spot of high conductance, until the gap is closed again. These sites appear morphologically as apoptotic rosettes in the epithelium and also allow larger molecules to pass the epithelium, e.g. lactulose[7]. Furthermore, and no less important, apoptotic sites are much more conductive if stimulated by proinflammatory cytokines than apoptoses which occur spontaneously. This could be a consequence of cytokine effects on the tight junction of the surrounding cells[8]. As a further important point in this respect, the formerly 'tight' epithelium of HT-29/B6 becomes 'leaky' at a rate of 12% apoptosis, as obtained from experiments in which apoptoses were selectively induced by camptothecin[7]. While PEG 4000 was not able to pass single apoptotic sites in the epithelium[7], it is possible that larger molecules including macromolecules could penetrate the epithelium when apoptotic events are so frequent that apoptotic foci appear in which several apoptotic cells are in direct contact with each other. However, this point needs further experimental exploration, and so far macromolecular transfer through the epithelium has to be assumed to take place mainly transcellularly by transcytosis or through epithelial lesions (e.g. erosions or ulcer-type lesions).

EPITHELIAL BARRIER FUNCTION IN IBD

Epithelial barrier function and tight junction structure in ulcerative colitis (UC)

UC is an autoimmune disease of unknown origin with inflammation of the colonic mucosa followed by profuse diarrhoea. Possible mechanisms for this epithelial dysfunction comprise reduced absorption and a defect in epithelial barrier function. Therefore, epithelial barrier function and tight junction structure were studied in inflamed sigmoid colon from UC patients undergoing colectomy[9]. Specimens were chosen which exhibited only mild to moderate histological disease activity (i.e. no erosions or ulcer-type lesions). Histologically, the epithelial cell lining was intact and the properties of this diseased tissue refer to a mucosa which endoscopically appears hyperaemic, oedematous, granular and vulnerable. Alternating-current impedance analysis was applied to determine the epithelial (R^e) and subepithelial (R^{sub}) components of R^t. In-vivo R^{sub} is no part of the barrier, because the majority of the subepithelial tissues is situated below the blood capillaries. The discrimination between R^e and R^{sub} is crucial if both figures change in opposing directions as in UC (Table 3). Epithelial resistance (R^e) decreased by 79%, which in the conventional Ussing technique would have been masked by the increase of the subepithelial resistance (R^{sub}) due to inflammatory cell infiltration and submucosal oedema. Thus, the inflamed colonic mucosa in ulcerative colitis is characterized by a very pronounced loss of barrier function.

It has been shown for several epithelia that large differences in resistance are associated with only small differences in the number of horizontally oriented strands[10]. This was also proven true in UC-altered tissues where the pronounced decrease in epithelial resistance was paralleled by a rather small reduction in epithelial cell tight junction complexity (Table 3). From the distribution of the strand counts[9] it can be seen that tight junctions of UC tissues often had only one or two strands while control tissues had at least five strands, although strand number retained its Gaussian distribution in UC, suggesting an orderly interference with the assembly/disassembly process of tight junction formation.

Table 3 Electrical resistance and tight junction morphometry in ulcerative colitis

	Electrical resistance ($\Omega \cdot cm^2$)		TJ strand count	
	Epithelium	Subepithelium	Surface	Crypt
Control	95 ± 5 (10)	14 ± 1 (10)	6.9 ± 0.3 (9)	7.3 ± 0.3 (9)
Mild–moderate UC	20 ± 3 (11)***	36 ± 3 (11)***	4.8 ± 0.5 (9)***	5.5 ± 0.4 (9)**
Severe UC	22 ± 4 (7)	54 ± 4 (7)††	–	–

In sigmoid colon of controls and patients with ulcerative colitis (UC), epithelial and subepithelial resistance were measured by alternating-current impedance analysis and the numbers of horizontally oriented strands in the main compact meshwork (TJ strand count) of the tight junction were evaluated by freeze–fracture electron microscopy. All values are means ± SEM; numbers of patients are given in parentheses. **$p < 0.01$ versus control; ***$p < 0.001$ versus control; ††$p < 0.01$ versus mild–moderate UC.

The appearance of tight junction sites with very low strand count may be functionally even more important than mean strand number during inflammation and could – together with other phenomena which influence mucosal barrier function, e.g. epithelial apoptotic rate – explain Claude's observation. Strand discontinuities were not more frequent in ulcerative colitis than in controls[9]. On a first view this may go against a contribution of strand discontinuities to the barrier defect. In reality, strand discontinuities may become functionally important at sites with only one or two strands. At these sites strand discontinuities may enable macromolecules, including food antigens and bacterial lipopolysaccharides, to pass the epithelial barrier.

Contribution of epithelial apoptoses and epithelial lesions to the barrier disturbance in UC

In addition to changes in epithelial tight junctions there is evidence for an up-regulation of epithelial apoptoses in ulcerative colitis[11] as well as for the appearance of epithelial lesions such as erosions. Therefore we applied a refined technique for spatial resolution of the increased conductance in UC, namely the conductance scanning technique. This technique allowed us to quantify the contribution of these barrier defects to the increased colonic ion permeability in UC[12]. The sigmoid colon of UC patients undergoing colectomy and control tissue were stripped off the muscularis propria and the spatial distribution of a current clamped across this viable epithelium was recorded by a scanning microelectrode. Local leaks were marked, and structural changes were investigated histologically. The overall conductivity was elevated from $8.4 \pm 0.7 \, mS/cm^2$ in controls to $11.7 \pm 0.6 \, mS/cm^2$ in mild inflammation and to $34.4 \pm 6.2 \, mS/cm^2$ in moderate-to-severe inflammation. Only partly was this caused by increased basal conductivity ($12.2 \pm 1.5 \, mS/cm^2$ in moderate-to-severe UC vs. 8.3 ± 0.7 in controls). The spatial distribution of conductivity, which was even in controls, showed leaks in UC. Leaks found in mild inflammation without an epithelial lesion proved to be foci of epithelial apoptoses. In moderate-to-severe inflammation, leaks correlated with epithelial erosion/ulcer-type lesions or crypt abscesses. Thus, in early UC the seemingly intact epithelium had leaks at apoptotic foci. In more intensive inflammation, erosions/ulcer-type lesions are highly conductive, even if covered with fibrin. Local leaks contributed 19% to the overall epithelial conductivity in mild and 65% in moderate-to-severe inflammation.

Epithelial barrier function in collagenous colitis

In order to characterize epithelial barrier function in collagenous colitis, biopsies of sigmoid colon were obtained endoscopically[13]. In miniaturized Ussing chambers, alternating-current impedance analysis was performed to discriminate epithelial (R^e) from subepithelial resistance (R^{sub}). Since mucosal surface area and apoptotic rate were not altered, we concentrated on the characterization of tight junction proteins occludin and claudin-1 to -5 in membrane fractions by Western blotting (Table 4). In collagenous colitis, subepithelial resistance increased from 7 ± 1 to $18 \pm 2 \, \Omega/cm^2$ due to subepithelial collagenous bands. R^e was diminished from 44 ± 3 to $29 \pm 2 \, \Omega/cm^2$ and this was accompanied by a decrease in occludin and claudin-4 expression, while claudin-1 remained

Table 4 Electrical resistance and tight junction protein expression in collagenous colitis

	R^e	Occludin	Claudin-1	Claudin-4
Control	$44 \pm 3\ \Omega/cm^2$ (7)	100% (5)	100% (5)	100% (5)
Collagenous colitis	$29 \pm 2\ \Omega/cm^2$ (8)	47% (5)	90% (5)	43% (5)
p	<0.01	<0.05	n.s.	<0.05

In sigmoid colon of controls and patients with collagenous colitis (UC), epithelial resistance was measured by alternating-current impedance analysis and the tight junction strand proteins occludin, claudin-1 and claudin-4 were quantified densitometrically by Western blots. All values are means $\pm$ SEM; numbers of patients are given in parentheses.

unchanged. In addition, there was higher claudin-2 expression in four of five patients with collagenous colitis. In conclusion, regulation of tight junction molecules but not epithelial apoptoses are structural correlates of barrier dysfunction contributing to diarrhoea by a leak flux mechanism in collagenous colitis.

Transcytotic macromolecule transfer through the epithelium may contribute to antigen uptake in CD

There is increasing evidence in the past few years that antigens can be taken up to a significant amount through the transcellular route by endocytosis. This mechanism seems to be up-regulated in CD, as indicated by electron microscopy studies using ovalbumin and horseradish peroxidase[14]. The mechanisms which stimulate this transport during inflammation, however, are still unknown.

EFFECT OF THERAPEUTIC AGENTS ON INTESTINAL BARRIER FUNCTION

The increasing amount of information on epithelial barrier features at cellular and molecular levels, as well as on their disturbance and regulation during inflammation, has raised the expectation that defined tools could be designed to repair barrier function in IBD. However, this is at present only partly the case, namely when an anti-inflammatory therapy strategy is successful and the mucosa has healed. On the other hand, several distinct agents have been proposed to improve barrier function. The conclusion on their efficacy in IBD, however, is usually either lacking or was arrived at in other models or conditions. The latter group of agents comprises, e.g., glutamine, butyrate and probiotics. Before discussing their effects and limitations, a brief comment should be made on anti-inflammatory long-term effects on barrier function.

Anti-inflammatory therapy strategies can improve epithelial barrier function

That anti-inflammatory therapy can improve epithelial barrier function is in principle true for every therapeutic agent, and can be assumed to directly correlate with its anti-inflammatory efficacy. Data to support this have usually been obtained using *in-vivo* permeability tests with drinking solutions containing various permeability markers including lactulose/rhamnose-ratio, PEG 400 or [^{51}Cr]EDTA. On the one hand this is indicated by a correlation of CD activity and intestinal permeability[15,16]. On the other hand this is supported by data from patients with active CD either before and after steroid therapy or before and after application of elemental diets[17,18]. Having this in mind, it seems reasonable to assume also that anti-TNF-α antibody therapy is a good candidate in this respect. Preliminary data from our own group seem to definitely support an early effect of infliximab on barrier function after only 2 weeks (data not shown).

Lack of evidence for a direct barrier effect of glutamine, butyrate and probiotics in IBD

Glutamine has been shown to have direct short-term effects on increased bacterial translocation in animal models, including mice after a skin burn injury[19], and in rats on total parenteral nutrition[20]. However, no effect was observed in CD patients with total parenteral nutrition when supplemented with glutamine[21]. A possible explanation for this discrepancy could be that glutamine acts as an important source of energy for the enterocytes, and that there is, in contrast to the other experimental conditions, no metabolic deficiency in IBD.

The same line of argument could be relevant for butyrate. Butyrate enemas are effective in diversion colitis and have significant anti-inflammatory effects in ulcerative colitis[22] as well as in the rat TNBS-colitis model[23]. Again, though, there is so far no evidence for a direct short-term effect on barrier dysfunction in IBD.

Another therapeutic approach in IBD which has been hypothesized to affect epithelial barrier function comprises probiotics. This assumption is mainly based on experimental studies performed in animal or cell line models. For example, *Saccharomyces boulardii* improved epithelial barrier function and diminished the translocation of enteropathogenic *Escherichia coli* in infected T84 cell monolayers[24] and the probiotic compound VSL#3 normalized epithelial barrier function of the inflamed intestine in IL-10-deficient mice and attenuated *Salmonella* invasion in T84 cells[25]. Although this seems to support the hypothesis of a barrier-preserving effect, direct experimental evidence for a short-term influence on the disturbed intestinal barrier function in IBD and putative inherent mechanisms has not yet been obtained.

References

1. Schmitz H, Barmeyer C, Fromm M et al. A decrease in tight junction complexity contributes to the severely impaired epithelial barrier function in ulcerative colitis. Gastroenterology. 1999;116:301–9.
2. Mankertz J, Tavalali S, Schmitz H et al. Expression from the human occludin promoter is affected by tumor necrosis factor alpha and interferon gamma. J Cell Sci. 2000;113:2085–90.
3. Saitou M, Furuse M, Sasaki H et al. Complex phenotype of mice lacking occludin, a component of tight junction strands. Mol Biol Cell. 2000;11:4131–42.
4. Inai T, Kobayashi J, Shibata Y. Claudin-1 contributes to the epithelial barrier function in MDCK cells. Eur J Cell Biol. 1999;78:849–55.
5. Van Itallie C, Rahner C, Anderson JM. Regulated expression of claudin-4 paracellular conductance through a selective decrease in sodium permeability. J Clin Invest. 2001;107:1319–27.
6. Furuse M, Furuse K, Sasaki H, Tsukita S. Conversion of zonulae occludentes from tight to leaky strand types by introducing claudin-2 into Madin-Darby canine kidney I cells. J Cell Biol. 2001;153:263–72.

7. Bojarski C, Gitter AH, Bendfeldt K *et al.* Permeability of HT-29/B6 colonic epithelium as a function of apoptosis. J Physiol (Lond.) 2001;535:541–52.

8. Gitter AH, Bendfeldt K, Schulzke JD, Fromm M. Leaks in the epithelial barrier caused by spontaneous and TNFα-induced single-cell apoptosis. FASEB J. 2000;14:1749–53.

9. Schmitz H, Fromm M, Bentzel CJ *et al.* Tumor necrosis factor-alpha (TNFα) regulates the epithelial barrier in the human intestinal cell line HT-29/B6. J Cell Sci. 1999;112:137–46.

10. Claude P. Morphological factors influencing transepithelial permeability: a model for the resistance of the zonula occludens. J Membrane Biol. 1978;39:219–32.

11. Straeter J, Wellisch I, Riedl S *et al.* CD95 (APO-1/Fas)-mediated apoptosis in colon epithelial cells: a possible role in ulcerative colitis. Gastroenterology. 1997;113:160–7.

12. Gitter AH, Wullstein F, Fromm M, Schulzke JD. Epithelial barrier defects in ulcerative colitis: characterization and quantification by electrophysiological imaging. Gastroenterology. 2001;121:1320–8.

13. Bürgel N, Bojarski C, Mankertz J, Zeitz M, Fromm M, Schulzke JD. Mechanisms of diarrhea in collagenous colitis. Gastroenterology. 2002;123:433–43.

14. Schurmann G, Bruewer M, Klotz A, Schmidt KW, Senninger N, Zimmer KP. Transepithelial transport processes at the intestinal mucosa in inflammatory bowel disease. Int J Colorect Dis. 1999;14:41–6.

15. Andre F, Andre C, Emery Y, Forichon J, Descos L, Minaire Y. Assessment of the lactulose–mannitol test in Crohn's disease. Gut. 1988;29:511–15.

16. Adenis A, Colombel JF, Lecouffe P *et al.* Increased pulmonary and intestinal permeability in Crohn's disease. Gut. 1992;33:678–82.

17. Sanderson IR, Boulton P, Menzies I, Walker-Smith JA. Improvement of abnormal lactulose/rhamnose permeability in active Crohn's disease of the small bowel by an elemental diet. Gut. 1987;28:1073–6.

18. Zoli G, Care M, Parazza M *et al.* A randomized controlled study comparing elemental diet and steroid treatment in Crohn's disease. Aliment Pharmacol Ther. 1997;11:735–40.

19. Gennari R, Alexander JW. Arginine, glutamine, and dehydroepiandrosterone reverse the immuno-suppressive effect of prednisone during gut-derived sepsis. Crit Care Med. 1997;25:1207–14.

20. Li J, Langkamp-Henken B, Suzuki K, Stahlgren LH. Glutamine prevents parenteral nutrition-induced increases in intestinal permeability. J Parent Ent Nutr. 1994;18:303–7.

21. Akobeng AK, Miller V, Stanton J, Elbadri AM, Thomas AG. Double-blind randomized controlled trial of glutamine-enriched polymeric diet in the treatment of active Crohn's disease. J Pediatric Gastroenterol Nutr. 2000;30:78–84.

22. Scheppach W, Sommer H, Kirchner T *et al.* Effect of butyrate enemas on the colonic mucosa in distal ulcerative colitis. Gastroenterology. 1992;103:51–6.

23. Butzner JD, Parmar R, Bell CJ, Dalal V. Butyrate enema therapy stimulates mucosal repair in experimental colitis in the rat. Gut. 1996;38:568–73.

24. Czebrucka D, Dahan S, Mograbi B, Rossi B, Rampal P. *Saccharomyces boulardii* preserves the barrier function and modulates the signal transduction pathway induced in enteropathogenic *E. coli* infected T84 cells. Infect Immun. 2000;68:5998–6004.

25. Madsen K, Cornish A, Soper P *et al.* Probiotic bacteria enhance murine and human intestinal epithelial barrier function. Gastroenterology. 2001;121:580–91.

Section III
Alternative concepts –
new targets in the making

8
The adipose tissue as a source of proinflammatory signals in Crohn's disease?

J.-F. COLOMBEL, L. DUBUQUOY, W. J. SANDBORN and P. DESREUMAUX

INTRODUCTION

Although considerable variation exists in the presentation of the disease in surgical specimens, Crohn's disease (CD) is often recognized solely on the appearance of the macroscopic lesions. Surgical assessment of the intestine in CD reveals that the mesentery is often thickened, stiff, with white adipose tissue (WAT) hypertrophy[1–3]. Fat-wrapping, defined as WAT hypertrophy extending from the mesenteric attachment and covering partially the intestinal circumference in association with loss of the bowel-mesentery angle, is common in both small and large intestine and is also considered as a hallmark of CD[4]. Adipose tissue is now accepted as having a much wider involvement in the immune system than was believed a few years ago[5,6]. The older anatomical literature repeatedly mentions intimate associations between adipose tissue and lymph nodes in various mammals including humans. More recent research suggests functional interactions between lymphoid cells and adipose tissue[5,6]. The link between adipose tissue and immunity has been reinforced by the demonstration that adipocytes could actually function as macrophage-like cells expressing molecules related to the innate immune system and secreting major mediators of inflammation such as tumour necrosis factor alpha (TNF-α)[7–12].

In spite of this circumstantial evidence, adipose tissue has not featured prominently in the extensive research into CD pathology. This chapter attempts to redress the lack of interest in a component which may play an important role in the inflammatory process of CD.

ACCUMULATION OF FAT IN THE MESENTERY IS A HALLMARK OF CD

The connective tissue changes that accompany intestinal CD and particularly fat hypertrophy have long been recognized by surgeons and used to delineate the extent of active disease[13]. Dr Burrill B. Crohn himself mentioned this characteristic appearance of mesenteric adipose tissue as a consistent symptom of the disease that bears his name[14]. Fat wrapping has been defined on a transverse section of the intestine and regarded as being present when more than 50% of the intestinal circumference is affected[4]. Fibrous strands are present in the mesenteric fat irradiating from the intestine and surrounding thickened, hypertrophied fat lobules[4]. Prevalence of fat abnormalities in CD has not been formally assessed in population-based studies. In a consecutive, unselected series of 27 intestinal resections performed on 25 patients for histologically confirmed CD, fat-wrapping was identified in 12 of 16 ileal resections and in seven of 11 large bowel resections[4]. There was no evidence of bowel wall shrinkage in the presence of increased mesenteric thickness and fat wrapping did not correlate with disease duration or extent. A retrospective review of 225 small intestinal resections suggested that fat-wrappping is a feature peculiar to CD. In that series there was evidence of fat-wrapping in 31/58 cases of CD but it was never seen in other conditions, including ischaemia or infarction, Meckel's diverticulum, carcinoma or lymphoma, perforation of various cases, radiation enteritis and carcinoid. Furthermore, fat-wrapping is not observed in intestinal tuberculosis and other chronic granulomatous disease such as yersiniosis.

Computed tomography (CT) gives unique information about the margins of the intra-abdominal organs and the mesentery. At CT, fibrofatty proliferation appears as an increased quantity of mesenteric fat, producing a mass effect on adjacent loops, with strand-like areas of increased attenuation and hypervascularity within the mesentery (giving the so-called aspect of vascular jejunization of the ileum or the comb sign)[15–17]. The increased attenuation coefficient of fat and stranding have been assigned to the influx of inflammatory cells and fluid which have a higher CT number than fat. Fibrofatty proliferation is often associated with regional lymphadenopathy. In a series of 25 children with CD, adenopathy and focal fatty proliferation were seen in 11 and 18 patients respectively and it was concluded that identification of these mesenteric abnormalities on CT scan may support the diagnosis of CD in paediatric patients[18].

Magnetic resonance imaging is a reliable non-invasive method for measurement of regional adiposity. We used magnetic resonance imaging to quantify the intra-abdominal and subcutaneous fat in CD patients and controls. CD patients and controls had similar areas of total abdominal fat, intra-abdominal fat and subcutaneous fat. However, the ratio of intra-abdominal fat area to total abdominal fat area was significantly higher in patients with CD than in controls[19].

MESENTERIC FAT IS AN IMPORTANT SOURCE OF PROINFLAMMATORY SIGNALS IN CD, WHICH MAY EXPLAIN OTHER CLINICAL CHARACTERISTIC FEATURES OF THE DISEASE

Recent findings suggest that adipocytes may play an important physiological role in the regulation of both the innate and adaptive immune response. Adipocytes actively secrete and respond to inflammatory cytokines such as tumour necrosis factor alpha (TNF-α), interleukin-1β (IL-1β) and IL-6[12]. Intra-abdominal WAT has been linked with the development of metabolic disorders and insulin resistance, possibly related to its capacity to synthesize mediators such as TNF-α[20,21].

Desreumaux *et al.* showed that mesenteric WAT in CD specifically expressed TNF-α mRNA, but not the mRNA of other proinflammatory cytokines[19]. TNF-α mRNA concentrations in the mesentery were comparable to the quantity of TNF-α mRNA detected in stimulated peripheral blood mononuclear cells isolated from CD patients. Using immunohistochemical analysis and *in-situ* hybridization, adipocytes were identified as the main source of TNF-α.

As in unstimulated monocytes and macrophages, TNF-α release from human adipose tissue and isolated adipocytes occurs at low levels under controlled conditions[7]. In the study by Desreumaux *et al.* the lack of TNF-α mRNA in the mesentery from controls suggests that this cytokine is not constitutively expressed in this site[19]. Adipocytes express recognition receptors for bacterial lipopolysaccharides (LPS) such as CD14 and toll-like receptor 4 (TLR4)[7,8]. Adipocytes are also susceptible to being infected or to capture viral particles[9]. It may be hypothesized that, in CD, stimulation of adipocytes in the mesentery may occur as a result of the increased penetration of foreign antigens through a compromised mucosal barrier[22].

TNF-α synthesis by mesenteric tissues may contribute to other clinical characteristic features of CD. In CD, transmural inflammation and patchy or linear mucosal ulcerations are located prominently along the mesenteric attachment, the severity of the lesions being more pronounced along the mesenteric border[1–3]. This is in contrast with other infectious and inflammatory bowel disorders: in intestinal tuberculosis, ulcerations are usually oriented transversely rather than longitudinally; in infectious conditions mimicking CD (*Salmonella typhi*, *Shigella* or *Yersinia pseudotuberculosis* and *enterocolitica*) mucosal ulcerations are linear, near Peyer's patches, parallel with the long axis of the intestine along the anti-mesenteric border[1,2]. Thus, the axial polarity and the predominance of the ulcerations beneath the attachment of the mesentery are characteristic of CD. Two studies have shown that the extent of connective tissue changes and fat wrapping nicely correlate with transmural inflammation and mucosal ulcerations[4,23]. A causal link between these observations and TNF-α synthesis by the mesentery may thus be suggested.

THE ORIGIN OF ABNORMAL FAT DISTRIBUTION IN CD IS UNKNOWN

The origin of excessive intra-abdominal fat in CD is unknown, and occurred despite a normal body mass index and absence of metabolic disease.

It is generally believed that the serosal connective tissue abnormalities in CD develop as the long-term consequence of chronic inflammation and result from the local effects of substances released by the inflammatory changes in the outer layers of the bowel wall[23]. Adipocyte hyperplasia results from the recruitment of new adipocytes from pluripotent precursor cells. This may occur as a consequence of chronic stimulation of adipocytes by bacterial and/or viral antigens to which they are equipped to respond[7–9]. Levine *et al.* have shown that macrophage colony-stimulating factor (MCSF) promotes human adipose tissue hyperplasia and that adipocytes isolated from creeping fat in patients with CD showed up-regulation of MCSF expression compared to mesenteric fat distant to the site of bowel inflammation[24].

Mesenteric fat accumulation in CD may implicate preferential interactions between the immune system and perinodal adipocytes. The mesenteric lymph nodes which are commonly swollen in CD are embedded in fat and there is an intimate relationship between perinodal adipocytes and lymphoid tissue. *In-vitro* and *in-vivo* experiments have shown that adipose tissue that encloses lymph nodes has the capacity to respond to stimuli from activated lymphoid cells[25,26]. Pond and colleagues demonstrated that, when a lymph node is activated with LPS, lipolysis in the adipocytes immediately surrounding it increases within 1 h and remains elevated for at least 9 h[22]. The portion of the adipose tissue surrounding the activated lymph node that displays this property increases if stimulation of lymph node is repeated. In other words, a prolonged and intensifying bacterial attack recruits more of the adipocytes to respond to the local stimulation of the enclosed lymph node. According to their hypothesis, the intraabdominal WAT in CD may respond to chronic activation of immune cells by forming more adipocytes. Since CD affects only the lymphoid tissue of the gut, selective growth of perinodal tissue would be limited to the mesenteric depot.

Alternatively, mesenteric fat accumulation in CD may be a primary event. WAT hypertrophy is often identified at the onset of the disease and is not affected by its duration or activity. Several determinants of visceral fat accumulation, such as smoking, high sucrose intake and low rate of physical activity, have been associated with CD in epidemiological studies[27-29]. Peroxisome proliferator-activated receptor gamma (PPARγ) is a member of the nuclear hormone receptor superfamily, which is predominantly expressed in adipocytes and is involved in critical steps of lipogenesis and lipid homeostasis[30-32]. Desreumaux *et al.* found that mesenteric PPARγ mRNA expression in CD patients was higher relative to controls and confined to the mesenteric WAT[19]. A dysregulation of PPARγ expression, confined to the mesentery, could thus contribute to intra-abdominal WAT hypertrophy in CD.

CONCLUSION

Mesenteric fat accumulation is a unique feature of CD. Previous studies suggested that it represented a secondary phenomenon resulting from chronic intestinal inflammation. It is now becoming apparent that adipocytes from the mesenteric tissue do not simply represent innocent bystander cells but that they act as effectors involved in sustaining the inflammatory process through the release of TNF-α. Further studies are needed in order to know whether the adipose tissue may exert an inflammatory role in other regions where it accumulates, such as the anoperineum. Interestingly, a recent study has noted that obese CD patients had an increased frequency of anoperineal lesions at onset and a particular propensity of anoperineal lesions to abscess and fistula formation[33]. The specific effect of medical treatments such as steroids, immunosuppressants and anti-TNF agents on fat proliferation also needs to be documented.

References

1. Mottet NK. Intestinal histopathology of regional enteritis. In: Mottet NK, editor. Histopathologic Spectrum of Regional Enteritis and Ulcerative Colitis. Philadelphia: Saunders, 1971:63–107.

2. Thompson H. Histopathology of Crohn's disease. In: Allan RN, Keighley MRB, Alexander-Williams J, Hawkins C, editors. Inflammatory Bowel Disease. New York: Churchill-Livingstone, 1990:263–85.

3. Geboes K. Histopathology of Crohn's disease and ulcerative colitis. In: Satsangi J, Sutherland LR, Colombel JF, Fiocchi C, Lofberg R, Pemberton, editors. Inflammatory Bowel Disease. New York: Churchill Livingstone, 2003 (In press).

4. Sheehan AL, Warren BF, Gear MW, Shepherd NA. Fat-wrapping in Crohn's disease: pathological basis and relevance to surgical practice. Br J Surg. 1992;79:955–8.

5. Pond CM. Adipose tissue: quartermaster to the lymph node garrisons. Biologist (London). 2000;47:147–50.

6. Pond CM. Adipose tissue, the anatomists' Cinderella, goes to the ball at last, and meets some influential partners. Postgrad Med J. 2000;76:671–3.

7. Sewter CP, Digby JE, Blows F, Prins J, O'Rahilly S. Regulation of tumour necrosis factor-alpha release from human adipose tissue *in vitro*. J Endocrinol. 1999;163:33–8.

8. Lin Y, Lee H, Berg AH, Lisanti MP, Shapiro L, Scherer PE. The lipopolysaccharide-activated toll-like receptor (TLR)-4 induces synthesis of the closely related receptor TLR-2 in adipocytes. J Biol Chem. 2000;275:24255–63.

9. Hazan U, Romero IA, Cancello R *et al*. Human adipose cells express CD4, CXCR4, CCR5 and receptors: a new target cell type for the immunodeficiency virus-1? FASEB J. 2002;16:1254–6.

10. Hotamisligil GS, Shargill NS, Spiegelman B. Adipose tissue expression of tumor necrosis factor-alpha: direct role in obesity-linked insulin resistance. Science. 1993;259:87–91.

11. Mattacks CA, Pond CM. Interactions of noradrenalin and tumour necrosis factor alpha, interleukin 4 and interleukin 6 in the control of lipolysis from adipocytes around lymph nodes. Cytokine. 1999;11:334–46.

12. Mohamed-Ali V, Pinkney JH, Coppack SW. Adipose tissue as an endocrine and paracrine organ. Int J Obes Relat Metab Disord. 1998;22:1145–8.

13. Weakley FL, Turnbull RB. Recognition of regional ileitis in the operating room. Dis Colon Rectum. 1971;14:17–23.

14. Crohn BB, Ginsburg L, Oppenheimer GD. Regional ileitis: a clinical and pathological entity. J Am Med Assoc. 1932;99:1323–9.

15. Goldberg HI, Gore RM, Margulis AR, Moss AA, Baker EL. Computed tomography in the evaluation of Crohn disease. Am J Radiol. 1983;140:277–82.

16. Meyers MA, McGuire PV. Spiral CT demonstration of hypervascularity in Crohn disease: 'vascular jejunization of the ileum' or the 'comb sign'. Abdom Imag. 1995;20:327–32.

17. Wills JS, Lobis IF, Denstman FJ. Crohn disease: state of the art. Radiology. 1997;202:597–610.

18. Jabra AA, Fishman EK, Taylor GA. Crohn disease in the pediatric patient: CT evaluation. Radiology. 1991;179:495–8.

19. Desreumaux P, Ernst O, Geboes K *et al*. Inflammatory alterations in mesenteric adipose tissue in Crohn's disease. Gastroenterology. 1999;117:73–81.

20. Hotamisligil GS, Arner P, Caro JF, Atkinson RL, Spiegelman B. Increased adipose tissue expression of tumor necrosis factor-a in human obesity and insulin resistance. J Clin Invest. 1995;95:2409–15.

21. Kern PA, Saghidazeh M, Ong JM, Bosch RJ, Deem R, Simsolo RB. The expression of tumor necrosis factor in human adipose tissue: regulation by obesity, weight loss, and relation to lipoprotein lipase. J Clin Invest. 1995;95:2111–19.

22. Pond CM. Long-term changes in adipose tissue in human disease. Proc Nutr Soc. 2001;60:365–74.

23. Borley NR, Mortensen NJ, Jewell DP, Warren BF. The relationship between inflammatory and serosal connective tissue changes in ileal Crohn's disease: evidence for a possible causative link. J Pathol. 2000;190:196–202.

24. Levine JA, Jensen MD, Eberhardt NL, O'Brien T. Adipocyte macrophage colony-stimulating factor is a mediator of adipose tissue growth. J Clin Invest. 1998;101:1557–64.

25. Pond CM, Mattacks CA. Interactions between adipose tissue around lymph nodes and lymphoid cells *in vitro*. J Lipid Res. 1995;36:2219–31.

26. Pond CM, Mattacks CA. *In vivo* evidence for the involvement of the adipose tissue surrounding lymph nodes in immune responses. Immunol Lett. 1998;63:159–67.

27. Calkins BM. A meta-analysis of the role of smoking in inflammatory bowel disease. Dig Dis Sci. 1989;34:1841–54.

28. Thornton JR, Emmet PM, Heaton KW. Diet and Crohn's disease: characteristics of the preillness diet. Br Med J. 1979;2:762–4.
29. Loudon CP, Corroll V, Butcher J, Rawsthorne P, Bernstein CN. The effects of physical exercise on patients with Crohn's disease. Am J Gastroenterol. 1999;94:697–703.
30. Walczak R, Tontonoz P. PPARadigms and PPARadoxes: expanding roles for PPARgamma in the control of lipid metabolism. J Lipid Res. 2002;43:177–86.
31. Fajas L, Debril MB, Auwerx J. The pleiotropic functions of peroxisome proliferator-activated receptor gamma. J Mol Med. 2001;79:30–47.
32. Dubuquoy L, Dharancy S, Nutten S, Pettersson S, Auwerx J, Desreumaux P. PPARg/RXR in inflammatory digestive diseases: a new therapeutic target in hepatogastroenterology. Lancet. 2002;360:1410–18.
33. Blain A, Cattan S, Beaugerie L, Carbonnel F, Gendre JP, Cosnes J. Crohn's disease clinical course and severity in obese patients. Clin Nutr. 2002;21:51–7.

9
Intraluminal targets in Crohn's disease: the possible role of bile acids

A. F. HOFMANN

INTRODUCTION

In this chapter the luminal events in Crohn's disease (CD) will be considered. The chapter will also include a discussion of bile acid metabolism as it pertains to CD, and discuss the possibility that conjugated bile acid administration might be efficacious.

CD is considered to be an autoimmune disease in which there is an excessive response of the ileum to bacteria and/or bacterial antigens in the lumen[1,2]. An alternative aetiology would be a normal inflammatory response to an abnormal bacterial stimulus. This belief that CD is an autoimmune disease with intraluminal stimuli serving as a *sine qua non* is based on the response of CD to steroids, as well as the improvement observed when the intestinal stream is diverted. The very recent report of a dramatic response in disease activity to granulocyte–macrophage colony-stimulating factor provides further evidence for an innate immune defect contributing to the pathogenesis of this disease[3]. Additional support for intestinal flora playing a key role in the pathogenesis of inflammation has come from the observation that in two interleukin knockout models (genetic ablation of IL-2 or IL-10), intestinal inflammation has required the presence of intraluminal bacteria[4,5]. Nonetheless, the not-infrequent occurrence of CD in the proximal intestine, stomach, or oesophagus indicates that the inflammatory response can occur at sites quite far removed from the ileum. Thus, ileal bacteria appear to initiate an inappropriate inflammatory response that becomes self-sustaining and translocates to distant gastrointestinal sites.

THE COMPLEX MILIEU OF THE LUMEN OF THE TERMINAL ILEUM

General considerations

The terminal ileum lumen may be considered a 'bioreactor', in that it is the final common path of endogenous and exogenous secretions as well as inflammatory

Table 1   The complex mixture of substances in the lumen of the terminal ileum of patients with Crohn's disease

---

Endogenous constituents
Salivary, gastric and pancreatic enzymes
Conjugated and unconjugated bile acids
Conjugated and unconjugated bilirubin
Immunoglobulins and defensins
Mucosal lymphocytes that migrate into the lumen
Inflammatory exudates from inflamed mucosa
Oral bacteria, fungi, and viruses
Colonic bacteria, viruses, and fungi refluxing across the ileocaecal valve

Exogenous constituents
Unabsorbed nutrients (fatty acids, peptides, amino acids)
Other dietary lipids and phytochemicals
Dietary fibre
Food additives (e.g. polyethylene glycol, methylcellulose, carrageenan, guar gum)
Microparticles (titanium oxide, silica, precipitated calcium phosphate)
Conjugates of phytochemicals and drugs secreted in bile
Drugs and their metabolites that are incompletely absorbed and/or secreted in bile
Ingested bacteria, fungi and viruses

---

secretions. In addition, bacteria and caecal contents reflux across the ileocaecal valve. The constituents that are likely to be present in the lumen of the terminal ileum are listed in Table 1.

Endogenous secretions

Endogenous secretions (besides inorganic electrolytes) reaching the terminal ileum comprise digestive secretions, immune secretions, growth factors, sloughed epithelial cells, and bacteria.

Digestive secretions include salivary and pancreatic enzymes. Pancreatic enzymes are destroyed by the endo- and exo-peptidases present in pancreatic juice, but the process is incomplete and pancreatic enzymes such as elastase and phospholipase are still active in the terminal ileum[6]. The alkaline pH of the terminal ileum precludes pepsin activity. The other major digestive secretion is a group of conjugated bile acids, whose chemical and physical forms are discussed below. Conjugates of bilirubin will be present and, if glucuronidase activity is present, unconjugated bilirubin will be formed.

Immune secretions include IgA, which is secreted in bile and by transcytosis across the small intestinal epithelium. In addition, there is likely to be movement of intraepithelial lymphocytes into the intestinal lumen. Presumably these cells are digested by pancreatic enzymes, liberating their contents.

Small intestinal enterocytes have a very rapid turnover. Although for many years, the intact cell was considered to be sloughed into the intestinal lumen, the current view is that cell loss may involve several different mechanisms, some of which alter the barrier function of the small intestinal epithelium and some of which do not[7].

Exogenous constituents

A still more complex mixture of exogenous constituents reaches the terminal ileum. These include incompletely absorbed dietary constituents – fatty acids, as well as amino acids and peptides. Dietary fibre by definition is not absorbed, and what is ingested passes to the ileum.

Today's processed food contains numerous additives for flavouring, appearance, consistency, and preservation. These include thickening agents such as polyethylene glycol, methylcellulose, and carrageenan[8]. Another class of food additives is a variety of microparticles such as titanium dioxide and silicates. In addition, dietary calcium and phosphate precipitate in the intestinal lumen to form another type of microparticle[9]. Phytochemicals are present in vegetables and fruits; these may be absorbed, and then secreted in bile as glucuronic acid conjugates[10].

In addition to dietary constituents, drug metabolites may be secreted in bile, generally in conjugated form. The usual modes of conjugation – sulphate, glucuronate, amino acids such as glycine or taurine, and glutathione – are linked to the 'aglycone' by covalent linkages that are resistant to digestion by pancreatic or brush-border enzymes. Thus such conjugates pass down the small intestine without undergoing hydrolysis or absorption until hydrolytic enzymes of non-pancreatic origin are encountered in the lumen.

Bacteria are ingested in the diet and are present in the oral cavity. In individuals with bacterial overgrowth in the proximal small intestine, bacteria will be released that will also pass to the distal intestine. Bacterial proliferation in the small intestine is considered uncommon, occurring only when there is a deficiency in immunoglobulins or an anatomical abnormality causing intestinal stasis. Nonetheless, a large part of the population ingest proton pump inhibitors, and there is some evidence that bacterial colonization is greater in the proximal small intestine in such individuals[11]. Bacterial overgrowth as inferred from hydrogen breath tests is present in a subset of patients with CD[12]. In addition to bacteria, food also contains fungi and viruses.

Inflammatory exudates

In patients with active CD, leucocytes and other constituents of the inflammatory process are likely to pass into the intestinal lumen[13]. White cells, for example, might be digested by pancreatic enzymes and liberate glucuronidases that would in turn hydrolyse glucuronides that were secreted in bile.

Regurgitation of caecal content

The ileocaecal sphincter acts similarly to the lower oesophageal sphincter in blocking reflux of caecal contents into the ileum. Based on autopsy studies the angle of the ileocaecal junction is important; if ileal entry is at a suboptimal angle increased reflux may result[14]. Caecal content is rich in bacteria and bacterial enzymes. Moreover, since caecal content contains short-chain fatty acids, caecal content might acidify ileal contents, although there is no evidence that this occurs in CD. Whether ileocaecal reflux is greater in CD is not known but, as noted, there is a subset of patients with bacterial overgrowth, and it is reasonable to propose that reflux contributes. Operations in which ileocaecal sphincter competency is preserved are claimed to result in less disease recurrence than is observed for operations in which a simple end-to-end anastomosis is performed.

The above discussion has considered the ileal lumen. Detailed chemical analysis of ileal contents in CD does not seem to have been performed. Such an analysis could be done using the analytical techniques of 'proteomics', but it is certainly unclear whether such a fishing expedition would yield useful information.

The sampling of luminal contents by aspiration might not provide information on the composition of the unstirred layer or the surface of ileal enterocytes. It is entirely possible that there are commensal bacteria that would escape sampling. Elevated antibody levels to *Bacteroides ovatus*, a well-known commensal bacterial species, have been reported for patients with CD[15].

BILE ACID METABOLISM IN CD

Bile acid metabolism and bile acid functions in health

Bile acids are formed in the hepatocyte from cholesterol by a multienzyme process. After synthesis is completed the bile acid molecules are conjugated in N-acyl linkage with glycine or taurine, and secreted into the biliary canaliculus. Conjugated bile acids are stored in the gall bladder, and emptied into the duodenum when a meal is ingested. Efficient small intestinal absorption occurs mostly in the ileum and is carrier-mediated. The efficient intestinal conservation leads to the accumulation of a 'pool' of bile acids whose mass is equivalent to the synthesis of bile acids occurring in about a week. The pool circulates about twice during digestion of a normal meal[16].

In the duodenum and proximal jejunum, bile acids form mixed micelles with fatty acids (and monoglycerides), thereby promoting fat absorption. In addition, conjugated bile acids are likely to act as intestinal antibiotics, based on *in-vitro* studies[17–19] and on one recent study, in which conjugated bile acid feeding to cirrhotic rats reduced bacterial translocation (to lymph nodes) and endotoxaemia[20]. Thus the high concentration of conjugated bile acids in the jejunum and proximal ileum may contribute to their relative sterility.

Intestinal bacteria act on bile acids in the distal ileum. Bile acids are deconjugated in part, the glycine conjugates undergoing deconjugation to a greater extent than taurine conjugates. The unconjugated bile acids that are formed are soluble at the alkaline pH of the terminal ileum[21], but binding to bacteria or formation of insoluble calcium salts might render a fraction insoluble. Dihydroxy-bile acids that are in solution are likely to be rapidly absorbed passively as chenodeoxycholic acid (CDCA) and deoxycholic acid (DCA) are fully membrane-permeable[22]. Cholic acid (CA), being less membrane permeable than dihydroxy-bile acids, may be absorbed both passively and via the ileal bile acid transport system[23]. The unconjugated bile acids return to the liver and are 'reconjugated'. There is thus a process of deconjugation and reconjugation in health[24].

A small fraction of secreted bile acids passes into the colon. Here bile acids undergo further deconjugation if not already deconjugated, with the result that caecal bile acids are likely to be completely in unconjugated form. In addition, primary bile acids undergo bacterial 7-dehydroxylation, a process that converts CA to DCA, and CDCA to lithocholic acid. A variable fraction of these 'secondary' bile acids is passively absorbed. In the liver, DCA and lithocholic acid are conjugated with glycine or taurine. In some species, but not in humans, there is 7-rehydroxylation. Deoxycholyl conjugates are secreted into bile and circulate with the primary bile acid conjugates. Lithocholic acid, in contrast, is not only conjugated on the side chain with glycine or taurine, but is also sulphated at the C-3 position to form sulpholithocholyl amidates. These compounds are secreted into bile, but are not substrates for the ileal bile acid transport system. As a result, lithocholic acid that is absorbed from the colon is rapidly lost from the bile acid pool and never constitutes more than a small percentage of biliary bile acids. As noted, the deconjugation–dehydroxylation process generates bile acids that have very limited solubility at caecal pH (pH 5–6)[21]. Thus, the concentration of bile acids in the caecum should be less than 1 mmol and there is some experimental evidence in support of this assertion[25].

The concentration and physical state of bile acids in the terminal ileum has not been well defined. Bile acid concentrations appear to decrease as one moves distally in the ileum[26,27]. The apparent bile acid concentration depends on the rate of bile acid absorption in relation to the rate of water absorption. As noted, unconjugated bile acids formed by bacterial deconjugation should be fully soluble at the alkaline pH of the terminal ileum, but whether binding to bacteria or food constituents or formation of insoluble salts results in the formation of an insoluble fraction has not been defined.

Alteration of the circulating bile acids by bile acid feeding

Mixtures of bovine bile have been used for centuries to treat constipation, but the modern era of bile acid feeding began with the discovery that CDCA feeding would decrease the cholesterol saturation of bile and induce the gradual dissolution of cholesterol gallstones[28]. CDCA suppresses primary bile acid synthesis, and the circulating bile acids become considerably enriched (50–70%) in CDCA[29]. CDCA has mild hepatotoxicity and also increases plasma levels of low density lipoprotein (LDL) cholesterol, presumably because CDCA down-regulates LDL receptors[30]. CDCA was replaced by ursodeoxycholic acid (UDCA), its 7-beta isomer, as UDCA also induces desaturation of biliary cholesterol and gallstone dissolution. UDCA is devoid of hepatotoxicity and is now used widely to treat chronic cholestatic liver disease such as primary biliary cirrhosis and primary sclerosing cholangitis. Both CDCA and UDCA undergo bacterial 7-dehydroxylation in the colon so that most administered CDCA or UDCA is converted to lithocholic acid[31]. Nonetheless the proportion of lithocholic acid in biliary bile acids increases little, presumably because what lithocholic acid is absorbed is efficiently sulphated, secreted into bile, and not reabsorbed from the small intestine. The possibility has been raised that lithocholic acid is also sulphated in the colonic enterocyte[32].

There have been a small number of studies in which conjugated bile acids have been administered for therapeutic purposes such as gallstone dissolution[33–39]. Use of conjugated bile acids for therapeutic purposes has raised little enthusiasm because administered unconjugated bile acids are efficiently absorbed and conjugated in the liver. A limitation of administering a given conjugated bile acid is that conjugated bile acids undergo deconjugation and reconjugation during enterohepatic cycling. Moreover, chemical synthesis of conjugated bile acids of high purity is difficult, with the result that conjugated bile acids are much more costly than unconjugated bile acids.

Cholylsarcosine is a conjugated bile acid analogue in which cholic acid is conjugated to sarcosine (*N*-methylglycine). The methyl group that is present on the nitrogen atom prevents bacterial deconjugation and dehydroxylation, with the result that cholylsarcosine undergoes little bacterial metabolism[40]. Cholylsarcosine has been shown to be useful as a bile acid replacement in a patient with a short bowel syndrome, but it did not differ in efficacy from a mixture of natural conjugated bile acids isolated from ox bile[41]. In ascitic cirrhotic rats, cholylsarcosine abolishes bacterial overgrowth, reduces bacterial translocation, and diminishes endotoxaemia. However, the same effect was obtained with cholylglycine, suggesting that resistance to deconjugation–dehydroxylation is not important in this animal model[20].

Bile acid metabolism in CD

Two abnormalities of bile acid metabolism have been identified in CD. First, an increased proportion of UDCA in biliary bile acids has been reported[42,43]. UDCA is formed from CDCA by bacterial epimerization, and this finding is likely to indicate the presence of an abnormal ileal flora. Second, patients with CD have mild bile acid malabsorption that is fully compensated for by increased hepatic biosynthesis[44–47]. The mechanism of this malabsorption has not been defined, but it could result from inflammation influencing the expression of the apical or the basolateral transporter involved in the ileal bile acid transport system. If the apical transporter has decreased function, bile acid malabsorption occurs, with the possible clinical consequence of diarrhoea. If the function of the basolateral transporter is impaired, then bile acids might accumulate in the ileal enterocyte where they could induce apoptosis or necrosis.

If the ileum is resected, a greater degree of bile acid malabsorption occurs. If this is compensated for by increased hepatic biosynthesis, the major clinical manifestation is diarrhoea, and fat malabsorption is mild. When the resection exceeds 100 cm in length, hepatic biosynthesis cannot compensate for severe bile acid malabsorption, and decreased secretion, together with loss of the anatomical reserve of the intact ileum, results in severe steatorrhoea. If malabsorption is sufficiently severe to jeopardize nutrition, the patient may be considered to have a short bowel syndrome[48].

Possible contribution of bile acids to the pathogenesis of CD

Perturbed bile acid metabolism could contribute to the pathogenesis of CD in three ways: (1) a deficiency of bile acids in the lumen promoting bacterial proliferation, (2) increased concentrations in the ileal enterocyte causing apoptosis/necrosis or promotion of the synthesis of inflammatory mediators, and (3) increased concentrations of bile acids in the submucosa causing mast cell activation. Any or all of these might occur simultaneously.

If bile acids were extensively deconjugated in the distal ileal lumen they might be rapidly absorbed, lowering their aqueous concentration. This in turn would promote bacterial proliferation, that in turn would cause increased deconjugation. This vicious cycle is likely to occur in the jejunum in patients with cirrhosis[20,49], but there is no evidence for its occurrence in CD.

Bile acids are transported from the ileal enterocyte via *mrp3*, an ATP-stimulated pump[50,51]. If for some reason, e.g. an ATP deficiency in the ileal enterocyte, bile acids were to accumulate in the epithelial cell they would induce apoptosis and/or necrosis. Bile acids might also induce inflammatory mediators in the ileal enterocyte[52]. In primary human colonic epithelial cells, bile acids induce inflammatory mediators such as IL-8, AP-1, and NF-κB (poster presented at this meeting by C. Hellebrand *et al.*).

If the blood supply to the ileal epithelium were impaired by the inflammatory process, bile acids might accumulate in the submucosa. Here they could activate mast cells[53] and thereby promote the liberation of potent inflammatory mediators. Bile acids could also enter the mucosa via paracellular absorption, if paracellular permeability were increased. Increased paracellular permeability has been reported to occur in CD (reviewed in ref. 54), but at least one thorough study[55] has challenged this finding.

Bile acid feeding and CD

Many thousands of patients have received CDCA for gallstone dissolution or UDCA for gallstone dissolution or cholestatic disease. To date there have been no claims that ingestion of either bile acid caused improvement in either CD or ulcerative colitis. It seems likely that, if these compounds had efficacy, it would have been noted, because with any disease that fluctuates in intensity there would be improvement while bile acids were ingested which would occur solely by chance. Thus, it seems likely to the author that neither CDCA nor UDCA alters the natural history of CD or ulcerative colitis. In animal models of induced inflammation by indomethacin, results are contradictory. One group observed improvement[56] whereas another reported that UDCA actually exacerbated the inflammation[52].

If a bile acid deficiency in the terminal ileal lumen led to bacterial proliferation, and if such bacterial proliferation contributed to the evolution of CD, it should be possible to correct the deficiency by cholylsarcosine administration. Cholylsarcosine would be absorbed by the ileal transport system, suppress primary bile acid synthesis in the liver, and thus accumulate in the circulating bile acids. Trihydroxy-bile acids such as cholylsarcosine activate mast cells at much higher concentrations than dihydroxy-bile acids and are less apoptotic/necrotic[53]. Therefore administration of cholylsarcosine should eliminate any possible effects of a diminished bile acid concentration in the terminal ileal lumen and simultaneously decrease the cytotoxic and proinflammatory effects of dihydroxy-bile acids.

DIETARY CONSTITUENTS IN THE PATHOGENESIS OF CD

There is no evidence to suggest that a change in the proportion of nutrients – fat, carbohydrate, protein – would be beneficial in CD[57], although diets rich in polyunsaturated fatty acids appear to have some efficacy as compared to diets containing more monounsaturated acids[58]. Ingestion of microparticles was advanced as a causal factor in CD by Lomer *et al.*[9], but a recent placebo-controlled, double-blind study has failed to show efficacy in CD patients receiving a low microparticle diet (RPH Thompson, personal communication).

EPILOGUE

This brief survey has suggested that luminal composition is not well defined in CD. There is evidence that commensal bacteria are involved in the pathogenesis of CD. There are modest bile acid abnormalities in CD, and bile acid deficiency in the terminal ileal lumen might contribute to bacterial proliferation that in turn could contribute to the pathogenesis of CD. Increased paracellular permeability and/or impaired capillary blood flow could promote the accumulation of bile acids at pathological levels in the submucosa. Were such to occur, mast cells would be activated, releasing inflammatory mediators. As noted, the postulated conjugated bile acid deficiency in the terminal ileal lumen could be remedied by cholylsarcosine administration, which in turn should abolish bacterial proliferation. Such administration of cholylsarcosine might also reduce the cytotoxicity of the circulating bile acid pool that in turn would lead to less mast cell activation. Assessment of efficacy of therapeutic agents in CD is not simple, and the arguments presented here may not be sufficiently persuasive to bring about the initiation of a clinical trial. Let us hope this is not the case. However, the striking improvement induced by granulocyte–macrophage colony-stimulating factor[3] suggests that controlled studies of this new agent should take the highest priority.

Acknowledgements

The author's work is supported in part by NIH Grant 37172 (PI: Dr John S. Fordtran, Baylor University Medical Center, Dallas, Texas), and a grant-in-aid from the Falk Foundation e.V., Freiburg, Germany.

References

1. Podolsky DK. Inflammatory bowel disease. N Engl J Med. 2002;347:417–29.
2. Hendrickson BA, Gokhale R, Cho JH. Clinical aspects and pathophysiology of inflammatory bowel disease. Clin Microbiol Rev. 2002;15:79–94.
3. Dieckgraefe BK, Korzenik JR. Treatment of active Crohn's disease with recombinant human granulocyte–macrophage colony-stimulating factor. Lancet: 2002;360:1478–80.
4. Contractor NV, Bassiri H, Reya T et al. Lymphoid hyperplasia, autoimmunity, and compromised intestinal intraepithelial lymphocyte development in colitis-free gnotobiotic IL-2-deficient mice. J Immunol. 1998;160:385–94.
5. Sellon RK, Tonkonogy S, Schultz M et al. Resident enteric bacteria are necessary for development of spontaneous colitis and immune system activation in interleukin-10-deficient mice. Infect Immun. 1998;66:5224–31.
6. Holtmann G, Kelly DG, Sternby B, DiMagno EP. Survival of human pancreatic enzymes during bowel transit: effect of nutrients, bile acids, and enzymes. Am J Physiol. 1997;273:G553–8.
7. Mayhew TM, Myklebust R, Whybrow A, Jenkins R. Epithelial integrity, cell death and cell loss in mammalian small intestine. Histol Histopathol. 1999;14:257–67.
8. Green S. Research activities in toxicology and toxicological requirements of the FDA for food and color additives. Biomed Environ Sci. 1988;1:424–30.
9. Lomer MCE, Thompson RPH, Powell JJ. Fine and ultrafine particles of the diet: influence on the mucosal immune response and association with Crohn's disease. Proc Nutr Soc. 2002;61:123–30.

10. Nutrition and cancer prevention: new insights into the role of phytochemicals. Adv Exp Med Biol. 2001;492:1–347.
11. Shindo K, Machida M, Fukumura M, Koide K, Yamazaki R. Omeprazole induces altered bile acid metabolism. Gut. 1998;42:266–71.
12. Castiglione F, Del Vecchio Blanco G, Riso P et al. Orocecal transit time and bacterial overgrowth in patients with Crohn's disease. J Clin Gastroenterol. 2000;31:63–6.
13. Saverymuttu SH, Camilleri M, Rees H, Lavender JP, Hodgson HJ, Chadwick VS. Indium 111-granulocyte scanning in the assessment of disease extent and disease activity in inflammatory bowel disease. A comparison with colonoscopy, histology, and fecal indium 111-granulocyte excretion. Gastroenterology. 1986;90:1121–8.
14. Kumar D, Phillips SF. The contribution of external ligamentous attachments in function of the ileocecal junction. Dis Colon Rectum. 1987;30:1410–16.
15. Saitoh S, Noda S, Aiba Y et al. *Bacteroides ovatus* as the predominant commensal intestinal microbe causing a systemic antibody response in inflammatory bowel disease. Clin Diag Lab Immunol. 2002;9:54–9.
16. Hofmann AF. Intestinal absorption of bile acids and biliary constituents: the intestinal component of the enterohepatic circulation and the integrated system. In: Johnson LR, Alpers DH, Christensen J, Jacobson ED, Walsh JH, editors. Physiology of the Gastrointestinal Tract, 3rd edn. Volume 2. New York: Raven Press, 1994:1845–65.
17. Floch MH, Gershengoren W, Elliott S, Spiro HM. Bile acid inhibition of the intestinal microflora – a function for simple bile acids. Gastroenterology. 1971;61:228–33.
18. Binder HJ, Filburn B, Floch M. Bile acid inhibition of intestinal anaerobic organisms. Am J Clin Nutr. 1975;28:119–25.
19. Sung JY, Shaffer EA, Costerton JW. Antibacterial activity of bile salts against common pathogens. Effects of hydrophobicity of the molecule and in the presence of phospholipids. Dig Dis Sci. 1993;38:2104–12.
20. Lorenzo-Zuniga V, Bartoli R, Planas R et al. Oral bile acid administration reduces endotoxemia and bacterial translocation in ascitic cirrhotic rats. Hepatology. 2003;37:551–7.
21. Hofmann AF, Mysels KJ. Bile acid solubility and precipitation *in vitro* and *in vivo*: the role of conjugation, pH and Ca^{2+} ions. J Lipid Res. 1992;33:617–26.
22. Gurantz D, Hofmann AF. Influence of bile acid structure on bile flow and biliary lipid secretion in the hamster. Am J Physiol. 1984;247:G736–48.
23. Craddock AL, Love MW, Daniel RW et al. Expression and transport of the human ileal and renal sodium-dependent bile acid transporter. Am J Physiol. 1998;274:G157–69.
24. Hofmann AF. Enterohepatic circulation of bile acids. In: Schulz SG, editor. Handbook of Physiology: The Gastrointestinal System, Vol. II: Salivary, Gastric, Pancreatic, and Hepatobiliary Secretion. Bethesda, MD: American Physiological Society, 1989:567–96.
25. McJunkin B, Fromm H, Sarva RP, Amin P. Factors in the mechanism of diarrhoea in bile acid malabsorption: fecal pH – a key determinant. Gastroenterology. 1981;80:1454–64.
26. Northfield TC, McColl I. Postprandial concentrations of free and conjugated bile acids down the length of the normal human small intestine. Gut. 1973;14:513–18.
27. Mallory A, Kern F Jr, Smith J, Savage D. Patterns of bile acids and microflora in the human small intestine I. Bile acids. Gastroenterology. 1973;64:26–33.
28. Thistle JL, Hofmann AF. Efficacy and specificity of chenodeoxycholic acid therapy for dissolving gallstones. N Engl J Med. 1973;289:655–9.
29. Danzinger RG, Hofmann AF, Thistle JL, Schoenfield LJ. Effect of oral chenodeoxycholic acid on bile acid kinetics and biliary lipid composition in women with cholelithiasis. J Clin Invest. 1973;52:2809–21.
30. Schoenfield LJ, Lachin JM, the Steering Committee, and the National Cooperative Gallstone Study Group: Chenodiol (chenodeoxycholic acid) for dissolution of gallstones: the National Cooperative Gallstone Study. Ann Intern Med. 1981;95:257–82.
31. Bachrach WH, Hofmann AF. Ursodeoxycholic acid in the treatment of cholesterol cholelithiasis: a review. Dig Dis Sci. 1982;27:737–61, 27:833–56.
32. Makashima M, Lu TT, Xie W et al. Vitamin D receptor as an intestinal bile acid sensor. Science. 2002;296:1313–16.
33. Hardison WG, Grundy SM. Effect of ursodeoxycholate and its taurine conjugate on bile acid synthesis and cholesterol absorption. Gastroenterology. 1984;87:130–5.

34. Muraca M, Vilei MT, Cianci V, Liu XT. Effect of tauroursodeoxycholic acid on biliary lipid composition. Ital J Gastroenterol. 1995;27:439–40.
35. Crosignani A, Budillon G, Cimino L *et al*. Tauroursodeoxycholic acid for the treatment of HCV-related chronic hepatitis: a multicenter placebo-controlled study. Hepatogastroenterology. 1998;45:1624–9.
36. Invernizzi P, Setchell KD, Crosignani A *et al*. Differences in the metabolism and disposition of ursodeoxycholic acid and of its taurine-conjugated species in patients with primary biliary cirrhosis. Hepatology. 1999;29:320–7.
37. Angelico M, Tisone G, Baiocchi L *et al*. One-year pilot study on tauroursodeoxycholic acid as an adjuvant treatment after liver transplantation. Ital J Gastroenterol Hepatol. 1999;31:462–8.
38. Larghi A, Crosignani A, Battezzati PM *et al*. Ursodeoxycholic and tauro-ursodeoxycholic acids for the treatment of primary biliary cirrhosis: a pilot crossover study. Aliment Pharmacol Ther. 1997;11:409–14.
39. Peled Y, Bar-Meir S, Rotmensch HH, Tiomny A, Gilat T. Effect of tauroursodeoxycholic acid on patients with ileal resection. Isr J Med Sci. 1982;18:812–14.
40. Schmassmann A, Fehr HF, Locher J *et al*. Cholylsarcosine, a new bile acid analogue: metabolism and effect on biliary secretion in humans. Gastroenterology. 1993;104:1171–81.
41. Gruy-Kapral C, Little KH, Fordtran JS, Hagey LR, Hofmann AF. Conjugated bile acid replacement therapy for short bowel syndrome: a comparison of cholylsarcosine and a natural bile acid mixture. Gastroenterology. 1999:116:15–21.
42. Vantrappen G, Ghoos Y, Rutgeerts P, Janssens J. Bile acid studies in uncomplicated Crohn's disease. Gut. 1977;18:730–5.
43. Lapidus A, Einarsson C. Bile acid composition in patients with ileal resection due to Crohn's disease. Inflamm Bowel Dis. 1998;4:89–94.
44. Farivar S, Fromm H, Schindler D, McJunkin B, Schmidt FW. Test of bile-acid and vitamin B12 metabolism in ileal Crohn's disease. Am J Clin Pathol. 1980;73:69–74.
45. Tougaard L, Giese B, Pedersen BH, Binder V. Bile acid metabolism in patients with Crohn's disease in terminal ileum. Scand J Gastroenterol. 1986;21:627–33.
46. Rutgeerts P, Ghoos Y, Vantrappen G. Kinetics of primary bile acids in patients with non-operated Crohn's disease. Eur J Clin Invest. 1982;12:135–43.
47. Nyhlin H, Merrick MV, Eastwood MA. Bile acid malabsorption in Crohn's disease and indications for its assessment using SeHCAT. Gut. 1994;35:90–3.
48. Hofmann AF. Bile acid malabsorption caused by ileal resection. Arch Intern Med. 1972;130: 597–605.
49. Hofmann AF, Hagey LR. Bile acids and biliary disease: peaceful coexistence versus deadly warfare. In: Blum HE, Bode C, Bode JC, Sartor RB, editors. Gut and Liver. Lancaster: Kluwer, 1998:85–103.
50. Rost D, Mahner S, Sugiyama Y, Stremmel W. Expression and localization of the multidrug resistance-associated protein 3 in rat small and large intestine. Am J Physiol. 2002;282:G720–6.
51. Scheffer GL, Kool M, de Haas M *et al*. Tissue distribution and induction of human multidrug resistant protein 3. Lab Invest. 2002;82:193–201.
52. Uchida A, Yamada T, Hayakawa T, Hoshino M. Taurochenodeoxycholic acid ameliorates and ursodeoxycholic acid exacerbates small intestinal inflammation. Am J Physiol. 1997;272: G1249–57.
53. Quist RG, Ton-Nu H-T, Lillienau J, Hofmann AF, Barrett KE. Activation of mast cells by bile acids. Gastroenterology. 1991;101:446–56.
54. DeMeo MT, Mutlu EA, Keshavarzian A, Tobin MC. Intestinal permeation and gastrointestinal disease. J Clin Gastroenterol. 2002;34:385–96.
55. Mulkholm P, Langholz E, Hollander D *et al*. Intestinal permeability in patients with Crohn's disease and ulcerative colitis and their first degree relatives. Gut. 1994;35:1675–6.
56. Kullmann F, Gross V, Ruschoff J *et al*. Effect of ursodeoxycholic acid on the inflammatory activity of indomethacin-induced intestinal inflammation in rats. Z Gastroenterol. 1997;35: 171–8.
57. Leiper K, Woolner J, Mullan MM *et al*. A randomized controlled trial of high versus low long chain triglyceride whole protein feed in active Crohn's disease. Gut. 2001;49:790–4.
58. Gassull MA, Fernandez-Banares F, Cabre E *et al*. Fat composition may be a clue to explain the primary therapeutic effect of enteral nutrition in Crohn's disease: results of a double blind randomized multicentre European trial. Gut. 2002;51:164–8.

10
Therapeutic targets in rheumatoid arthritis: is there a lesson to be learned for gastroenterologists?

U. MÜLLER-LADNER

INTRODUCTION

Rheumatoid arthritis (RA) is a disease of very complex pathophysiology, combining genetic factors, alterations of cellular and humoral immune responses, potential involvement of infectious agents, and various mechanisms of tissue destruction. In addition, extra-articular organs can be secondarily affected. Molecular biology has provided numerous new aspects in the pathophysiology of the disease (Fig. 1). When compared to inflammatory bowel diseases (IBD), remarkable similarities in pathophysiological mechanisms as well as in management of therapy exist, which may allow the development of novel strategies for each of these disease entities derived from the knowledge of the counterpart (Table 1).

THE DEVELOPMENT OF TREATMENT STRATEGIES

Since the beginning of drug-based approaches to target rheumatoid arthritis in the first half of the twentieth century (Table 2), every decade faced a 'new' disease-modifying drug (DMARD), and sometimes decades had to pass from the first application of a DMARD to its validation by controlled studies (Table 2). However, in the last decade, basic research as well as clinical studies revealed numerous novel aspects and approaches in all fields of RA therapy. The spectrum of NSAIDs (non-steroidal anti-inflammatory drugs) has been extended by the development of specific cyclooxygenase-2 (COX-2) inhibiting drugs, and DMARD combination therapy has been proven to be both safe and effective. The inhibition of pyrimidine synthesis by leflunomide has been added to the spectrum of DMARDs, and targeting 'biological' molecules such as proinflammatory cytokines including tumour necrosis factor alpha (TNF-α) and interleukin-1 (IL-1) has generated a new class of drugs bearing the potential of

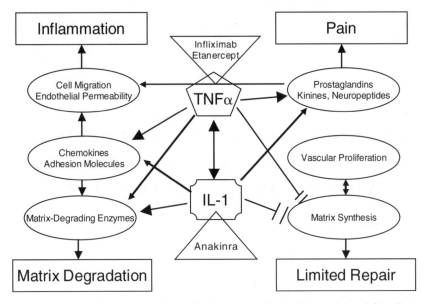

Fig. 1 Advances in RA pathophysiology: the impact of molecular biology. Adapted from Dayer, J Rheumatol Suppl. 2002;65:10–15.

Table 1 Similarities between RA and IBD

	RA	IBD
HLA association	✓	✓
Microorganisms	?	✓
Autoimmunity	✓	✓
Cytokines	✓	✓
Tissue destruction	✓	✓
Fibrosis	✓	✓
Extrafocal manifestations	✓	✓

= common targets?

Table 2 Disease-modifying drugs

Year (used first in RA patients)	DMARD	(Primary) mechanism of action
1930 (1927)	Gold	Cellular immunomodulation
1970 (1964)	Azathioprine	Purine antagonist, cellular immunomodulation
1980 (1948)	Sulphasalazine	T-cell inhibition
1990 (1951)	Methotrexate	Folate inhibitor, inhibition of cellular proliferation
1995 (1979)	Cyclosporine A	T-cell inhibition
2000 (1993)	Biologics	Specific inhibition of cytokines

steroid replacement in flares as well as providing a new component for long-term combination therapy[1].

However, recent clinical trials have confirmed the efficacy and clinical advantage of DMARD combination therapy (including methotrexate (MTX) by improvement of the majority of standard disease variables[2,3], e.g. the number of swollen and tender joints, duration of morning stiffness, and the erythrocyte sedimention rate. Among the patients receiving a DMARD combination therapy (MTX, sulphasalazine, hydroxychloroquine) 77% reported at least 50% improvement in disease parameters at 9 months until completion of the study after 24 months, whereas in the other groups (sulphasalazine/hydroxychloroquine and MTX monotherapy) only up to 40% of patients showed this extent of improvement after 24 months. Combination of three DMARDs together with steroids even resulted in remission in 36 of 97 patients after 2 years. Thus it is most likely that combination of different immunosuppressive agents might also be beneficial for IBD. Therefore, studies should be performed which evaluate the potential of combination therapy not only in long-term or 'refractory' stages but also in highly active early disease.

PROS AND CONS OF COX-2 INHIBITION

As the hitherto-used NSAIDs are not selective for inhibition of one of the two Cox isoforms, side-effects such as induction of gastrointestinal ulcers (especially in combination with steroids) and inhibition of platelet aggregation are identical for all currently available NSAIDs. Thus, development of COX-2-specific inhibitors is a desirable goal for RA treatment. Two highly specific COX-2 inhibitors, rofecoxib and celecoxib, have been approved for RA, osteoarthritis, and pain. Although trial data indicate that up to a 4-fold analgesic effect can be achieved when compared to the maximum dosage of COX-1/2 inhibitors, the most important benefit of specific COX-2 inhibitors might be the approximately 50% reduction of gastrointestinal ulcers[4]. In contrast, recent data indicate that they most likely will not resolve the sequelae of currently used COX-1/2 inhibitors in treatment of arthritic symptoms in IBD, which frequently deteriorate intestinal inflammation or even trigger a flare, as COX-2 appears to be crucial for anti-inflammatory mechanisms in the intestinal mucosa[5].

COMPLICATIONS OF LONG-TERM DMARD TREATMENT

As well as the potential decrease of clinical efficiency during long-term DMARD therapy, there are other complications that may force modification or alteration to the therapeutic regimen. The majority of side-effects arise from the use of immunosuppressive and immunomodulating drugs. In RA the classical drugs are corticosteroids, MTX, azathioprine, cyclosporine, sulphasalazine, gold, and hydroxychloroquine[6]. In addition, in recent years a completely new class of antirheumatic drugs has been introduced into the therapeutic armamentarium, the so-called 'biologics'. A number of different monoclonal antibodies and soluble cytokine receptors have been developed to inhibit the effects of proinflammatory cytokines. Among them, TNF-α-targeted substances and inhibition of the proinflammatory cytokine IL-1 by soluble IL-1 receptor antagonist have been shown to be the most promising[1]. Inhibition of TNF-α has been achieved by two antibody-based 'biologic' approaches and by application of soluble TNF-α receptors, which both 'capture' circulating TNF-α. Interestingly, the anti-TNF-α antibody infliximab also induces apoptosis in activated T cells in the mucosa. All biologics require subcutaneous or intravenous application, ranging from twice a week to one infusion every 8 weeks. Current studies show a very rapid decrease in clinical and serological inflammation parameters, and patients report amelioration of joint swelling and pain, mostly within a few days. There is also a rationale for combination of biologics with DMARDs. Infliximab in combination with MTX showed a higher number of patients reaching at least 50% reduction in clinical activity criteria than patients receiving either MTX or infliximab alone[7].

However, at present these potent drugs cannot be recommended unrestrictedly for first-line therapy, mainly due to a number of side-effects and unanswered questions in long-term therapy: (a) patients subjected to receive anti-TNF-α and anti-IL-1 biologics should not show signs of active infection, as additional immunosuppression may be deleterious in this situation; (b) definite application schemes for biologics still need to be established; (c) a decrease in efficacy might be due to development of neutralizing antibodies, especially when anti-TNF-α antibodies are used; and (d) development of secondary malignancies due to reduced TNF-α activity needs to be monitored closely in long-term follow-up studies. A distinct problem that has arisen since the beginning of the era of anti-TNF therapy is the reactivation of tuberculosis. At present approximately 25 out of 100 000 patients receiving anti-TNF therapy will develop active tuberculosis (Table 3); therefore, additional recommendations for prophylaxis and therapy of tuberculosis in anti-TNF-treated patients have been established[8]. In summary, biologics should be used only in patients with persistent active disease in addition to DMARD therapy, or to limit or replace the amount of steroids usually

Table 3 Tuberculosis following TNF inhibition
(70 reported patients out of 147 000 treated patients)

Demographics	Value*
Median age	57 (18–83) years
Number of infliximab doses	3 (1–9)
Mean duration to onset	12 (1–52) weeks
USA	17
Europe	45
Indication	
RA	47
IBD	18
Recent use of immunosuppressants	55
Recent combination therapy	31
Extrapulmonary	57% of all cases

Adapted from Keane et al., N Engl J Med. 2001;345: 1098–104; Weismann, J Rheumatol Suppl. 2002;65:33–8.
*n if not otherwise stated.

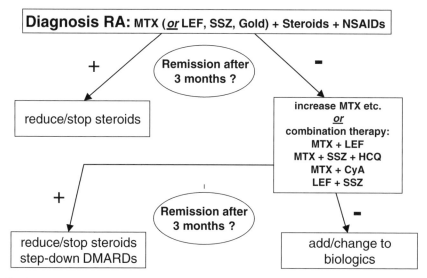

Fig. 2 Recommendations of the German Rheumatology Society. Adapted from Gromnica-Ihle, Z. Rheumatol. 2002; 61:II/37.

needed to control a flare. These recommendations are reflected by the algorithm of the German Rheumatology Society (Fig. 2), which is in line with international recommendations addressing this problem. Intensive follow-up should accompany these therapies, especially until the questions regarding whether anti-TNF-α therapies are also able to reduce long-term joint destruction and/or support the development of malignancies and autoimmune diseases are sufficiently answered. In addition, detailed molecular analysis of the effects of anti-TNF-α therapy will also help to answer the question of why rheumatic diseases appear to show a better general response to biologics and combination therapies than do IBD. At present it can be speculated that this effect is due to differences in pathophysiology between the two disease groups, and to differences in the binding pattern of anti-TNF-α antibodies and soluble TNF receptors, e.g. the potential to bind to lymphotoxin[9], which is illustrated by the fact that treatment of spondylarthropathies with etanercept ameliorates only the arthritic and not the gastrointestinal symptoms[9]. Moreover, anti-TNF-α antibodies – in contrast to soluble TNF receptors – are capable of inducing macrophage apoptosis by direct binding to surface-bound TNF-α[10].

SUMMARY

The development of novel drugs for long-term treatment, as well as for acute flares of RA, allows us to support more intensive therapeutic regimens at an earlier stage of the disease in order to prevent joint destruction and avoid disability. These developments replaced the former therapeutic 'pyramid' strategy, which implied an increase in drug dosage and number when increase in activity was noted, by a modern 'hit-early-and-hard' regimen to suppress inflammation and joint destruction early in the course of the disease (Fig. 2) – an approach which might also be feasible for the treatment of IBD.

References

1. Furst DE, Breedveld FC, Kalden JR *et al*. Updated consensus statement on biological agents for the treatment of rheumatoid arthritis and other rheumatic diseases (May 2002). Ann Rheum Dis. 2002;61(Suppl.2):ii2–7.
2. Möttönen T, Hannonen P, Leirisalo-Repo M *et al*. Comparison of combination therapy with single-drug therapy in early rheumatoid arthritis: a randomised trial. Lancet. 1999;353:1568–73.
3. O'Dell JR, Leff R, Paulsen G *et al*. Treatment of rheumatoid arthritis with methotrexate and hydroxychloroquine, methotrexate and sulfasalazine, or a combination of the three medications: results of a two-year, randomized, double-blind, placebo-controlled trial. Arthritis Rheum. 2002;46:1164–70.
4. Scheiman JM. Gastrointestinal outcomes: evidence for risk reduction in patients using coxibs. Am J Manag Care. 2002;17(Suppl.):S518–28.
5. Cipolla G, Crema F, Sacco S *et al*. Nonsteroidal anti-inflammatory drugs and inflammatory bowel disease: current perspectives. Pharmacol Res. 2002;46:1–6.
6. Koopman WJ, editor. Arthritis and Allied Conditions. A Textbook of Rheumatology, 15th edn. Baltimore: Lippincott, Williams & Wilkins, 2003.
7. Maini RN, Breedveld FC, Kalden JR *et al*. Therapeutic efficacy of multiple intravenous infusions of anti-tumor necrosis factor alpha monoclonal antibody combined with low-dose weekly methotrexate in rheumatoid arthritis. Arthritis Rheum. 1998;41:1552–663.
8. Furst DE, Cush J, Kaufmann S *et al*. Preliminary guidelines for diagnosing and treating tuberculosis in patients with rheumatoid arthritis in immunosuppressive trials or being treated with biological agents. Ann Rheum Dis. 2002;61(Suppl. 2):ii62–3.
9. Marzo-Ortega H, McGonagle D, O'Connor P, Emery P. Efficacy of etanercept for treatment of Crohn's related spondylarthritis but not colitis. Ann Rheum Dis. 2003;62:74–6.
10. Van Deventer SHJ. Transmembrane TNFα induction of apoptosis, and the efficacy of TNF-targeting therapies in Crohn's disease. Gastroenterology. 2001;121:1242–6.

Section IV
Learning from others

11
Interstitial lung diseases and inflammatory bowel diseases: pathophysiological parallels and differences

J. MÜLLER-QUERNHEIM

INTRODUCTION

Sarcoidosis (SAR) is a multiorgan disorder of unknown origin, characterized in the affected organs by T-lymphocyte–mononuclear phagocyte infiltration, granuloma formation, and distortion of the normal microarchitecture[1].The lung is the most commonly involved organ, and studies with lung inflammatory cells from the lower respiratory tract recovered by bronchoalveolar lavage (BAL), and from other sites of the body, revealed concepts regarding the immunopathogenesis of the disease.

These concepts exhibit some similarities with those of inflammatory bowel diseases (IBD). SAR is frequently insidious and discovered in asymptomatic individuals by routine chest X-rays or heralded by constitutional complaints. Involvement of the eye, heart, central nervous system, or the development of hypercalcaemia may require immediate action. Acute disease is characterized by constitutional complaints, cough, dyspnoea on exertion, erythema nodosum, and characteristic chest X-ray findings. More than 90% of sarcoid patients will eventually develop pulmonary abnormalities easily recognizable on chest X-ray or by tests of pulmonary function. The chest X-ray is rarely normal; most commonly it reveals bilateral hilar adenopathy and/or diffuse reticulonodular infiltrates in the parenchyma. SAR is best defined in histopathological terms as 'a disease characterized by the presence in all of several affected organs and tissues of non-caseating epitheloid-cell granulomas, proceeding either to resolution or to conversion into hyaline connective tissue'[2]. The clinical diagnosis, however, can only be supported by typical histopathological findings. Pathognomonic criteria or a diagnostic 'golden standard' are absent. Most authorities thus include several clinical, radiological, immunological, and histological features into their diagnostic criteria since other disease processes can simulate SAR in many ways. Occasionally, all of these features may suggest the diagnosis of SAR in patients later proven to have other diseases[3]. Therefore, rigorous efforts should be made to exclude alternative diagnoses, e.g. tuberculosis, lymphoma, berylliosis, etc., and patients diagnosed as suffering from SAR must regularly be subjected to review and further testing.

Thus, SAR is a systemic granulomatous disorder diagnosed by exclusion. Most interestingly, although it is a systemic disorder, sarcoid lesions are only rarely seen in the gut[4,5]. Similarly, chronic IBD are also diagnosed by exclusion[6] and systemic manifestations are observed[7,8]. Moreover, even alveolitis can be elicited by IBD[9,10]. Analyses of activated immune cells have demonstrated that both SAR and IBD are characterized by an alteration of the cytokine network. Moreover, clinical and immunopathological similarities and overlaps between SAR and Crohn's disease (CD) are reported[5,11]. An interesting difference between SAR and CD is the fact that smoking decreases the incidence of SAR but increases that of CD, and increases the severity of its manifestation[12–14].

CYTOKINE NETWORK

Due to a considerable increase in cellularity of bronchoalveolar lavage, the absolute number of alveolar macrophages and T lymphocytes expands in SAR. The percentage of alveolar macrophages with monocytic appearance is elevated in SAR, suggesting a recent immigration of monocytic precursors of alveolar macrophages from the blood. A number of cytokines chemotactic for monocytes and T cells are produced by alveolar cells in the course of inflammatory reactions of SAR and other interstitial lung diseases, supporting the notion of monocyte and T-cell immigration. The activated state of these cells has been demonstrated on the basis of their spontaneous *in-vitro* production of interleukins IL-1 and IL-2, tumour necrosis factor alpha (TNF-α), interferon-gamma (IFN-γ) and many other proinflammatory cytokines. This activation of the alveolar immune cells is compartmentalized, i.e. alveolar macrophages and T cells release these mediators spontaneously, whereas the corresponding cells of the peripheral blood are quiescent[1]. A similar phenomenon can be observed in CD with activated mucosal T cells in inflamed segments of the intestine producing IL-2 and quiescent T cells in the peripheral blood[15].

In SAR a study analysing spontaneous bronchoalveolar immune cell release of TNF-α, IL-8, and macrophage inflammatory protein (MIP)-1α revealed that, compared to controls, newly diagnosed SAR patients with progressive disease are characterized by an exaggerated release of these proinflammatory mediators. Interestingly, an asymptomatic subgroup of patients diagnosed by chance due to abnormal findings in routine chest X-rays who were categorized to have stable disease also exhibited increased cytokine release which proves active, 'smouldering' inflammation in these asymptomatic sarcoid patients (Fig. 1)[16]. Similarly, in tissue of both inflamed and un-inflamed Crohn's colitis proinflammatory cytokines such as IL-1 and IL-8 could be found (Fig. 2)[17]. Mononuclear cells within the lamina propria could be identified to be the producers of these cytokines in CD and in ulcerative colitis (UC). In a study by Reinecker *et al.* a lamina propria mononuclear cell IL-1 and IL-6 release was

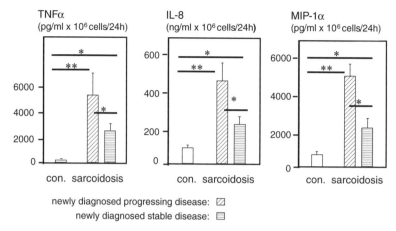

Fig. 1 Spontaneous release of proinflammatory cytokines of cultured alveolar macrophages in newly diagnosed sarcoidosis. The release of TNF-α, IL-8 and MIP-1α differed significantly between sarcoid patients with progressing disease compared to controls (**$p < 0.005$) and compared to sarcoid patients with stable disease (*$p < 0.05$). Interestingly, some sarcoid patients with stable disease showed an exaggerated release of these mediators, leading to a moderate increase compared with controls (*$p < 0.05$). (Adapted from ref. 16)

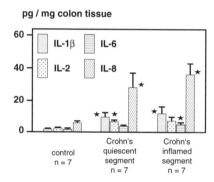

Fig. 2 Cytokines in tissue extractions of inflamed and un-inflamed intestine segments of Crohn's colitis (*$p < 0.05$ compared with control). (Adapted from ref. 17)

found in inflamed and un-inflamed segments of both CD and in UC. Interestingly, in both disorders TNF-α release was restricted to inflamed segments (Fig. 3)[18]. The pivotal role of TNF-α in SAR was demonstrated by the prognostic value of its exaggerated release by bronchoalveolar cells[19]. For both SAR and CD this notion was supported by the observation that drugs with anti-TNF-α capacity such as thalidomide are of some benefit[20-23].

In SAR and IBD a dysregulation of the cytokine network in favour of pro-inflammatory cytokines can be noted and immune-dampening mechanisms seem to be down-regulated or overburdened[24-26]. Spontaneous resolutions take place in SAR and counter-regulating, immune-dampening cytokines might be involved.

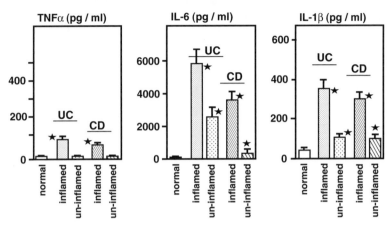

Fig. 3 Spontaneous cytokine release of lamina propria mononuclear cells from inflamed and un-inflamed intestine segments of ulcerative colitis and Crohn's disease ($*p < 0.05$ in comparison with control). (Adapted from ref. 3)

One candidate is IL-10, which inhibits cytokine production as well as proliferation of human monocytes and T cells[27]. Although several investigators have searched for this molecule its presence in the alveolitis of SAR could not be established[28,29], but equivocal results regarding its gene transcription by BAL cells have been obtained[30,31] and elevated serum levels have been recorded in SAR patients[32]. A gene polymorphism at position -1082 of the IL-10 gene influences the amount of this cytokine released by regulatory immune cells. However, comparisons of allele and genotype frequencies between clinically defined SAR groups and healthy blood donors revealed no significant differences, which demonstrates that this polymorphism does not influence the frequency of spontaneous resolution or progressing disease[33]. Most interestingly, IL-10 administered in active CD achieved a significant reduction of the CD activity index in the cohort treated with verum in comparison with placebo, which demonstrates that the therapeutic manipulation of the cytokine network is a feasible approach[34].

Transforming growth factor-beta (TGF-β) belongs to a superfamily of ubiquitous regulatory proteins which are necessary for cell growth, cell differentiation, and regulation of extracellular matrix production. Growing evidence also supports the role of TGF-β as an immunomodulator, exhibiting proinflammatory and anti-inflammatory activities[35] and stimulating the development of Th1 cells[36]. TGF-β was found in supernatants of patients with active disease and a spontaneous remission within 6 months after the investigation, whereas patients requiring therapy or suffering from chronic disease showed TGF-β levels not differing from controls (Fig. 4). Furthermore, a strong and significant negative correlation was found between IL-2 and TGF-β production by bronchoalveolar lavage cells[29]. This suggests an inhibiting role of TGF-β on the IL-2 production of T cells. In keeping with the literature we conclude from these data that the release of TGF-β by BAL cells is indicative of a mechanism which results in the cessation of inflammatory processes. Whether TGF-β is the key cytokine in

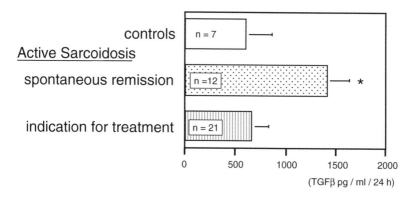

Fig. 4 Spontaneous transforming growth factor β release by bronchoalveolar cells of patients with active sarcoidosis in comparison with controls. A significant difference (*$p < 0.05$) was demonstrated between patients requiring corticosteroid treatment and patients who underwent spontaneous remission within 6 months after investigation. (Adapted from ref. 29)

down-regulating the alveolitis, or whether it acts together with other, still unknown mediators, requires further investigation.

The hypothesis can therefore be put forward that SAR and IBD result from a dysregulated Th1-cell response to ubiquitous antigens that is not appropriately controlled by normal counter-regulatory mechanisms[1,26]. These processes determine the clinical course of the diseases in as much as the predominance of proinflammatory cytokines heralds progression and anti-inflammatory cytokines a spontaneous resolution. From this concept several serological parameters, such as soluble IL-2 receptor, gauging disease activity and being of prognostic value, have been delineated for both SAR and IBD[1,19,37].

GENETICS

Numerous reports on familial SAR, HLA-linkages, and divergent prevalence rates and clinical appearances in different races point to the existence of genes predisposing for SAR[38,39]. Recently, maps of markers that cover the entire human genome have enabled the chromosome localization of many genes that predispose to autoimmunity in humans and animal models (reviewed in ref.[40]). Many autoimmune or immune-related diseases cluster in families, and the degree of familial clustering of diseases can be estimated from the ratio between the risk of siblings suffering from a given disease and the population prevalence. If the sibling's risk is equal to the general prevalence familial clustering is not observed and the ratio (λ_s) is close to 1.0. When the siblings are at greater risk of developing a given disease λ_s exceeds 1.0. For the diseases in Table 1, λ_s is greatly elevated. This is true for non-granulomatous diseases and granulomatous diseases such as CD and primary biliary cirrhosis, which share some immunological features with SAR. The clustering of diseases in families is caused by genetic factors, environmental factors, or both. The λ_s for the major histocompatibility

Table 1 Population frequencies and familial clustering of human autoimmune and immune-related diseases

Disease	Population frequency (%)	Sibling risk (%)	λs	MHC λs	Reference
Psoriasis	2.8	17	6		78
Rheumatoid arthritis	1	8	8	1.6	79
Ulcerative colitis	0.1	1.2	12	8.3	80
Type 1 diabetes	0.4	6	15	2.4	81
Lupus (SLE)	0.1	2	20		82
Multiple sclerosis	0.1	2	20	2.4	81
Crohn's disease	0.06	1.2	20	1.3	80
Primary biliary cirrhosis	0.008	0.8	100		83
Sarcoidosis	0.04	0.3–0.8	8–20		*

Modified from ref. 40.
*Estimated range from the literature and unpublished observations.

complex (MHC) is available for some diseases. If the overall λ_s equalled the MHC λ_s this would imply that only one MHC gene accounts for the clustering. It is evident from Table 1 that, in all diseases where data are available, λ_s greatly exceeds MHC λ_s, implying that the linkage of the MHC region cannot entirely account for the clustering. In CD ($\lambda_s = 20$, MHC $\lambda_s = 1.3$) genome scans have identified a susceptibility locus outside the MHC on chromosome 16[41,42]. Interestingly, the gene of Blau syndrome (familial granulomatosis), an autosomal, dominantly Mendelian-inherited disease characterized by multiorgan inflammation with granulomatous arthritis, skin rash, and uveitis, has been mapped to the same region[43]. Estimating the λ_s of SAR, from the numbers available for Germany[44,45], yields a range from 8 to 20 and points very strongly to the existence of predisposing genes (Table 1).

The human leucocyte antigen (HLA) complex plays a pivotal role in the immune response by presenting antigen for T-cell recognition and defining the self-epitopes tolerated by the immune system. Distinct HLA class II alleles confer both predisposition and resistance to immune-related disorders. In primary biliary cirrhosis distinct haplotypes confer resistance and others are significantly increased in patients with the disease[46]. For SAR loose positive and negative HLA-linkages have been observed in numerous studies, but a clear-cut linkage disequilibrium with a distinct HLA class II allele has not been found[47,48]. A Scandinavian study identified an association of distinct sarcoid phenotypes with certain HLA class II alleles[49]. There is a vast number of highly polymorphic microsatellites (i.e. short tandem DNA motifs) throughout the genome that are widely used to label chromosomes. Using a strategy of genotyping with 225 microsatellites and multipoint linkage analysis in a panel of 63 families with affected siblings a whole genome search was carried out, and several chromosomal candidate regions of predisposition to SAR could be identified[50]. Seven chromosomal regions of increased allele sharing in the panel of 63 families suggest a multigenetic nature of SAR susceptibility. The most prominent peak of the non-parametric-linkage (NPL) analysis yielded a score of

2.99 and is consistent with numerous reports on associations between gene variants of the region of the MHC on chromosome 6 and the risk of SAR[50,51]. Some of the other NPL-score peaks are in the vicinity of genes of the cytokine network, e.g. chemokine receptor genes (chromosome 3), the gene for the γ-chain of the IL-2 receptor (chromosome 10), or the TGF-β receptor (chromosome 9).

Another major candidate region was the centromeric part of chromosome 16. A major susceptibility gene of CD[41,42] and the gene causing Blau syndrome[43] have been mapped to this region. Blau syndrome is a rare inherited granulomatous disorder with granulomatous skin disease, synovitis, uveitis, and in some cases visceral manifestations. It is caused by a single dominant gene mapped close to the centromere of chromosome 16 and starts in early childhood, thus suggesting it to be a monogenic early-onset variant of SAR.

SAR and CD cluster in close relatives in approximately 5% of affected families. Coincidence of CD and SAR in one family or even in one individual is more frequently observed than expected by chance alone[52]. Concomitant affection of skin, eyes, and joints is common in SAR and can also be found in CD, which results in some overlap with Blau syndrome. Thus, an analysis of whether a common genetic background defines the susceptibility to these disorders is warranted. Three independent groups have recently shown that distinct alleles of the intracellular lipopolysaccharide receptor gene CARD15 predispose to CD[41,42,53].

Presumably a main function of CARD15 is the activation of the nuclear regulatory factor (NF)-κB pathway in response to microbial lipopolysaccharides binding to cellular pattern-recognition receptors. High NF-κB activity is a consistent feature in CD[54] and SAR[55]. More recently, mutations of the same gene, i.e. CARD15, have been detected in families with Blau syndrome[56]. Interestingly, different CARD15 mutations associate with CD and Blau syndrome, respectively, suggesting that alterations of different elements of the gene cause or contribute to different granulomatous disorders.

The similarities in phenotypes of SAR, Blau syndrome, and CD suggest that an analysis of CARD15 gene variations in the named disorders will contribute to the understanding of granuloma formation. Therefore, we have genotyped a SAR population and a control group for the three main CD-associated CARD15 polymorphisms SNP8, SNP12, and SNP13. No significant differences of allele frequencies were detected between 138 SAR patients in comparison with controls (Schürmann M et al., manuscript in preparation). Detailed studies on the pathophysiology of Blau syndrome do not exist. The mutations causing Blau syndrome are located in the nucleotide-binding domain (NBD) of the CARD15 gene and the SNPs associated with CD are located in the leucin-rich repeat region (LRR) of the gene. In a cohort of familial SAR in none of the affected siblings could the reported Blau syndrome mutations be detected, excluding a major contribution of this mutation to the immunopathogenesis of SAR (Schürmann M et al., manuscript in preparation).

Therefore, mutations of the NBD and LRR gene regions seem to be linked to different diseases within the spectrum of granulomatous disorders. In conclusion, our results of association, transmission and sequence analysis rule out a major role of CARD15 mutations in the pathogenesis of SAR. These results are consistent with our data from a previous genome-wide scan to localize predisposing genes in SAR[51] by linkage to a panel of microsatellite DNA polymorphisms of known chromosomal position. The DNA locus D16S3396 of the marker set used in that study is located close to the CARD15 gene, with a distance of approximately 0.6×10^6 base pairs between the sites. There was no evidence ($p = 0.21$) that siblings suffering from SAR tend to be identical by descent for this region of chromosome 16, as would be expected in the case of a major contribution of CARD15 to the aetiology of SAR.

By linkage analysis Rybicki et al. ruled out an influence of the NBD gene region of the CARD15 gene for African American siblings affected with SAR[57]. This study, and the results reported above, demonstrate a lack of association between CARD15 polymorphisms and the risk of SAR. Thus, although SAR, CD, and Blau syndrome show a considerable overlap in phenotype and patho-mechanisms they depend on different genetic backgrounds, and the regulation of NF-κB levels in SAR seems to involve other pathways which possibly employ different pathogen-recognition receptors (Toll-like receptors). Toll-like receptor 4 (TLR4) expressed on the surface of alveolar macrophages is one candidate since its gene is located on chromosome 9 in the vicinity of the polymorphic DNA marker D9S934. At the genome-wide search for predisposing genes of SAR this marker showed an increased portion of shared parental alleles in siblings suffering from SAR ($p = 0.033$)[50]. Thus, in the complex pathogenesis of the discussed disorders common pathogenetic pathways – such as elevated NF-κB levels – initiated by still-elusive aetiological agents, are influenced by different genes and a common genetic background of granulomatous disorders might not exist. This notion is supported by the finding of a putative gene locus associated with early-onset CD on chromosome 5 in the vicinity of genes encoding a variety of cytokine receptors[58]. It is noteworthy that on chromosome 5 no elevated NPL scores were observed in our genome-wide search in SAR[50]. A future goal of these genetic studies is to generate individual genetic risk profiles for patients and non-affected family members to enable individualized treatment or early diagnosis.

TREATMENT

TNF-α release by alveolar macrophages and lamina propria macrophages is a crucial feature in the immunopathogenesis of both SAR and IBD. Moreover, in SAR exaggerated TNF-α release heralds disease progression and in recalcitrant disease TNF-α release is corticosteroid-resistant (Fig. 5)[59]. The therapeutic regimen demonstrated to suppress alveolar macrophage TNF-α release in corticosteroid-resistant SAR exhibited effectiveness in these problematic cases[60]. In CD disease activity can be gauged by serological markers of immune cell activation which indicate exaggerated cytokine release[61]. Azathioprine and methotrexate are effective in corticosteroid-dependent active SAR[60,62] or CD[63] and induce remissions. Interestingly, although cyclosporine acts on pivotal patho-mechanisms of SAR and CD[64], its use is not suggested, due to limited clinical effectiveness to induce or to maintain remission[63,65,66].

The availability of anti-TNF agents, e.g. the chimaeric IgG infliximab, has extended the therapeutic options for CD[67,68]. Infliximab's mode of action is incompletely understood since the sole binding of soluble TNF-α is not sufficient

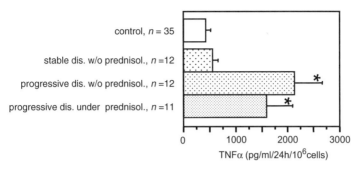

Fig. 5 Comparison of spontaneous alveolar macrophage TNF-α release in controls and patients with long-lasting, chronic sarcoidosis. TNF-α release was significantly higher in patients with progressive disease while not being on steroids and in those with a progressive disease under steroid therapy (corticosteroid-resistant disease) compared to controls (*$p < 0.05$). (Adapted from ref. 59)

to explain its effectiveness. TNF-α precursor expressed on the surface of macrophages and monocytes is thought to be bound by infliximab, and by its capability of complement fixation it might induce apoptosis of these TNF-α-producing cells[69,70]. Two studies demonstrated the effectiveness of infliximab in CD[67,68] and this mode of treatment is now used in routine practice.

In a preliminary study infliximab was used to treat three patients with progressive SAR despite treatment with corticosteroids and other immunosuppressive drugs. In these disparate cases, after a 16-week period of treatment, skin disease and lung function improved considerably without serious side-effects taking place[23]. A woman presenting with complex SAR, including severe protein-losing enteropathy, hypoalbuminaemia, and proximal myopathy, who had not responded sufficiently to corticosteroid therapy, was successfully treated with three courses of infliximab. However, the clinical course was complicated by the development of a hypercoagulable state associated with circulating anticardiolipin antibodies, which prompted discontinuation of infliximab therapy. This side-effect may possibly be caused by the manipulation of the cytokine network favouring a Th2 response with the development of autoantibodies[71].

Advances in the understanding of the immunopathophysiology of SAR and IBD, even if they are still incomplete, have led to much interest in the therapeutic manipulation of the cytokine network with established and new drugs. Pentoxifylline and thalidomide are drugs with anti-TNF-α effects which may be used alone or as corticosteroid-sparing drugs in a regimen. For both drugs some clinical effectiveness has been demonstrated for SAR and CD[22,72–77]. Cytokines and anticytokines shifting the immune response from Th1-cell domination to Th2-cell predominance are under investigation for restoration of the cytokine balance in CD. Among the tested agents are: IL-10, IL-11, anti-IL-12, anti-IFN-γ, and anti-integrins[63]. For SAR these studies are in their infancy.

The concept of the cytokine network is redundancy. Thus, it is surprising that the use of a single anticytokine such as infliximab is capable of inducing remissions, since other proinflammatory cytokines are supposed to substitute for the blocked effect. Whether the observed positive results are long-lasting, or maintenance therapy successful, remains to be established. A future combination therapy might increase effectiveness and reduce side-effects. It is reasonable to expect that genes conferring susceptibility to IBD and SAR will be identified. Unravelling the mechanisms through which they lead to inflammatory disorders will lead to more precise genetic-based diagnoses, including presymptomatic risk assesment in family members, and individualized treatment on the basis of genetic risk profiles.

CONCLUSION

Comparing SAR and IBD shows that the immunopathogenesis of these disorders employ common inflammatory effector mechanisms which are most likely initiated by the still-elusive aetiological agents of the named diseases. Although there are considerable overlaps of phenotypes and inflammatory mechanisms, differences in the genetic background defining the susceptibility of SAR and CD have been observed, which demonstrates that these disorders are independent entities and not different variants of a yet-unknown disease. Useful new therapies will be developed on the basis of the understanding of immuno-pathogenesis and genetic risk profiles.

References

1. Müller-Quernheim J. Sarcoidosis: immunopathogenetic concepts and their clinical application. Eur Respir J. 1998;12:716–38.
2. Mitchell D, Scadding J, Heard B, Hinson K. Sarcoidosis: histopathological definition and clinical diagnosis. J Clin Pathol. 1977;30:395–408.
3. Newman LS, Rose CS, Maier LA. Medical progress: sarcoidosis. N Engl J Med. 1997; 336: 1224–34.
4. Schultek T, Herbst EW, Otte M, Sack K. Epitheloidzellige Granulomatose des Peritoneums. Internist. 1986;27:331–5.
5. Gallwitz B, Janig U, Fölsch UR. Differentialdiagnose granulomatoser Erkrankungen–Epitheloidzellgranulome im Darm und in der Leber bei Morbus, Crohn. Z Gastroenterol. 1994; 32:252–5.
6. Vogelsang H, Granditsch G, Binder C et al. Konsensus der Arbeitsgruppe für chronisch-entzündliche Darmerkrankungen der, Oggh zum Thema Diagnostik und Therapie von chronisch-entzündlichen Darmerkrankungen im Adoleszenzalter. Z Gastroenterol. 2000;38:791–4.
7. Otto HF. Morbus Crohn: Morphologische Befunde zu extraintestinalen, Krankheitsmanifestationen. Z Gastroenterol. 1993;31:253–9.
8. Pierer M, Krause C, Hantzschel H. Extraintestinale Manifestationen chronisch-entzündlicher Darmerkrankungen. Z Gastroenterol. 2002;40(Suppl. 1):S92–4.
9. Mahadeva R, Walsh G, Flower CD, Shneerson JM. Clinical and radiological characteristics of lung disease in inflammatory bowel disease. Eur Respir J. 2000;15:41–8.
10. Bewig B, Manske I, Bottcher H, Bastian A, Nitsche R, Folsch UR. Crohn's disease mimicking sarcoidosis in bronchoalveolar lavage. Respiration. 1999;66:467–9.
11. Fellermann K, Stahl M, Dahlhoff K, Amthor M, Ludwig D, Stange EF. Crohn's disease and sarcoidosis: systemic granulomatosis? Eur J Gastroenterol Hepatol. 1997;9:1121–4.
12. Drent M, Jacobs JA, de Vries J, Lamers RJ, Liem IH, Wouters EF. Does the cellular bronchoalveolar lavage fluid profile reflect the severity of sarcoidosis? Eur Respir J. 1999; 13: 1338–44.
13. Lindberg E, Jarnerot G, Huitfeldt B. Smoking in Crohn's disease: effect on localisation and clinical course. Gut. 1992;33:779–82.
14. Lindberg E, Tysk C, Andersson K, Jarnerot G. Smoking and inflammatory bowel disease. A case control study. Gut. 1988;29:352–7.

15. Mullin GE, Lazenby AJ, Harris ML, Bayless TM, James SP. Increased interleukin-2 messenger RNA in the intestinal mucosal lesions of Crohn's disease but not ulcerative colitis. Gastroenterology. 1992;102:1620–7.
16. Ziegenhagen MW, Schrum S, Zissel G, Zipfel PF, Schlaak M, Müller-Quernheim J. Increased expression of proinflammatory chemokines in bronchoalveolar lavage cells of patients with progressing idiopathic pulmonary fibrosis and sarcoidosis. J Invest Med. 1998;46:223–31.
17. Sher ME, D'Angelo AJ, Stein TA, Bailey B, Burns G, Wise L. Cytokines in Crohn's colitis. Am J Surg. 1995;169:133–6.
18. Reinecker HC, Steffen M, Witthoeft T et al. Enhanced secretion of tumour necrosis factor-alpha, IL-6, and IL-1 beta by isolated lamina propria mononuclear cells from patients with ulcerative colitis and Crohn's disease. Clin Exp Immunol. 1993;94:174–81.
19. Ziegenhagen MW, Benner UK, Zissel G, Zabel P, Schlaak M, Müller-Quernheim J. Sarcoidosis: TNF-alpha release from alveolar macrophages and serum level of sIL-2R are prognostic markers. Am J Respir Crit Care Med. 1997;156:1586–92.
20. Vasiliauskas EA, Kam LY, Abreu-Martin MT et al. An open-label pilot study of low-dose thalidomide in chronically active, steroid-dependent Crohn's disease. Gastroenterology. 1999; 117:1278–87.
21. Ehrenpreis ED, Kane SV, Cohen LB, Cohen RD, Hanauer SB. Thalidomide therapy for patients with refractory Crohn's disease: an open-label trial. Gastroenterology. 1999;117:1271–7.
22. Carlesimo M, Giustini S, Rossi A, Bonaccorsi P, Calvieri S. Treatment of cutaneous and pulmonary sarcoidosis with thalidomide. J Am Acad Dermatol. 1995;32:866–9.
23. Baughman RP, Lower EE. Infliximab for refractory sarcoidosis. Sarcoidosis Vasc Diffuse Lung Dis. 2001;18:70–4.
24. Foley N, Lambert C, McNicol M, Johnson N, Rook GAW. An inhibitor of the toxicity of tumor necrosis factor in the serum of patients with sarcoidosis, tuberculosis and Crohn's disease. Clin Exp Immunol. 1990;80:395–9.
25. Ziegenhagen MW, Fitschen J, Martinet N, Schlaak M, Müller-Quernheim J. Serum level of soluble tumour necrosis factor receptor II (75 kDa) indicates inflammatory activity of sarcoidosis. J Intern Med. 2000;248:33–41.
26. Strober W, Kelsall B, Fuss I et al. Reciprocal IFN-gamma and TGF-beta responses regulate the occurrence of mucosal inflammation. Immunol Today. 1997;18:61–4.
27. de Waal Malefyt R, Haanen JBAG, Spits H et al. Interleukin 10 (IL-10) and viral IL-10 strongly reduce antigen-specific human T cell proliferation by diminishing the antigen-presenting capacity of monocytes via downregulation of class II major histocompatibility complex expression. J Exp Med. 1991;174:915–24.
28. Moller DR, Forman JD, Liu MC et al. Enhanced expression of IL-12 associated with Th1 cytokine profiles in active pulmonary sarcoidosis. J Immunol. 1996;156:4952–60.
29. Zissel G, Homolka J, Schlaak J, Schlaak M, Müller-Quernheim J. Anti-inflammatory cytokine release by alveolar macrophages in pulmonary sarcoidosis. Am J Respir Crit Care Med. 1996;154:713–19.
30. Marshall RP, McAnulty RJ, Laurent GJ. The pathogenesis of pulmonary fibrosis: is there a fibrosis gene? Int J Biochem Cell Biol. 1997;29:107–20.
31. Minshall EM, Tsicopoulos A, Yasruel Z et al. Cytokine mRNA gene expression in active and nonactive pulmonary sarcoidosis. Eur Respir J. 1997;10:2034–9.
32. Bansal AS, Bruce J, Hogan PG, Allen RK. An assessment of peripheral immunity in patients with sarcoidosis using measurements of serum vitamin D3, cytokines and soluble CD23. Clin Exp Immunol. 1997;110:92–7.
33. Muraközy G, Gaede KI, Zissel G, Schlaak M, Müller-Quernheim J. Analysis of gene polymorphisms in interleukin-10 and transforming growth factor-beta 1 in sarcoidosis. Sarcoidosis Vasc Diffuse Lung Dis. 2001;18:165–9.
34. van Deventer SJ, Elson CO, Fedorak RN. Multiple doses of intravenous interleukin 10 in steroid-refractory Crohn's disease. Crohn's Disease Study Group. Gastroenterology. 1997;113:383–9.
35. Wahl SM, McCartney-Francis N, Mergenhagen S. Inflammatory and immunoregulatory roles of TGF-β. Immunol Today. 1989;10:258–61.
36. Romagnani S. Th1 and Th2 in human diseases. Clin Immunol Immunopathol. 1996;80:225–35.
37. Van Kemseke C, Belaiche J, Louis E. Frequently relapsing Crohn's disease is characterized by persistent elevation in interleukin-6 and soluble interleukin-2 receptor serum levels during remission. Int J Colorectal Dis. 2000;15:206–10.

38. Rybicki BA, Maliarik MJ, Major M, Popovich J Jr, Iannuzzi MC. Epidemiology, demographics, and genetics of sarcoidosis. Semin Respir Infect. 1998;13:166–73.
39. Martinetti M, Tinelli C, Kolek V *et al.* 'The sarcoidosis map': a joint survey of clinical and immunogenetic findings in two European countries. Am J Respir Crit Care Med. 1995; 152:557–64.
40. Vyse TJ, Todd JA. Genetic analysis of autoimmune disease. Cell. 1996;85:311–18.
41. Hugot JP, Laurent P, Gower-Rousseau C *et al.* Mapping of a susceptibility locus for Crohn's disease on chromosome 16. Nature. 1997;379:821–3.
42. Hampe J, Grebe J, Nikolaus S *et al.* Association of NOD2 (CARD 15) genotype with clinical course of Crohn's disease: a cohort study. Lancet. 2002;359:1661–5.
43. Tromp G, Kuivaniemi H, Raphael S *et al.* Genetic linkage of familial granulomatous inflammatory arthritis, skin rash, and uveitis to chromosome 16. Am J Hum Genet. 1996;59:1097–107.
44. Jörgensen G. Die Genetik der Sarkoidose. Acta Med Scand. 1964;425(Suppl.):209–12.
45. Kirsten D. Sarkoidose in Deutschland. Pneumologie. 1995;49:378–82.
46. Begovich AB, Klitz W, Moonsamy PV, Van de Water J, Peltz G, Gershwin ME. Genes within the HLA class II region confer both predisposition and resistance to primary biliary cirrhosis. Tissue Antigens. 1994;43:71–7.
47. Odum N, Milman N, Jakobsen BK, Georgsen J, Svejgaard A. HLA class II (DR, DQ, DP) in patients with sarcoidosis: evidence of an increased frequency of DRw6. Exp Clin Immunogenet. 1991;8:227–32.
48. Lenhart K, Kolek V, Bartova A. HLA antigens associated with sarcoidosis. Dis Markers. 1990; 8:23–9.
49. Berlin M, Fogdell-Hahn A, Olerup O, Eklund A, Grunewald J. HLA-DR predicts the prognosis in Scandinavian patients with pulmonary sarcoidosis. Am J Respir Crit Care Med. 1997; 156: 1601–5.
50. Schürmann M, Reichel P, Müller-Myhsok B, Schlaak M, Müller-Quernheim J, Schwinger E. Results from a genome-wide search for predisposing genes in sarcoidosis. Am J Respir Crit Care Med. 2001;164:840–6.
51. Schürmann M, Reichel P, Müller-Myhsok B *et al.* Angiotensin-converting enzyme (ACE) gene polymorphisms and familial occurrence of sarcoidosis. J Intern Med. 2001;249:77–83.
52. Wirnsberger RM, de Vries J, Wouters EF, Drent M. Clinical presentation of sarcoidosis in The Netherlands: an epidemiological study. Neth J Med. 1998;53:53–60.
53. Ogura Y, Bonen DK, Inohara N *et al.* A frameshift mutation in NOD2 associated with susceptibility to Crohn's disease. Nature. 2001;411:603–6.
54. Schreiber S, Nikolaus S, Hampe J. Activation of nuclear factor kappa B inflammatory bowel disease. Gut. 1998;42:477–84.
55. Drent M, van den Berg R, Haenen GR, van den Berg H, Wouters EF, Bast A. NF-kappaB activation in sarcoidosis. Sarcoidosis Vasc Diffuse Lung Dis. 2001;18:50–6.
56. Miceli-Richard C, Lesage S, Rybojad M *et al.* CARD15 mutations in Blau syndrome. Nat Genet. 2001;29:19–20.
57. Rybicki BA, Maliarik MJ, Bock CH *et al.* The Blau syndrome gene is not a major risk factor for sarcoidosis. Sarcoidosis Vasc Diffuse Lung Dis. 1999;16:203–8.
58. Rioux JD, Daly MJ, Silverberg MS *et al.* Genetic variation in the 5q31 cytokine gene cluster confers susceptibility to Crohn's disease. Nat Genet. 2001;29:223–8.
59. Ziegenhagen M, Rothe M, Zissel G, Müller-Quernheim J. Exaggerated TNF-alpha release of alveolar macrophages in corticosteroid resistant sarcoidosis. Sarcoidosis Vasc Diffuse Lung Dis. 2002 (In press).
60. Müller-Quernheim J, Kienast K, Held M, Pfeifer S, Costabel U. Treatment of chronic sarcoidosis with an azathioprine/prednisolone regimen. Eur Respir J. 1999;14:1117–22.
61. Louis E, Belaiche J, van Kemseke C *et al.* A high serum concentration of interleukin-6 is predictive of relapse in quiescent Crohn's disease. Eur J Gastroenterol Hepatol. 1997;9:939–44.
62. Lower EE, Baughman RP. Prolonged use of methotrexate for sarcoidosis. Arch Intern Med. 1995;155:846–51.
63. Podolsky DK. Inflammatory bowel disease. N Engl J Med. 2002;347:417–29.
64. Martinet Y, Pinkston P, Saltini C, Spurzem J, Müller-Quernheim J, Crystal RG. Evaluation of the *in vitro* and *in vivo* effects of cyclosporine on the T-lymphocyte alveolitis of active pulmonary sarcoidosis. Am Rev Respir Dis. 1988;138:1242–8.

65. Rebuck A, Sander B, MacFadden D, Man S, Cohen R. Cyclosporin in pulmonary sarcoidosis. Lancet. 1987;1:1486.

66. Wyser CP, van Schalkwyk EM, Alheit B, Bardin PG, Joubert JR. Treatment of progressive pulmonary sarcoidosis with cyclosporin A. A randomized controlled trial. Am J Respir Crit Care Med. 1997;156:1371–6.

67. Targan SR, Hanauer SB, van Deventer SJ et al. A short-term study of chimeric monoclonal antibody cA2 to tumor necrosis factor alpha for Crohn's disease. Crohn's Disease cA2 Study Group. N Engl J Med. 1997;337:1029–35.

68. Present DH, Rutgeerts P, Targan S et al. Infliximab for the treatment of fistulas in patients with Crohn's disease. N Engl J Med. 1999;340:1398–405.

69. ten Hove T, van Montfrans C, Peppelenbosch MP, van Deventer SJ. Infliximab treatment induces apoptosis of lamina propria T lymphocytes in Crohn's disease. Gut. 2002;50:206–11.

70. Lugering A, Schmidt M, Lugering N, Pauels HG, Domschke W, Kucharzik T. Infliximab induces apoptosis in monocytes from patients with chronic active Crohn's disease by using a caspase-dependent pathway. Gastroenterology. 2001;121:1145–57.

71. Yee AM, Pochapin MB. Treatment of complicated sarcoidosis with infliximab anti-tumor necrosis factor-alpha therapy. Ann Intern Med. 2001;135:27–31.

72. Wettstein AR, Meagher AP. Thalidomide in Crohn's disease. Lancet. 1997;350:1445–6.

73. Moller DR, Wysocka M, Greenlee BM et al. Inhibition of IL-12 production by thalidomide. J Immunol. 1997;159:5157–61.

74. Wolkenstein P, Latarjet J, Roujeau JC et al. Randomised comparison of thalidomide versus placebo in toxic epidermal necrolysis. Lancet. 1998;352:1586–9.

75. MacDonald TT. Oxpentifylline, tumour necrosis factor-alpha and Crohn's disease. Gut. 1997;40:559.

76. Zabel P, Entzian P, Dalhoff K, Schlaak M. Pentoxifylline in treatment of sarcoidosis. Am J Respir Crit Care Med. 1997;155:1665–9.

77. Oliver SJ, Kikuchi T, Krueger JG, Kaplan G. Thalidomide induces granuloma differentiation in sarcoid skin lesions associated with disease improvement. Clin Immunol. 2002;102:225–36.

78. Elder JT, Nair RP, Guo SW, Henseler T, Christophers E, Voorhees JJ. The genetics of psoriasis. Arch Dermatol. 1994;130:216–24.

79. Wordsworth P. Genes and arthritis. Br Med Bull. 1995;51:249–66.

80. Satsangi J, Welsh KI, Bunce M et al. Contribution of genes of the major histocompatibility complex to susceptibility and disease phenotype in inflammatory bowel disease. Lancet. 1996;347:1212–17.

81. Risch N. Assessing the role of HLA-linked and unlinked determinants of disease. Am J Hum Genet. 1987;40:1–14.

82. Hochberg MC. The application of genetic epidemiology to systemic lupus erythematosus. J Rheumatol. 1987;14:867–9.

83. Gregory WL, Bassendine MF. Genetic factors in primary biliary cirrhosis. J Hepatol. 1994; 20: 689–92.

12

A functional genomics approach to study wound repair: the roles of activin and S100A8/S100A9 in the healing process

I. S. THOREY, M. WANKELL, A. GOPPELT and S. WERNER

INTRODUCTION

Injury to the skin initiates a series of biological events directed at the reconstruction of the damaged area. Among them are the migration, proliferation, and differentiation of various cell types; the production and deposition of extracellular matrix; as well as the removal of irreversibly destroyed tissue[1]. These processes are well described at the histological level, but the underlying molecular mechanisms have been poorly defined. A series of studies from us and from others have revealed that most genes, which are up- or down-regulated after injury, are of functional importance for the wound healing process. These genes encode, for example, various growth factors, cytokines and their receptors, extracellular matrix proteins, transcription factors, enzymes and also structural proteins. Based on this observation we attempted to identify novel genes involved in the healing response. For this purpose we performed differential display reverse transcriptase polymerase chain reaction and subtractive hybridization to compare the gene expression profile between non-wounded and wounded mouse skin[2–4]. To minimize the risk of detecting differences in gene expression levels that are based on changes in the cellular composition rather than on transcriptional regulation, we compared normal skin with early (24 h) wounds, since only a few changes in cell type composition occur during this initial healing period.

Here we report on the expression and function of two wound-regulated genes, which encode the growth and differentiation factor activin and the Ca^{2+}-binding protein S100A8, respectively.

ACTIVIN

Activins are members of the transforming growth factor β (TGF-β) family of growth and differentiation factors. In mammals this family also includes, for example, three types of TGF-β (TGF-β1, β2 and β3), various bone morpho-genetic proteins (BMPs), Mullerian inhibiting substance, and the inhibins[5]. Like most other TGF-β family members, activins are dimeric proteins, the monomeric polypeptides of which are connected by disulphide linkage. Three different forms of activin, the homodimeric activin A (βAβA) and activin B (βBβB), as well as the heterodimeric activin AB (βAβB) have been described[5]. βC, βD, and βE chains have also been discovered, but little is as yet known about the corresponding proteins. Activins exert their biological functions by binding to heteromeric receptor complexes consisting of a type I (ActRIA and ActRIB) and a type II receptor (ActRII and ActRIIB), which are all characterized by the presence of an intracellular serine/threonine kinase domain[6]. Besides these transmembrane receptors, soluble activin-binding proteins, follistatins, have been discovered, which bind to activins and thereby inhibit their biological effects[7].

Recent studies from our laboratory revealed a novel role of activin in skin wound healing. In a first set of experiments we determined the expression of activins and their receptors in normal and wounded mouse skin. Interestingly, expression levels of both the activin βA and βB chains were very low in normal skin. However, we found a strong induction of activin βA and βB expression in the granulation tissue and in suprabasal keratinocytes of the hyperproliferative wound epithelium after skin injury (Fig. 1). In addition to the ligands, all known activin receptors were expressed in normal and wounded skin, although their expression was not induced after injury[8]. A similar expression pattern of activin and its receptors was also observed in human wounds (Werner S, unpublished; Fig. 1, right panel).

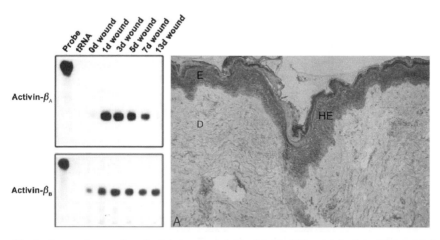

Fig. 1 Increased expression of activin in wounded skin. A total of 20 μg total cellular RNA isolated from normal and wounded back skin of BALB/c mice was analysed by RNase protection assay for the expression of activin βA and βB; 1000 cpm of the hybridization probes were loaded in the lanes labeled 'probe' and used as size markers; 20 μg tRNA was used as a negative control. The time after injury is indicated on top of the autoradiograms. A frozen section from a 4-day-old human incisional wound was stained with an antibody directed against activin. D: Dermis, E: epidermis, HE: hyper-proliferative wound epithelium

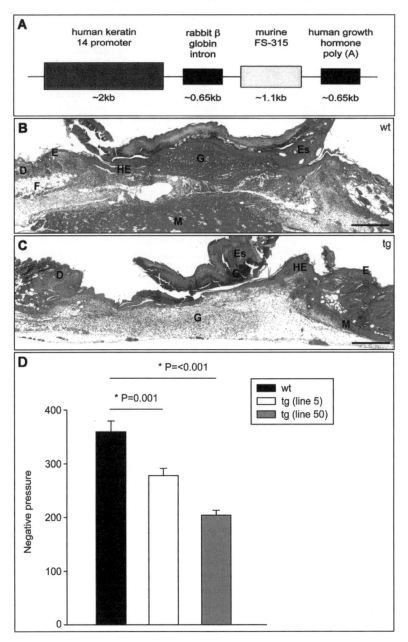

Fig. 2 Impaired wound healing in transgenic mice overexpressing the activin antagonist follistatin in the epidermis. The construct used for the generation of transgenic mice is shown in (**A**). Functional elements include the human K14 promoter, the rabbit β-globin intron, the murine follistatin cDNA, and the human growth hormone poly-A. **B, C**: Full-thickness excisional wounds were made on the back of transgenic mice (tg) and control littermates (wt). Paraformaldehyde-fixed paraffin sections from the middle of 5-day wounds were stained by the Masson trichrome procedure.

To determine the activities of activin in the skin we generated transgenic mice overexpressing the activin βA chain in the basal keratinocytes of the epidermis as well as in hair follicle keratinocytes under the control of a keratin 14 promoter[9]. The transgenic mice were characterized by remarkable abnormalities in the skin. The thickness of the epidermis was greatly increased, due to an increased proliferation rate of the basal keratinocytes and abnormalities in keratinocyte differentiation. The morphological abnormalities of the epidermis were similar to those seen in hyperproliferative human skin disease, e.g. in psoriasis, although no signs of inflammation were observed in our transgenic animals. Surprisingly, we also observed fibrosis in the dermis where the transgene is not expressed, most likely due to diffusion of activin from the basal keratinocytes to the underlying connective tissue[9].

The most striking result of our study was the strongly enhanced healing rate of full-thickness excisional skin wounds in the activin-overexpressing mice. In particular, the process of granulation tissue formation was enhanced[9]. Although the enhancement of wound healing appears beneficial, first analyses of late wounds revealed a strongly extended area of the scar tissue, indicating that the increased levels of activin in the healing wound induce connective tissue deposition and subsequent scarring (our unpublished data). Taken together, the results obtained with the activin-overexpressing mice revealed novel activities of this factor in the regulation of keratinocyte proliferation and differentiation, as well as in dermal fibrosis and wound healing. However, the roles of endogenous activin in these processes remained to be determined.

To address this question we attempted to block the endogenous activin in the skin. Since activin βA knockout mice die within the first day after birth from multiple abnormalities[10], it was not possible to analyse the wound healing process in these mice. Furthermore, a tissue-specific deletion of the activin βA gene in the skin was not suitable for the analysis of activin function in the wound, because activin is expressed by different cell types in the wound, which as yet cannot be targeted by suitable promoters. Therefore, we generated transgenic mice overexpressing the activin antagonist follistatin in the epidermis and in hair follicle keratinocytes[11] (Fig. 2A). Since follistatin is a secreted, soluble protein, it is likely to diffuse from the basal keratinocytes and hair follicles to the interfollicular dermis and to the granulation tissue of wounded skin.

Transgenic mice that express high levels of follistatin were smaller than their control littermates, but they were viable and fertile. In the skin a minor thinning of both the dermis and the epidermis was observed, and the dermal matrix was less dense. In contrast to the activin-overexpressing mice, however, no obvious abnormalities in keratinocyte proliferation or differentiation were found.

D, dermis; Es, eschar; F, fatty tissue; G, granulation tissue; HE, hyperproliferative epithelium; HF, hair follicle; M, muscle (panniculus carnosus). Bar indicates 500 μm. **D**: Tensile strength of full-thickness incisional wounds in follistatin transgenic (high-expressing line = line 50, $n = 9$; low-expressing line = line 5, $n = 5$) and wild-type mice ($n = 7$) was measured on day 5 after wounding according to the manufacturer's protocol for the non-human disruptive linear incision analysis. *In-situ* wound strength was measured as maximum amount of negative pressure (mmHg) required for failure. Bars represent mean values ± SEM within each group of animals; p-values are derived from Student's *t* test. (Reprinted with permission from ref. 11; copyright Oxford University Press, UK)

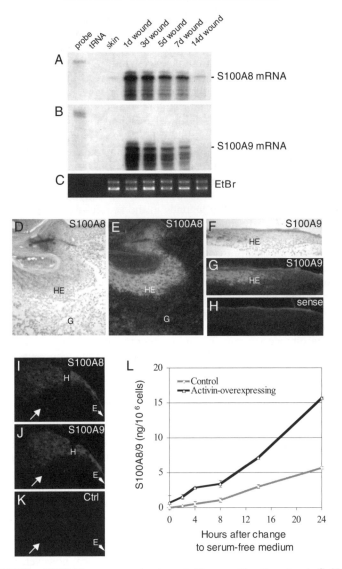

Fig. 3 S100A8 and S100A9 are expressed and secreted by wound keratinocytes. **A–C**: 20 μg RNA aliquots prepared from murine skin wounds at different times after injury were analysed by RNase protection for the expression of S100A8 (panel **A**) or S100A9 (panel **B**); 1 μg RNA aliquots were separated on an agarose gel and stained with ethidium bromide (panel **C**). 1000 cpm of the hybridization probes were used as a standard for size and intensity of signal, 20 μg of tRNA was used as a negative control. Panels **D–H**: 6 μm frozen sections of murine 5-day-old full-thickness excisional wounds were hybridized to ^{35}S-labelled antisense probes, which recognized coding sequences of murine S100A8 (panels **D, E**) or murine S100A9 (panels **F, G**), or to a murine S100A9 probe transcribed in the sense direction (panel **H**). Sections were exposed for 3 weeks, counter-stained with Mayer's haemalum and eosin, and viewed at a magnification of ×200. Specific hybridization is indicated by dark grains in the bright field views (panels **D, F**) and by bright grains in the dark field views (panels **E, G, H**). G, granulation tissue; HE, hyperproliferative epithelium

However, a remarkable phenotype was observed after injury to these mice. Thus the animals had a thinner hyperproliferative wound epithelium, and a strongly reduced granulation tissue was found at day 5 after injury (Fig. 2B and C). These histological abnormalities correlated with a reduced wound breaking strength, demonstrating that the overexpression of follistatin results in functional deficits[11] (Fig. 2D).

Analysis of late wounds in these animals revealed that the area of scar tissue was reduced and the epidermis had returned to the normal thickness of unwounded skin. These results suggest that the levels of bioactive activin in a wound determine not only the speed of the repair process, but also the quality of healing. Therefore, modification of the levels of bioactive activin could be therapeutically explored for the treatment of wound healing disorders. Thus, overexpression of activin or inhibition of follistatin might be useful to enhance the speed of healing, whereas inhibition of activin action could be used for the prevention of scarring in patients suffering from hypertrophic scars and keloids or other types of fibrotic disease.

Besides its role in skin wound healing, recent studies from us and from others have provided evidence for a general role of activin in tissue repair. For example, activin was shown to enhance fracture healing in the rat fibula fracture model[12]. By contrast, it inhibited tubular regeneration after renal ischaemia in rats[13], indicating that activin affects healing processes in a tissue-specific manner. Most interestingly, several results suggest a role of activin in various types of inflammatory disease, since it is overexpressed in lung fibrosis, liver cirrhosis, inflammatory bowel disease, atherosclerosis, and inflammatory arthropathies[14]. Finally, we recently demonstrated a novel role of activin in neuroprotection after lesion to the central nervous system[15], suggesting that the development of substances that influence activin expression or receptor binding might offer new strategies to fight neuronal loss in stroke and brain trauma.

S100A8 AND S100A9

S100A8 (also called calgranulin A, MRP8, leukocyte protein L1 or cytokine CP10) and its dimerization partner S100A9 (MRP14) are members of the S100 protein family. These proteins bind Ca^{2+} with high affinity and mediate various

Panels I–K: Serial paraffin sections of 5-day-old murine wounds were stained with specific polyclonal antisera directed against S100A8 (panel I) or S100A9 (panel J), followed by Cy-3-conjugated anti-rabbit IgG. In panel K the specific first antibody was omitted. Shown is a view of the hyperproliferative epithelial tongue at the wound edge at original $\times$ 250 magnification. H, position of a hair shaft; E with an arrow, direction towards normal epidermis. The arrows indicate the position of the basal keratinocyte layer. Panel L: Aliquots of cell culture supernatant were taken from duplicate confluent plates of activin-overexpressing HaCaT human keratinocytes and cells transfected with a vector containing only the neomycin resistance gene (control) at different time points after switching to serum-free medium. The content of S100A8/9 was measured by a sandwich enzyme-linked immunosorbent assay for S100A9[27]. The absolute values were determined by interpolating a standard curve prepared with defined concentrations of the purified human S100A8/9 complex. Numbers were normalized to 10^6 cells and plotted against time. (Reprinted with permission from ref. 3; copyright American Society for Biochemistry and Molecular Biology)

Ca^{2+}-dependent cellular functions such as cell growth and differentiation, energy metabolism and cytoskeletal–membrane interactions. Some S100 proteins, including S100A8/S100A9, can also be secreted by certain cell types and exert extracellular functions[16,17]. S100A8 and S100A9 are constitutively expressed by neutrophils and monocytes. Their expression is hardly detectable in normal murine and human skin, but a strong up-regulation was observed in the epidermis and also in other tissues at sites of inflammation, e.g. in psoriatic skin and in inflammatory bowel disease[18].

Having identified the gene encoding S100A8 in a subtractive hybridization experiment, we first confirmed the differential expression of S100A8 and its dimerization partner S100A9 in normal and wounded skin of Balb/c mice. A strong increase in the levels of S100A8 and S100A9 mRNAs and proteins was observed within 1 day after skin injury. Expression remained high during the first 7 days after wounding and declined to basal levels after the wounds were fully healed (14 days after injury; Fig. 3A–C). In-situ hybridization and immunohistochemistry with mouse wounds revealed that inflammatory cells of the granulation tissue, and in particular suprabasal keratinocytes of the hyperproliferative wound epidermis, are the major producers of S100A8/S100A9 (Fig. 3D–K). A similar expression pattern was also seen in acute and chronic human wounds[3]. The increased expression of these proteins in wound keratinocytes is most likely a result of the activated state of the keratinocytes and not secondary to the presence of an inflammatory infiltrate in the skin, since we also found up-regulation of S100A8 and S100A9 in the non-wounded, non-inflamed hyperthickened epidermis of activin-overexpressing mice (see above)[3].

As a next step we determined whether S100A8/S100A9 is only present intracellularly in keratinocytes or whether it can also be secreted and exert extracellular functions. Therefore, we determined the concentrations of the S100A8/S100A9 dimer in cell lysates and in conditioned medium of HaCaT keratinocytes using a quantitative sandwich immunosorbent assay. Interestingly, we found that the S100A8/S100A9 dimer is secreted at substantial levels by the HaCaT cells, since the amount accumulating within 24 h in the culture supernatant corresponds to 35–40% of the intracellular content of an equal number of the cells at the beginning of the experiment[3] (Fig. 3L). This finding suggests that S100A8/S100A9 might also be secreted by wound keratinocytes, and the staining pattern observed by immunofluorescence of wound epidermis supports this hypothesis. Furthermore, we recently detected S100A8/S100A9 in human wound fluid (Goppelt A, unpublished data).

The role of S100A8/S100A9 in the wound repair process is as yet unknown. However, S100A8/S100A9 is likely to exert intracellular functions in keratinocytes such as modulation of cytoskeletal reconstruction upon differentiation of wound keratinocytes. The latter hypothesis is supported by the observed binding of S100A8/S100A9 to keratin filaments in squamous carcinoma cells[19] and by the fact that other S100 proteins, S100A and S100B, are capable of inhibiting the polymerization of glial intermediate filaments by binding to the subunit glial fibrillary acid protein[20]. In addition, there are possible extracellular functions. First, S100A8/S100A9 was shown to have antimicrobial activity[21], suggesting that these proteins could control microbial infection at the wound site. In addition, murine S100A8 was shown to act as a potent chemoattractant for myeloid cells[22], indicating a role of this protein in inflammation *in vivo*. The moiety performing this function is a non-covalent homodimer of two S100A8 molecules. The latter is oxidized to a non-functional disulphide-linked homodimer by hypochlorite under conditions similar to those prevailing in an inflamed tissue. This process may not only limit leukocyte recruitment to the site of inflammation, but may also protect cells from excessive oxidative damage by neutralizing reactive oxygen species[23]. Analysis of mice lacking S100A8 and/or S100A9 in keratinocytes, as well as overexpression of these proteins at the wound site, will help to clarify the role of S100A8/S100A9 in the healing response.

Taken together, our results demonstrate that the identification of genes that are regulated by skin injury is a powerful strategy for the identification of novel players involved in cutaneous wound repair. Most interestingly, these genes are likely to play similar roles in repair processes of other organs, as demonstrated for example by the overexpression of both activin and S100A8/S100A9 in inflammatory bowel disease[24-26]. Thus, this approach will help to identify the key regulators of repair in a wide range of tissues and organs. These genes are likely to be useful targets for the development of therapeutics for the treatment of healing impairments.

Acknowledgements

The work described in this chapter was supported by the ETH Zürich (to S.W.), the Swiss National Science Foundation (to S.W.), the German Ministry for Education and Research (BMBF, to S.W.) and by a Boehringer Ingelheim pre-doctoral fellowship (to M.W.).

References

1. Martin P. Wound healing – aiming for perfect skin regeneration. Science. 1997;276:75–81.
2. Munz B, Wiedmann M, Lochmüller H, Werner S. Cloning of novel injury-regulated genes. Implications for an important role of the muscle-specific protein skNAC in wound repair. J Biol Chem. 1999;274:13305–10.
3. Thorey JS, Roth J, Regenbogen J et al. The Ca^{2+}-binding proteins S100A8 and S100A9 are encoded by novel injury-regulated genes. J Biol Chem. 2001;276:35818–25.
4. Kaesler S, Regenbogen J, Durka S, Goppelt A, Werner S. The healing skin wound: a novel site of action of the chemokine C10. Cytokine. 2002;17:157–63.
5. Massague J. The transforming growth factor-β family. Annu Rev Cell Biochem. 1990;6: 597–641.
6. Mathews LS, Vale WW. Molecular and functional characterization of activin receptors. Receptor. 1993;3:173–81.
7. Sugino H, Sugino K, Hashimoto O, Shoji H, Nakamura T. Follistatin and its role as an activin-binding protein. J Med Invest. 1997;44:1–14.
8. Hübner G, Hu Q, Smola H, Werner S. Strong induction of activin expression after injury suggests an important role of activin in wound repair. Dev Biol. 1996;173:490–8.
9. Munz B, Smola H, Engelhardt F et al. Overexpression of activin in the epidermis of transgenic mice reveals new activities of activin in keratinocyte differentiation, cutaneous fibrosis and wound repair. EMBO J. 1999;18:5205–15.
10. Matzuk MM, Kumar TR, Vassalli A et al. Functional analysis of activins during mammalian development. Nature. 1995;374:354–6.
11. Wankell M, Munz B, Hübner G et al. Impaired wound healing in transgenic mice overexpressing the activin antagonist follistatin in the epidermis. EMBO J. 2001;19:5361–72.
12. Sakai R, Miwa M, Eto Y. Local administration of activin promotes fracture healing in the rat fibula fracture model. Bone. 1999;25:191–6.

13. Maeshima A, Zhang YQ, Nojima Y, Naruse T, Kojima, I. Involvement of the activin–follistatin system in tubular regeneration after renal ischemia in rats. J Am Soc Nephrol. 2001;12:1685–95.
14. Munz B, Hübner G, Tretter Y, Alzheimer C, Werner S. A novel role of activin in inflammation and repair. J Endocrinol. 1999;161:187–93.
15. Tretter YP, Hertel M, Munz B, ten Bruggencate G, Werner S, Alzheimer C. Induction of activin A is essential for the neuroprotective action of basic fibroblast growth factor *in vivo*. Nature Med. 2000;6:812–15.
16. Donato R. S100: a multigene family of calcium-modulated proteins of the EF-hand type with intracellular and extracellular functional roles. Int J Biochem Cell Biol. 2001;33:637–68.
17. Heizmann CW, Fritz G, Schafer BW. S100 proteins: structure, functions and pathology. Front Biosci. 2002;7:1356–68.
18. Passey RJ, Xu K, Hume DA, Geczy CL. S100A8: emerging functions and regulation. J Leukoc Biol. 1999;66:549–56.
19. Goebeler M, Roth J, van den Bos C, Ader G, Sorg C. Increase of calcium levels in epithelial cells induces translocation of calcium-binding proteins, migration inhibitory factor-related protein 8 (MRP8) and MRP14 to keratin intermediate filaments. Biochem J. 1995;309:419–24.
20. Garbuglia M, Verzini M, Sorci G *et al*. The calcium-modulated proteins, S100A1 and S100B, as potential regulators of the dynamics of type III intermediate filaments. Braz J Med Biol Res. 1999;32:1177–85.
21. Brandtzaeg P, Gabrielsen TO, Dale I, Muller F, Steinbakk M, Fagerhol MK. The leucocyte protein L1 (calprotectin): a putative nonspecific defence factor at epithelial surfaces. Adv Exp Med Biol. 1995;371A:201–6.
22. Lackmann M, Rajasekariah P, Iismaa SE *et al*. Identification of a chemotactic domain of the pro-inflammatory S100 protein CP-10. J Immunol. 1993;150:2981–91.
23. Harrison CA, Raftery MJ, Walsh J *et al*. Oxidation regulates the inflammatory properties of the murine S100 protein S100A8. J Biol Chem. 1999;274:8561–9.
24. Hubner G, Brauchle M, Gregor M, Werner S. Activin A: a novel player and inflammatory marker in inflammatory bowel disease? Lab Invest. 1997;77:311–18.
25. Schmid KW, Lugering N, Stoll R *et al*. Immunohistochemical demonstration of the calcium-binding proteins MRP8 and MRP14 and their heterodimer (27E10 antigen) in Crohn's disease. Hum Pathol. 1995;26:334–7.
26. Lugering N, Stoll R, Kucharzik T *et al*. Immunohistochemical distribution and serum levels of the Ca(2+)-binding proteins MRP8, MRP14 and their heterodimeric form MRP8/14 in Crohn's disease. Digestion. 1995;56:406–14.
27. Frosch M, Strey A, Vogl T *et al*. Myeloid-related proteins 8 and 14 are specifically secreted during interaction of phagocytes and activated endothelium and are useful markers for monitoring disease activity in pauciarticular-onset juvenile rheumatoid arthritis. Arthritis Rheum. 2000;43:628–37.

13
Neuroendocrine–immune interactions – a novel therapeutic approach in inflammatory bowel disease?

S. M. COLLINS

OVERVIEW

The notion that there is significant interaction between the neuroendocrine and immune systems is not new. Initially, ulcerative colitis was considered a psychosomatic disease and early studies focused on the role of behaviour and stress in the generation of this condition. Animal studies also supported this view. In a study by Lium, stimulation of motor activity by cholinergic nerves produced a clinical and histopathological response identical to colitis in dogs[1]. This was not due to ischaemia secondary to increased motor activity, as when the authors infused vasopressin, no colitis was produced.

Early studies used surgical denervation of the colon to treat refractory ulcerative colitis and even used truncal vagotomy in a similar manner[2]. However, the notion that the neuroendocrine system might influence disease activity in IBD lost its popularity for several decades. Interest was resurrected when receptors for neuropeptides were demonstrated on a variety of immune cells including mast cells and lymphocytes[3,4] Crohn's disease[5,6]. Interestingly, these receptors were clustered in lymphoid tissue and on blood vessels. A more recent observation supporting the neuromodulation of inflammation comes from a case report in which a patient with neuralgic pain in the upper limb was treated by stimulation of the dorsal horn of the spinal cord in an attempt to override painful sensation[7]. At the time this treatment was introduced, the patient was in remission from ulcerative colitis but it was found that the use of electrical stimulation was accompanied by relapse of the colitis. This provides a direct demonstration of the ability of the nervous system to influence the natural history of IBD. It remains to be seen whether this can be therapeutically exploited to manage IBD. Several observations from animal as well as human work suggest that this may be possible, although the data also provide a reason for caution in the development of such a strategy.

BASIC SCIENTIFIC OBSERVATIONS

A broad literature provides evidence that there are directional communications between the neuroendocrine and immune systems in the gut. Much of this work focused initially on nerve–mast cell interactions. Receptors for several neuropeptides were discovered on the surface of mast cells and simulation of these receptors induced mast cell degranulation. In addition, nerves have been found in close juxtaposition with mucosal mast cells in models of inflammation, providing an anatomical correlate of these functional studies. A more intriguing finding has been the observation that low concentrations of substance P reduced the threshold for mast cell degranulation; this provides a more plausible scenario by which nerves might modulate inflammatory responses. Subsequent work has been expanded to other cell types including lymphocytes, which possess receptors for a variety of neuropeptides including vasoactive intestinal peptide (VIP) and substance P. As already mentioned, increased substance P binding sites have been demonstrated in patients with Crohn's disease, implying a neuroimmune component to the pathophysiology of IBD.

The mechanism by which a sensory neuropeptide such as substance P modulates immune function is unclear. The concept of 'neurogenic inflammation' has been invoked in this context. Neurogenic inflammation was first described in the skin and airways where stimulation of sensory nerves results in the antidromal release of tachykinins such as substance P[8,9]. Tachykinins and bradykinins cause extravasation of plasma and leucocytes from postcapillary venules and enhance the inflammatory response. It is proposed that in pathological conditions, such as asthma[9], tissue damage results in the release of mediators that stimulate sensory nerves; hence the antidromal release of proinflammatory neuropeptides such as substance P.

Recent work has demonstrated neurogenic inflammation in the murine intestine[10]. Support for the involvement of this process during inflammatory conditions arises from studies showing that antagonists to substance P ameliorate inflammation, and from studies in which the bioavailability of substance P is altered. In the latter studies it has been shown that the main degrading enzyme for substance P, namely neutral endopeptidase, is down-regulated during inflammation, resulting in markedly increased bioavailability of the peptide[11]. Furthermore, in animals with a genetic deficiency of neutral endopeptidase (NEP), inflammation is more severe and prolonged compared to that in animals with normal NEP activity[12]. Taken together, these observations support a proinflammatory role for substance P in intestinal inflammation and predict that substance P antagonists might be beneficial in reducing the inflammatory response.

Afferent nerves not only relay painful sensations from the gut, but are also components of local reflexes that modulate intestinal physiology. Interruptions of this circuitry will therefore alter gut physiology. Studies using capsaicin to abolish substance P-containing sensory nerves have shown that ablation of these primary afferent nerves results in an increased susceptibility to inflammation[13–15].

These findings suggest that sensory nerves are part of a neural circuit that protects against inflammation. Hence, the use of antagonists for sensory neurotransmitters might produce changes in intestinal physiology that promote inflammation. Serotonin or 5-hydroxytryptamine (5-HT) sensitizes afferent nerves and has been implicated in chronic pain in functional bowel disorders[16,17]. Antagonism of the 5-HT$_3$ receptor by alosetron has been accompanied by reports of 'ischaemic' colitis. Theoretically, this could be a manifestation of increased intestinal susceptibility to inflammation following interruption of normal neural sensory function. Attempts to modulate intestinal inflammation using substance P antagonists have been disappointing and the lack of clear-cut benefit may reflect offsetting effects of substance P receptor blockade[18]. That is, reduction of neurogenic inflammation is compromised by the interruption of neural circuitry that increases susceptibility to inflammation. This point illustrates the complexity of therapeutically harnessing neuroimmune interactions to treat IBD. The apparent benefit of lidocaine in the treatment of refractory ulcerative proctitis may reflect a systemic anti-inflammatory effect of the drug rather than a reflection of its attenuation of sensory input[19,20].

THE AUTONOMIC NERVOUS SYSTEM

Changes in autonomic balance have been documented in patients with ulcerative colitis as well as in patients with Crohn's disease[21,22]. The contribution of this imbalance to the natural history of IBD remains, however, unclear. The apparent benefit of cigarette smoking or nicotine treatment for ulcerative colitis, and the deleterious effect of smoking in Crohn's disease[23], suggest that autonomic function influences the inflammatory process in patients with IBD. Studies in animals have shown, for example, that sympathectomy is protective against experimental colitis, suggesting that sympathetic nerves are proinflammatory and may aggravate intestinal inflammation. In an animal model of a Th1-mediated model of colitis, cigarette smoking aggravated the inflammation, in keeping with the documented adverse effects of cigarette smoking in patients with Crohn's disease[24]. In addition, nicotine has a bell-shaped dose–response relationship with inflammation in animal studies; while low doses of nicotine appeared protective, supramaximally effective doses were clearly deleterious[25,26]. This observation urges caution in the development of nicotinic analogues to treat colitis. Recent work from our laboratory has suggested that autonomic imbalance in colitis is variable and may reflect the extent of disease activity. Ganguli et al. have shown that there is sympathetic dominance only in patients with left-sided or distal colitis and that there may be parasympathetic dominance in those patients with more extensive disease (Ganguli et al., unpublished observation). If confirmed, these studies suggest that the development of nicotinic analogues to treat colitis might be reserved for patients with left-sided or distal disease, and again urge caution in extrapolating the use of parasympathomimetic drugs to the entire ulcerative colitis population. If patients can be subgrouped according to their degree of sympathetic/parasympathetic dominance, then the development of drugs that modulate the autonomic nervous system holds promise for the therapy of IBD.

ENDOCRINE FUNCTION IN IBD

There has been recent interest in the role of leptin in intestinal inflammation. Leptin is a hormone produced by adipose cells among other cell types, and exerts a variety of effects including modulation of food intake. Studies examining leptin function in IBD patients have suggested that there may be an increase in leptin activity[27] and there is speculation that this may be a mechanism for the anorexia observed in active IBD[28,29]. This subject remains controversial. Nevertheless, more recent studies have shown that leptin has definite proinflammatory properties. Studies in *ob/ob* mice, which are leptin-deficient, have shown that these animals have some resistance to inflammation[30]. Pharmacological inhibition of leptin using CCK antagonists has shown that there is a substantial improvement during the early phases of intestinal inflammation in an animal model[31]. From these studies it is possible to conceive of an endocrine component to the modulation of intestinal inflammation via the increased production of leptin from adipose tissue in mesentery surrounding the inflamed gut. Inhibition of leptin release or blockade of its receptor may hold promise in terms of reducing inflammation in IBD, and may have the added benefit of improving nutrition by increased food intake. This promising area requires further study.

CONCLUSION

Neuroendocrine–immune interactions offer therapeutic potential in IBD. However, because communication between these systems is bidirectional, attempts, for example, to improve symptoms by attenuating neuroendocrine function in the gut may be compromised by increasing the susceptibility to inflammation. There is more promise in exploiting neuroendocrine influences that have a definite proinflammatory property, and the blockage of which will not compromise host function; an example of this is leptin. The contribution of the autonomic nervous system to IBD needs careful evaluation, but preliminary data suggest that patients may be subtyped according to their sympathetic or parasympathetic predominance, and this in turn may provide a basis for rationally stratifying patients for selected therapies.

References

1. Lium R. Etiology of ulcerative colitis. II. Effects of induced muscular spasm on colonic explants in dogs with comment on relation of muscular spasm to ulcerative colitis. Arch Intern Med. 1939;63:210–17
2. Thorek P. Vagotomy for idiopathic ulcerative colitis and regional enteritis. J Am Med Assoc. 1951;145:140–6.
3. Ottaway CA, Greenberg GR. Interaction of VIP with mouse lymphocytes: Specific binding and the modulation of mitogen responses. J Immunol. 1984;132:417–23.
4. Payan DG, Brewster DR, Goetzi EJ. Specific stimulation of human T lymphocytes by substance P. J Immunol. 1983;131:1613–15.
5. Mantyh CR, Gates TS, Zimmerman RP *et al.* Receptor binding sites for substance P, but not substance K or neuromedin K, are expressed in high concentrations by arterioles, venules, and lymph nodules in surgical specimens obtained from patients with ulcerative colitis and Crohn's disease. Proc Natl Acad Sci USA. 1988;85:3235–9.

6. Mantyh PW, Catton MD, Boehmer CG *et al.* Receptors for sensory neuropeptides in human inflammatory diseases: implications for the effector role of sensory neurons. Peptides. 1989;10: 627–45.

7. Kemler MA, Barendse GA, Van Kleef M. Relapsing ulcerative colitis associated with spinal cord stimulation [In process citation]. Gastroenterology. 1999;117:215–17.

8. Ansel JC, Armstrong CA, Song I *et al.* Interactions of the skin and nervous system. J Invest Dermatol Symp Proc 1997. 1998;2:23–6.

9. Belvisi MG, Barnes PJ, Rogers DF. Neurogenic inflammation in the airways: characterisation of electrical parameters for vagus nerve stimulation in the guinea pig. J Neurosci Meth. 1990;32: 159–67.

10. Figini M, Emanueli C, Grady EF *et al.* Substance P and bradykinin stimulate plasma extravasation in the mouse gastrointestinal tract and pancreas. Am J Physiol. 1997;272:G785–93.

11. Hwang L, Leichter R, Okamoto A, Payan D, Collins SM, Bunnett NW. Downregulation of neural endopeptidase (EC 3.4.24.11) in the inflamed rat intestine. Am J Physiol. 1993;264: G735–43.

12. Sturiale S, Barbara G, Qiu B *et al.* Neutral endopeptidase (EC 3.4.24.11) terminates colitis by degrading substance P. Proc Natl Acad Sci USA. 1999;96:11653–8.

13. Evangelista S, Meli A. Influence of capsaicin-sensitive fibres on experimentally-induced colitis in rats. J Pharm Pharmacol. 1989;41:574–5.

14. McCafferty DM, Wallace JL, Sharkey KA. Effects of chemical sympathectomy and sensory nerve ablation on experimental colitis in the rat. Am J Physiol. 1997;272:G272–80.

15. Swain MG, Agro A, Blennerhassett P, Stanisz A, Collins SM. Increased levels of substance P in the myenteric plexus of *Trichinella*-infected rats. Gastroenterology. 1992;102:1913–19.

16. Gershon MD. Review article: Roles played by 5-hydroxytryptamine in the physiology of the bowel. Aliment Pharmacol Ther. 1999;13(Suppl.):15–30.

17. Humphrey PP, Bountra C, Clayton N, Kozlowski K. Review article: The therapeutic potential of 5-HT3 receptor antagonists in the treatment of irritable bowel syndrome. Aliment Pharmacol Ther. 1999;13(Suppl.2):31–8.

18. Wallace JL, McCafferty DM, Sharkey KA. Lack of beneficial effect of a tachykinin receptor antagonist in experimental colitis. Regul Pept. 1998;73:95–102.

19. Bjorck S, Dahlstrom A, Johansson L, Ahlman H. Treatment of the mucosa with local anaesthetics in ulcerative colitis. Agents Actions. 1992;10:C61–72.

20. McCafferty DM, Sharkey KA, Wallace JL. Beneficial effects of local or systemic lidocaine in experimental colitis. Am J Physiol. 1994;266:G560–7.

21. Lindgren S, Stewenius J, Sjölund K, Lilja B, Sundkvist G. Autonomic vagal nerve dysfunction in patients with ulcerative colitis. Scand J Gastroenterol. 1993;28:638–42.

22. Lindgren S, Lilja B, Rosén I, Sundkvist G. Disturbed autonomic nerve function in patients with Crohn's disease. Scand J Gastroenterol. 1991;26:361–6.

23. Rubin DT, Hanauer SB. Smoking and inflammatory bowel disease. Eur J Gastroenterol Hepatol. 2000;12:855–62.

24. Galeazzi F, Blennerhassett PA, Qiu B, O'Byrne PM, Collins SM. Cigarette smoke aggravates experimental colitis in rats (See comments). Gastroenterology. 1999;117:877–83.

25. Eliakim R, Karmeli F, Cohen P, Heyman SN, Rachmilewitz D. Dual effect of chronic nicotine administration: augmentation of jejunitis and amelioration of colitis induced by iodoacetamide in rats. Int J Colorectal Dis. 2001;16:14–21.

26. Qiu B, Collins SM. Nicotine improves experimental colitis in rats. Gastroenterology. 1997; Qui B, Deng YK, Galeazzi F, Collins S. Neural involvement in the bivalent action of nicotine on experimental colitis in rats. Gastroenterology 112.A 1065, 1997.

27. Barbier M, Cherbut C, Aube AC, Blottiere HM, Galmiche JP. Elevated plasma leptin concentrations in early stages of experimental intestinal inflammation in rats. Gut. 1998;43:783–90.

28. Hoppin AG, Kaplan LM, Zurakowski D, Leichtner AM, Bousvaros A. Serum leptin in children and young adults with inflammatory bowel disease. J Pediatr Gastroenterol Nutr. 1998; 26:500–5.

29. Stein RB, Lichtenstein GR, Rombeau JL. Nutrition in inflammatory bowel disease. Curr Opin Clin Nutr Metab Care. 1999;2:367–71.

30. Siegmund B, Lehr HA, Fantuzzi G. Leptin: a pivotal mediator of intestinal inflammation in mice. Gastroenterology. 2002;122:2011–25.

31. Barbier M, Attoub S, Joubert M *et al.* Proinflammatory role of leptin in experimental colitis in rats: benefit of cholecystokinin-B antagonist and beta3-agonist. Life Sci. 2001;69:567–80.

Aims of treatment in daily practice

14
State of the art lecture: Evolution of treatment from the 1930s to the end of the 1980s

P. RIIS

INTRODUCTION

The term chronic inflammatory bowel disease (IBD) has today acquired an idiomatic status, even if it linguistically covers much more than ulcerative colitis and Crohn's disease. In other words it represents a *toto pro parte* term, i.e. a broad meaning, but a narrow taxonomic precision. Dealing with terminology is crucial, because a near-historic survey of therapeutic modalities in IBD from the 1930s to the 1980s *must* reflect the diagnostic uncertainties early in the period, as one of the main reasons for the large therapeutic diversity that the present analysis will disclose.

Improved diagnostic and differential diagnostic precision acquired during the six decades is only one of three important factors behind the changes found in both shift of therapies and the reasons given, if any, by the clinicians involved. Another is the paradigmatic shift in testing and evaluating therapeutic interventions in the form of the controlled clinical trial, also named the randomized clinical trial (RCT) in the middle of the period. The third factor is the gradual, but ultimately strong, shift from therapeutic strategies in medicine as a whole (thereby also including treatment of IBD), starting with strategic mini-universes, i.e. *a* hospital, *a* university, or even *one* chief – the Geheimerat phenomenon – and spreading to the present day's fast global exchange of results of evidence-based therapeutic information.

Due to the strong influence of these three factors they will be dealt with in more detail and consequently exemplified by the shifting trends in the treatment of IBD.

THE CHANGING DIAGNOSTICS OF IBD

The first description of ulcerative colitis (UC) as a disease entity traditionally refers to Wilks and Moxon's publication from 1875[1] but, due to the small number of diagnostic procedures available, this priority setting depends greatly on additional clinical features, when compared to earlier descriptions.

The appearance of Crohn's disease (CD) can be dated more precisely (but still with competitive comparisons to earlier descriptions in history). The year 1932 is well known for Crohn, Ginzburg and Oppenheimer's description[2]. In other words we are historically situated in the first decade of the period being surveyed, but still far away from the recognition of CD of the colon, that must have interfered seriously with UC and therapeutic evaluations of this disease until Wells in 1952[3] and Brooke in 1959[4] made it possible in most cases to distinguish UC from CD of the colon.

Adding to the late impact of this separation on clinical work with gastrointestinal patients was the inertial tradition at that time of extrapolating diagnostic strategies of a department or hospital from generation to generation of clinicians. In other words one made the diagnoses within a universe of well-known diseases, most often in a vicarage perspective. This continued during the 1930s in most European countries, with the Second World War as a zero period in the pre-war global exchange of evidence-based clinical practices and concepts.

The postwar appearance of better diagnostic equipment, double-contrast X-ray barium enemas, biopsy tools, etc., was a slow process, at least in Europe; and the systematic growth of gastroenterology in Europe, including elaboration of diagnostic terms and specialist training plans, was also rather slow, resulting in the first cohesive diagnostic strategies for IBD in the 1950s and early 1960s.

THE NEW PARADIGM: THE RANDOMIZED CONTROLLED TRIAL

The twentieth century's most remarkable shift of paradigms was the introduction of systematic variation control as a central part of therapeutic evaluations, in its methodological format named *the randomized controlled trial*. This evolution, with an almost revolutionary impact on clinical science, was not confined to gastroenterology or any other clinical discipline, but in accordance with its paradigmatic nature it influenced *all* medical specialties from around the midpoint of the period in focus here, 1930–90. The running-in period of the controlled clinical trial was long; attempts aimed at formulating an overall new paradigm covered a couple of centuries.

The first complete design based on bias control was introduced just before the turn of the nineteenth to the twentieth century by Fibiger, in a trial of serum therapy for diphtheria[5]. Due to the publication in Danish, however, the lack of an informative boost in the form of follow-up publications by Fibiger, and the paralysing effect on medical internationalization by the First World War, it was not until Bradford-Hill described the new paradigm in detail[6], and later applied it in the epoch-making trial on streptomycin treatment of pulmonary tuberculosis[7].

From a personal viewpoint, with medical university studies from 1945 to 1952 and with postgraduate training in internal medicine just after, it has been a surprise to see the interval between Bradford-Hill's publication in 1948 and the first appearances of the new approach to clinical judgements in pre- and postgraduate education, and in articles published in national medical journals.

Based on a personal analysis in Denmark this did not happen before the early 1960s, and at that time still in very bias-containing forms[8]. For the IBDs the delay was even longer because the necessary platform for applying the controlled clinical trial was just starting to appear in Europe.

Further based on personal experiences the new scientific *methodology*, defined as the art of planning, carrying through, interpreting and publishing a clinical research project, had also to be adopted by the new specialists, the gastroenterologists. In its rather slow introductory phase the controlled clinical trial was considered more cookbook-like and dominated by statistical *figures*, instead of the underlying *logic*. The result was a lack of consideration of technical bias sources, for instance interpretation of a non-significant *p*-level as the equivalent for non-difference between two therapies without a necessary calculation of statistical power and high risks of type 2 errors[9].

The creation and application of the paradigm of variation and bias controlling methodology in the 1950s and 1960s started three revolution-like changes in European gastroenterology.

The first one was a showdown with the hierarchical structure of the clinical department, not primarily its administrative prerogatives, but more importantly its inborn illusion that chiefs of departments are, via a natural law, equipped with a pseudo-divine ability to judge what is effective and non-effective in the vast armamentarium of suggested therapeutics. I have named the necessary cleaning of the Augean stables 'From clevidence to evidence'.

The second one was a whole new way of planning a clinical scientific study, formulated in a detailed protocol and introducing new terms such as randomization, blinding, stratification, statistical power, MIREDIF (minimal relevant difference), type 1 and type 2 errors, and many others. Not only new drugs and other therapies were now subjected to these new principles of judgement, but also established, 'in University X we always learned', methods were tested by these new critical principles, adding to a way of critical thinking even in very self-centred university departments.

The third evolution was editors' general application of the new methodology for analytic purposes, not only by their own staff but also by the editorial advisers (referees), later followed by the general readers of scientific journals.

In clinical gastroenterology the new paradigm even permitted an evidence-based end to the illusion that new therapies can only be based on laboratory experiments in patients, and from here transferred to clinical application, as emphasized by Claude Bernard[10] and until the 1960s and 1970s still claimed by medical laboratory scientists. As will be mentioned later in the line of therapeutic suggestions from the 1930s to the 1990s, we now have at our disposal effective drugs, tested in controlled clinical trials, without any knowledge of the way they interfere with the chronic IBDs. Examples are salazosulphapyridine and its derivatives, azathioprine and prednisolone.

The third paradigmatic leap was the creation of gastroenterology as an academic specialty and the many new centres for clinical, epidemiological and basic gastroenterology forming a number of networks, comprising national and international conferences and meetings, training courses, own scientific journals, multicentre transnational trials and personal relationships. This development can be named 'From parochial isolation to globalization'.

The combined effects of these paradigmatic leaps can be illustrated by a brief survey of the prevalent therapeutic principles applied in IBD from the 1930s to the 1990s. (For the reader interested in reading further 'backwards' a brief introduction to the history of IBD can, for instance, be found in the historical review by Hawkins[11].) Due to the Second World War the 1930s concepts and treatment suggestions I encountered during the last half of the 1940s reasonably reflect the views of the 1930s, and this is also found in the textbooks on the national market[12].

CD, or regional ileitis, was well described, and consequently well diagnosed in cases of small bowel attacks. The therapy suggested was 'as large a resection as possible'. UC was suggested as connected to 'non-haemolytic streptococci' or 'nervous influences'. The therapeutic suggestions comprised 'constipating treatment', 'vitamins B and C', '12 apples a day' and a number of other fancy diets; and yet Salazopyrin is briefly mentioned. Local treatment is suggested as enemas with tannic acid, yatren, oil, starch, or silver nitrate, to mention a few. Surgery is mentioned only as colostomy, not colectomy.

Colectomy with ileostomy as a lifesaving intervention reached northern Europe around the 1950s and in some of the new gastroenterological departments, including my own, became a systematic and very aggressive approach in fulminant cases, according to the motto 'If no dramatic change has taken place within 2–3 days on medical treatment, then use colectomy'. Despite its shocking radicality for a *medical* gastroenterological approach, the policy soon showed itself to be life-saving and time-saving for the work taking place in parallel to find new and better medical treatments.

At the same time this meant an end to psychosomatic ways of treating UC. For CD surgery was still the best offer as the treatment of strictures, with fistulas as the most challenging complication. The observations of CD as a disease also involving the colon appeared around 1968–75[13,14], and represented a new challenge to both medical and surgical therapy of CD.

The three cornerstones of medical therapy – sulphasalazine, corticosteroids and immunosuppressive drugs – appeared around 1960 (for Salazopyrin it was a reappearance from partial oblivion[15]). Sulphasalazine was introduced as treatment of UC in 1960 and the first controlled trial appeared in 1962[16]. In CD our own Nordic study of Salazopyrin showed an effect in both ileocolic and colic cases but not in small bowel CD[17]. The results in post-resectomy cases and as a relapse-preventing drug have as a whole been disappointing, but inventive strategies have led to the use of 5-ASA drugs for controlled local release in CD.

The same development has led to the well-known use of 5-ASA in UC[18]. Corticosteroids as treatment of UC were introduced by Truelove and Witts in 1954–55[19,20], and shortly after our own group had started to test corticosteroids in rectal enemas innovatively, Truelove published his controlled study in 1958[21].

In active CD prednisone was tested in a controlled trial from 1979[22] and showed an effect compared to placebo in ileocolic and ileal disease, but not in colonic (which may be due to a weak power of the design). As with sulphasalazine no benefit is obvious in post-resectional and quiescent CD.

Azathioprine and the related 6-mercaptopurine have been used for a long time in UC after its introduction in 1962–74[23–25], not as a remission-inducing agent, but as a corticosteroid-saving drug in patients who cannot taper steroids. In many European centres the use of azathioprine has been more restrictive than in some US 'schools'. The many therapeutic ideas and attempts surrounding corticosteroids, salazosulphapyridine, 5-ASA and immunosuppressants, and surgery, have not held a lasting position in the treatment of IBD. Some will be mentioned here in order to emphasize the work-demanding ratio between ideas and lasting innovations. For UC the other suggestions and possibilities involve:

1. Cyclosporine[26]: Introduced at the end of the relevant historical period, evidence for its lasting beneficial effect has been controversial, especially when the potentially severe side-effects are considered[27].
2. Antibiotics have been used extensively, especially during the first part of the period surveyed, probably due to the common and false concept of identity between the terms inflammation and infection, enforced by the suffix -itis. For gastroenterologists demanding scientific evidence for choosing therapies (such as myself), antibiotics have never been used in UC as a treatment of the disease itself.
3. Nicotine has been suggested, after the clinical observation that smoking seemed to have a protective effect on UC. Neither smoking as such (!) nor nicotine gum nor plasters have obtained a therapeutic position in the treatment of UC.
4. Short-chain fatty acids have been tested in left-sided UC and in pouchitis, but their final therapeutic position is still doubtful.
5. Cytokines and chemokines were in focus in the minds of gastroenterologists during the last decades of the period ('Is UC a disease initiated by a special external agent in a normal bowel or is it initiated by a ubiquitous agent in a (genetically?) diverging bowel?'). It is, however, only in the 1990s that trials of such specific inflammatory pro- and antimessengers have appeared.

For CD the other therapeutic suggestions or possibilities comprise:

1. Cyclosporine has shown itself to be effective in short-term courses[28], but the long-term results were not significant[29].
2. Methotrexate was shown to be effective as a steroid-sparing drug in otherwise refractory CD[30]. Its ultimate role in long-term treatment was – and still is – unclear.
3. Antibiotics have often been used but, as for UC, not in departments considering evidence to be a *conditio sine qua non* in clinical decision-making.
4. Metronidazole was introduced in Sweden in the late 1970s[31], but has not passed the test of controlled trials, not even long term in fistulous cases.
5. Omega-3 fatty acids appeared as a therapeutic possibility around 1990, but their role is still controversial.
6. Ciprofloxacin and antimycobacterial drugs appeared as test drugs around 1990, but their therapeutic potentials are still unclear.
7. As for UC the same is true for cytokines, chemokines and agents of similar groups.

NEW ROADS TO THERAPEUTIC PROGRESS

From the 1960s large epidemiological studies have been based on comprehensive, complete regional groups of patients with IBD. In a therapeutic and preventive perspective this has paved the road to substantial progress. First it has created large cooperative groups of IBD patients, taken care of in subspecialized departments, and consequently accessible for consecutive and parallel clinical trials, large-scale genetic studies, studies of the influence of lifestyle factors, and socioeconomic and health-system administrative analyses (see refs 32, 33 and a long follow-up series).

WHAT CAN BE LEARNT FROM THE NEAR-HISTORY?

In a personal perspective much can be learnt, in accordance with the old statement that if we do not learn from history we are doomed to repeat the mistakes that it certifies.

One lesson is the surprising inertia of tradition, even in a scientifically based discipline such as academic medicine (here gastroenterology). Not only did it take 15–20 years before the paradigm of the controlled trial started to change the way clinicians evaluate *medical research*, but still outdated ways of reasoning when selecting therapies (not to mention sheer superstition in national cultures or in 'the alternative movement') exist around the world.

The next lesson is the delay in clinicians integrating *the principles behind* the methodology of the controlled clinical trial and extending it to diagnostics, surgical treatments, epidemiology and many other areas outside the classical drug trial. To integrate the two fundamental principles behind the axioms: 'all judgements rest on comparisons' and 'everything constantly moves or varies in the biology of medicine', leads to a mental revival in daily clinical practice. Further, it creates a much more fertile *cambrium* for new scientific ideas, whose nature is the combination of two masses of knowledge which have not previously been combined, with the aim of making a causal relationship probable or unlikely[34]. Judged in this way the 60 years of IBD treatment has not been a tiresome journey from porridge enemas to cytokines and chemokines, but has been a worthwhile passage to the 'molecular country' seen in dim morning light[35,36].

References

1. Wilks S, Moxon W. Lectures on Pathological Pathology, 2nd edn. Philadelphia: Lindsay & Blakiston, 1875:408–9.
2. Crohn BB, Ginzburg L, Oppenheimer GD. Regional ileitis: a pathologic and clinical entity. J Am Med Assoc. 1932;99:1323–9.
3. Wells C. Ulcerative colitis and Crohn's disease. Ann Roy Coll Surg Engl. 1952;11:105–20.
4. Brooke BN. Granulomatous diseases of the intestine. Lancet. 1959;2:745–9.
5. Fibiger J. Biography in Dansk Biografisk Leksikon. Copenhagen: Gyldendal, 1980.
6. Bradford-Hill AB. Principles of Medical Statistics, 1st edn. London: Lancet Ltd, 1937.
7. Bradford-Hill AB. Member of the Streptomycin in Tuberculosis Trials Committee. Streptomycin treatment in pulmonary tuberculosis. Br Med J. 1948;30 Oct.:769–82.
8. Riis P. When the controlled clinical trials arrived in Denmark. Dan Soc Hist Med. 11 Nov. 1998 (in Danish).

9. Anthonisen P, Barany F, Folkenborg O *et al*. The clinical effect of salazosulphapyridine (Salazopyrin) in Crohn's disease: a controlled double-blind study. Scand J Gastroenterol. 1974; 9:549–54.
10. Vandenbroucke JP. Clinical investigation in the 20th century: the ascendancy of numerical reasoning. Lancet. 1998;352:SII12–17.
11. Hawkins C. Historical review. In: Allan RH, Keighley MRB, Alexander-Williams J, Hawkins C, editors. Inflammatory Bowel Diseases. Edinburgh: Churchill Livingstone, 1983:1–7.
12. Bernth O, Hagens E. Medicinsk Kompendium, 4th edn. Copenhagen: Store Nordiske Videnskabsboghandel, 1944.
13. Farmer RG, Hawk WA, Turnbull RB. Regional enteritis of the colon: a clinical and pathological comparison with ulcerative colitis. Gastroenterology. 1968;13:501–14.
14. Farmer RG, Hawk WA, Turnbull RB. Clinical patterns in Crohn's disease: a statistical study of 615 cases. Am J Dig Dis. 1975;68:627–35.
15. Svartz N. Salazopyrin, a new sulfanilamide preparation. B. Therapeutic results in ulcerative colitis. Acta Med Scand. 1942;110:557–90.
16. Baron JH, Connell AM, Lennard-Jones JE, Jones A. Sulphasalazine and salizylazosulphadimidine in ulcerative colitis. Lancet. 1962;1:1094–6.
17. Anthonisen P, Barany F, Folkenborg O *et al*. The clinical effect of salazosulphapyridine (Salazopyrin) in Crohn's disease: a controlled double-blind study. Scand J Gastroenterol. 1974;9:549–54.
18. Hanauer SB. Medical therapy for ulcerative colitis. In: Kirsner JB, editor. Inflammatory Bowel Disease, 5th edn. Philadelphia: Saunders, 2000:529–56.
19. Truelove SC, Witts LJ. Cortisone in ulcerative colitis. Br Med J. 1954;2:375–8.
20. Truelove SC, Witts LJ. Cortisone in ulcerative colitis. Br Med J. 1955;2:1041–8.
21. Truelove SC. Treatment of ulcerative colitis with local hydrocortisone hemisuccinate sodium: a report on a controlled therapeutic trial. Br Med J. 1958;2:1072–7.
22. Summers RW, Switz DM, Sessions JT *et al*. National cooperative Crohn's disease study: results of drug treatment. Gastroenterology. 1979;77:847–69.
23. Bean RDH. The treatment of chronic ulcerative colitis with 6-mercaptopurine. Med J Aust. 1962;2:592.
24. Bowen GE, Irons GV, Rhodes JB *et al*. Early experiences with azathioprine in ulcerative colitis: a note of caution. J Am Med Assoc. 1960;195:460.
25. Jewell DP, Truelove SC. Azathioprine in ulcerative colitis: final report on controlled therapeutic trial. Br Med J. 1974;4:627.
26. Brynskov J. Cyclosporin for inflammatory bowel disease: mechanisms and possible actions. Scand J Gastroenterol. 1993;28:849.
27. Kornbluth A, Present DH, Lichtiger S *et al*. Cyclosporin for severe ulcerative colitis: a user's guide. Am J Gastroenterol. 1997;92:1424.
28. Brynskov J, Freund L, Rasmussen SN. A placebo-controlled, double-blind, randomized trial of cyclosporine in active chronic Crohn's disease. N Engl J Med. 1989;321:845.
29. Brynskov J, Freund L, Rasmussen SN *et al*. Final report on a placebo-controlled, double-blind, randomized, multicentre trial of cyclosporine treatment in active chronic Crohn's disease. Scand J Gastroenterol. 1991;26:689.
30. Kozarek RA, Patterson DJ, Gelfand MD *et al*. Methotrexate induces clinical and histological remission in patients with inflammatory bowel disease. Ann Intern Med. 1989;110:353.
31. Blichfeldt P, Blomhoff JP, Myhre E *et al*. Metronidazole in Crohn's disease: a double-blind, cross-over clinical trial. Scand J Gastroenterol. 1978;13:123.
32. Bonnevie O, Riis P, Anthonisen P. An epidemiological study of ulcerative colitis in Copenhagen County. Scand J Gastroenterol. 1968;3:432–8.
33. Höj L, Brix Jensen P, Bonnevie O, Riis P. An epidemiological study of regional enteritis and acute ileitis in Copenhagen County. Scand J Gastroenterol. 1973;8:381–4.
34. Riis P, Clausen T. Idé, problemformulering og forsøgsplanlægning. In: Andersen D, Havsteen B, Riis P, Almind G, Bock E, Hørder M, editors. Sundhedsvidenskabelig forskning: en introduktion. København, Aarhus, Odense: FADL, 1999:17–30.
35. Farrel RJ, Peppercorn MA. Ulcerative colitis. Lancet. 2002;359:331–40.
36. Elson C. Genes, microbes and F-cells: new therapeutic targets in Crohn's disease. N Engl J Med. 2002;346:614–16.

Section V
General targets

15
Extraintestinal manifestations – important target of treatment or just an expression of disease activity?

F. TAVARELA-VELOSO

CLINICAL ASPECTS

The clinical spectrum of extraintestinal manifestations varies from mild transitory to very severe lesions, sometimes more incapacitating than the underlying bowel disease. Several extraintestinal manifestations clinically appear related to the activity of bowel disease and, consequently, have been referred to as 'inflammatory'[1].

During the course of inflammatory bowel diseases (IBD) a significant number of patients may develop these extraintestinal manifestations[2,3]. They could appear isolated, but frequently occur simultaneously in the same patient overlapping joints, skin, eyes, and mouth, which suggest a common link in their pathogenesis[4,5].

In patients with Crohn's disease these systemic manifestations are less prevalent in those with ileal involvement (L1). In ulcerative colitis it is still controversial whether they are correlated with the extent of colonic involvement. Patients with one of these manifestations run a high risk not only of a repetition of the same manifestation, but also any of the other associated manifestations.

The great majority of these extraintestinal manifestations accompany the activity of intestinal disease and patients run a higher risk of a severe clinical course with a higher probability of steroid treatment[6].

There is agreement that these manifestations, which may be immune or inflammation-mediated, generally respond well to medical or surgical treatment targeted to the bowel disease.

COMMON INFLAMMATORY EXTRAINTESTINAL MANIFESTATIONS AND RESPONSE TO TREATMENT OF BOWEL DISEASE

Articular disease

Arthritis is the most common extraintestinal manifestation, symptomatically affecting about one-quarter of patients[7]. However, using articular scintigraphy, a sensitive indicator of active joint disease, asymptomatic forms of synovitis and sacroiliitis could be detectable, indicating that the prevalence of this complication could be much higher than generally believed[8]. Although its pathogenesis is unknown, it has been suggested that immunological events are likely to contribute to joint vulnerability. A link between enteritis and spondylarthropathy is well known, and there is strong evidence that intestinal inflammation may serve as an initiating event for chronic arthropathy. Clinical remission of articular symptoms has also been consistently associated with the normalization of gut histology, whereas persistence of locomotor inflammation is usually associated with persistence of gut inflammation[9]. Furthermore, it has been found that sulphasalazine has a beneficial effect on gastrointestinal and articular symptoms. These findings, together with the proven efficacy of infliximab therapy in Crohn's disease and rheumatoid arthritis, have led to the suggestion that anti-tumour necrosis factor alpha (TNF-α) treatment might also be a useful agent in the management of spondylarthropathies associated with Crohn's disease.

In two open studies infliximab was used in patients with ankylosing spondylitis, leading to clinical improvement[10,11]. The same was observed in patients studied with magnetic resonance imaging scans before and after infliximab infusions[12]. The use of etanercept in a randomized trial also resulted in an impressive improvement in clinical and laboratory abnormalities[13]. In four patients with spondylarthropathies associated with Crohn's disease a beneficial effect of anti-TNF-α treatment on intestinal disease and arthropathy has been reported[14]. Improvement of arthritis/arthralgia after treatment with infliximab has also been shown in a German prospective, multicentre trial in refractory Crohn's disease[15].

In a multicentre, randomized, double-blind international trial to evaluate the efficacy of infliximab maintenance therapy in patients with moderate to severe active Crohn's disease (ACCENT I), it has been reported that maintenance therapy with infliximab is superior to a single dose in resolving arthritis/arthralgia[16].

The treatment of arthritis in inflammatory bowel disease depends on the nature and duration of this complication. Using biologic drugs, more intensive therapeutic strategies could be tailored in the management of severe or refractory articular disease.

SKIN MANIFESTATIONS

There is a wide range of skin manifestations reported in patients with inflammatory bowel disease. Erythema nodosum is the most common skin lesion and clinically appears simultaneously with symptoms of active bowel disease. It is more common in females, patients with large intestine involvement and those with peripheral arthritis[2].

This skin disorder usually responds to systemic corticosteroids used to control the flare-up. Thalidomide has also been suggested as an agent that may be effective in the treatment of erythema nodosum leprosum[17]. Its action is associated with a decrease in serum concentrations of TNF-α. Consequently, infliximab could be effective in the treatment of refractory erythema nodosum associated with Crohn's disease. We have used this treatment in a patient with colonic Crohn's disease complicated by severe lesions of erythema nodosum and arthritis, refractory to high doses of steroids. Infliximab treatment resulted in rapid and complete resolutions of skin and articular manifestations. Infliximab has been successfully used in the treatment of six patients with steroid-refractory erythema nodosum, three of whom had ulcerative colitis[18].

Pyoderma gangrenosum is a severe and debilitating complication which sometimes parallels the activity of the bowel disease. High doses of oral prednisone and/or intralesional injections of corticosteroids are generally effective in the management. However, the best form of treatment, particularly in patients with inactive intestinal disease, has not yet been established. Several clinical cases have been successfully treated with intravenous cyclosporine, oral and topical tacrolimus, or mycophenolate-mofetil[20–22].

In an uncontrolled study, 11 patients with steroid-refractory pyoderma gangrenosum have been successfully treated with intravenous cyclosporine[22]. Although the duration of skin lesions was variable, most patients responded to treatment during the first month. The authors recommended this strategy as the treatment of choice for steroid-refractory pyoderma, followed by 6-mercaptopurine or azathioprine to maintain remission.

Biologic therapies, such as infliximab, are also effective in healing refractory pyoderma gangrenosum associated with inflammatory bowel disease[23]. In several reports patients treated with infliximab showed rapid healing of their pyoderma lesions. It has also been reported that severe peristomal pyoderma gangrenosum responds to infliximab[24]. Eight patients with Crohn's disease, complicated by refractory pyoderma gangrenosum, were treated with a single infusion or a series of infliximab infusions at 5 mg/kg. Some patients improved with a single infusion while others needed three or more maintenance infusions. We have successfully treated one patient in this way (Fig. 1). Nowadays infliximab is becoming the first choice in the treatment of pyoderma gangrenosum.

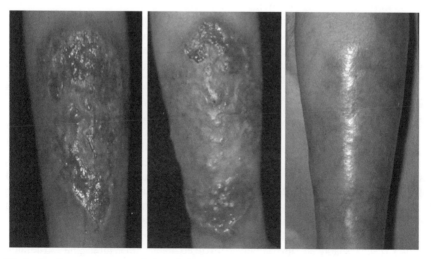

Fig. 1 Pyoderma gangrenosum before, during and after treatment with infliximab

MOUTH MANIFESTATIONS

Aphthous ulcers are the most common oral lesions in inflammatory bowel disease; they occur in about 10% of patients. Their onset is usually sudden, coinciding with the flare-up of intestinal disease and occurring simultaneously with other extraintestinal manifestations.

Oral ulceration may be painful and resistant to conventional therapy. Oral thalidomide has been reported to be beneficial in the treatment of aphthous stomatitis related to HIV infection, and could be tried for lesions in patients with inflammatory bowel disease[25]. Topical applications of tacrolimus have been effective in the treatment of three patients with oral Crohn's disease[26]. Infliximab has been used in the treatment of four patients with Crohn's disease complicated by gigantic oral ulcers which healed within 2 weeks after the administration of the third infusion[27].

Orofacial Crohn's disease includes granulomatous lesions of the face and the oral cavity with underlying bowel disease. The term Melkersson Rosenthal syndrome encompasses patients with recurrent orofacial oedema, peripheral facial palsy, and fissured tongue (lingua plicata). This disorder is difficult to treat as the response to treatment with steroids, immunossuppressants, or thalidomide is poor and slow. Although a patient with such a disorder has been treated satisfactorily with infliximab[28], our patient failed to respond with the same treatment.

EYE MANIFESTATIONS

The incidence of ocular lesions is approximately 6%, as observed in our series[2]. Uveitis is the most serious complication and may be the cause of significant morbidity. In two small studies etanercept was used in chronic active uveitis associated with rheumatic diseases[29]. One study performed prospectively on children reported an overall beneficial effect in 63%; the other study reviewed retrospectively 16 adult patients treated for joint disease who concurrently presented with uveitis/scleritis. All patients with active articular inflammation improved, and about 40% showed improvement in eye disease.

Infliximab has been reported to have a beneficial effect in a few patients suffering from Crohn's disease with uveitis and spondylarthropathy, as well as in patients treated in the ACCENT I study[16].

CONCLUSION

During the course of inflammatory bowel disease, extraintestinal manifestations are quite common (up to 40% in 10 years). Most of the extraintestinal complications are related to the activity of intestinal inflammation and significantly affect several organs concurrently. Phenotypic classification shows that certain subsets of patients are more susceptible to developing extraintestinal manifestations. They also have a higher probability of maintaining active disease during the clinical course.

Cytokines play important roles in the pathogenesis of inflammatory bowel diseases and are undoubtedly involved in immune/inflammation-related extraintestinal complications. That immune mechanisms are of the utmost importance in the development of many of these inflammatory extraintestinal manifestations is clinically evident from the favourable response to immunosuppressive treatment.

Since recent studies have supported the concept that inhibition of TNF-α leads to clinical improvement in patients with ankylosing spondylitis, infliximab is being successfully used in the management of refractory articular disease associated with Crohn's disease.

The efficacy of intravenous cyclosporine in the treatment of pyoderma gangrenosum is well established. Infliximab is also a good alternative as its administration leads to rapid healing of skin lesions.

A few patients with erythema nodosum, aphthous ulcers, orofacial Crohn's disease and uveitis have been treated with anti-TNF therapies with satisfactory results.

For most of the inflammatory extraintestinal manifestations the primary target of treatment is the bowel. However, earlier aggressive therapy with biologic drugs can minimize systemic complications, particularly severe or refractory manifestations. Maintenance treatment with these novel therapies could also prevent some devastating consequences.

Long-term studies with larger numbers of patients will be necessary to determine the patients who are most likely to benefit from specific treatment.

References

1. Greenstein AJ, Janowiz HD, Sachar PB. The extra-intestinal complications of Crohn's disease and ulcerative colitis. A study of 700 patients. Medicine. 1976;55:401–12.
2. Tavarela Veloso F, Carvalho S, Magro F. Immune-related systemic manifestations of inflammatory bowel disease. A prospective study of 792 patients. J Clin Gastroenterol. 1996;23:29–34.
3. Snook J, Jewell D. Management of the extraintestinal manifestations of ulcerative colitis and Crohn's disease. Semin Gastroenterol Dis. 1991;2:115–25.
4. Rankin GB, Watts HD, Melnyl CJ, Kelley ML. National Cooperative Crohn's Disease Study: Extra-intestinal manifestations and perianal complications. Gastroenterology. 1979;77:914–20.
5. Das KM. Relationship of extraintestinal involvements in inflammatory bowel disease. New insight into autoimmune pathogeneses. Dig Dis Sci. 1999;44:1–13.
6. Tavarela Veloso F, Ferreira JT, Barros L, Almeida S. Clinical outcome of Crohn's disease: analysis according to the Vienna classification and clinical activity. Inflamm Bowel Dis. 2001;7:306–13.
7. Mewissen SG, Crusius JB, Pena AS, Dekker S, Dijkmans B. Spondyloarthropathy and idiopathic inflammatory bowel diseases. Inflamm Bowel Dis. 1997;3:25–37.
8. Tavarela Veloso F. Inflammatory extraintestinal manifestations associated with IBD. In: Monteiro E, Tavarela Veloso F, editors. Inflammatory Bowel Diseases: new insight into mechanisms of inflammation and challenges in diagnosis and treatment. Lancaster: Kluwer, 1995:232–6.
9. De Vos M, Mielants H, Cuvelier C, Elewaut D, Veys E. Long-term evolution of gut inflammation in patients with spondylarthropathy. Gastroenterology. 1996;110:1696–703.
10. Brandt J, Haibel H, Cornely D et al. Successful treatment of active ankylosing spondylitis with the anti-tumour necrosis factor alpha monochemical antibody infliximab. Arthritis Rheum. 2000;43:1346–52.
11. Van den Bosch F, Kruithol E, Baeten D, De Keyser F. Effects of a loading dose regimen of three infusions of chimenic monoclonal antibody to tumour necrosis factor alpha (infliximab) in spondyloarthropaty: an open pilot study. Ann Rheum Dis. 2000;59:428–33.
12. Stone M, Salonen D, Lax, Payne V, Lapp V, Inman R. Clinical and imaging correlates of response to treatment with infliximab in patients with ankylosing spondylitis. J Rheumatol. 2001;28:1605–14.
13. Gordan JD, Sack KE, Davis JC. Treatment of ankylosing spondylitis by inhibition of tumor necrosis factor α. N Engl J Med. 2002;346:1349–56.

14. Van den Bosch F, Kruithof E, De Vos M, De Keyser F, Mielants H. Crohn's disease associated with spondyloarthropathy: effect of TNF-α blockade with infliximab on articular symptoms. Lancet. 2000;356:1821–2.
15. Andus T, Herfarth H, Obermeier F et al. Improvement of arthritis/arthralgia after treatment with infliximab (Remicade) in a German prospective open-label multicenter trial in refractory Crohn's disease. Gastroenterology. 2001;120(Suppl. 1):A621.
16. Hanauer SB, Lichstenstein GR, Mayer M, Keenan G, Rutgeerts P. Extraintestinal manifestations of Crohn's disease: response to infliximab (Remicade) in the ACCENT I trial through 30 weeks. Am J Gastroenterol. Suppl. 66th Annual Scientific Meeting, Las Vegas, 2001.
17. Sampaio EP, Kaplan G, Miranda A et al. The influence of thalidomide on the clinical and immunologic manifestation of erythema nodosum leprosum. J Infect Dis. 1993;168:408–14.
18. Fleisher M, Rubin S, Levine A, Burns A, Jacksonville FL. Infliximab in the treatment of steroid refractory erythema nodosum of IBD. Gastroenterology. 2002;122(Suppl. 1):A618.
19. Matis WL, Ellis CN, Griffiths C, Lazarus G. Treatment of pyoderma gangrenosum with cyclosporine. Arch Dermatol. 1992;128:1060–4.
20. D'Inca R, Fagiuoli SC. Tacrolimus to treat pyoderma gangrenosum resistant to cyclosporine. Ann Intern Med. 1998;128:783–4.
21. Hohenleutner U, Mohr VS, Michel S, Landthaler M. Mycophenolate mofetil and cyclosporine treatment for recalcitrant pyoderma gangrenosum. Lancet. 1997;350:1748.
22. Friedman S, Marison J, Scherl E, Rubin P, Present D. Intravenous cyclosporine in refractory pyoderma gangrenosum complicating inflammatory bowel disease. Inflamm Bowel Dis. 2001;7:1–7.
23. Hong JJ, Merel NH, Hanauer SB. Treatment of pyoderma gangrenosum complicating Crohn's disease with infliximab. Gastroenterology. 2001;120(Suppl. 1):A621.
24. Sheldon DG, Sawchuck L, Kozarek K, Thirlby R. Twenty cases of peristomal pyoderma gangrenosum. Diagnostic implications and clinical management. Arch Surg. 2000;135:564–9.
25. Alexander LN, Wilcox MD. A prospective trial of thalidomide for the treatment of HIV associated idiopathic esophageal ulcers. AIDS Res Hum Retroviruses. 1997;4:301–4.
26. Casson D, Eltumi M, Tomlin S. Topical tacrolimus may be effective in the treatment of oral and perineal Crohn's disease. Gut. 2000;47:436–40.
27. Jacksonville FL, Fleisher M, Rubin S et al. Remicade in the treatment of refractory extraintestinal manifestations of Crohn's disease. Gastroenterology. 2001;120(Suppl. 1):A.
28. Smith JR, Levinson RD, Holland GN et al. Differential efficacy of tumor necrosis factor inhibition in the management of inflammatory eye disease and associated rheumatic disease. Arthritis Care Res. 2001;45:252–7.
29. Fries W, Giofre MR, Catanoso M. Treatment of acute uveitis associated with Crohn's disease and sacroileitis with infliximab. Am J Gastrenterol. 2002;97:499–500.

16
What do patients want? Defining treatment goals from the 'other side'

J. MINCHEW

I am a typical inflammatory bowel disease (IBD) patient. I was diagnosed with Crohn's disease at age 19, nearly 20 years ago. During this span of time I have taken just about every drug available and experienced many side-effects associated with these treatments. IBD treatments impact patients' lives dramatically, affecting their daily routines and functions.

Eight thousand, seven hundred and sixty … this number represents the average number of pills that I take in 1 year. I take a large handful of pills every day (approximately 22–24). My local pharmacy gave me a small container to carry my daily medications in. It holds about four pills! I can't possibly fit all of my medications in that container, but it did make me think about several things that this container implies about future IBD treatments. First, it implies that there will only be a few drugs necessary to carry around; second, that a patient will only need to take one of each kind of drug; and third, that they will be stable in pill form. It goes without saying that the treatments should have minimal side-effects. These will all lead to less stress on the patients and to greater compliance.

A major 'stress' factor for patients is the efficacy of any one drug. Is this treatment going to work for me? Many times it is trial-and-error as to what works best for each patient. It is extremely frustrating and discouraging for patients to have to try several different medicines, or to frequently have to switch medicines because they have developed toxicity to a drug. This process exposes patients to more side-effects. I believe that the key to finding a drug of universal efficacy will be to target the cause, not just treat the symptoms of the disease. More research money needs to be channelled in that direction.

Another major problem for patients is the number of times per day that some medications must be taken and also the number of pills necessary per dose. To be able to take all of my medicines once a day would be a dream come true. Twice a day is certainly manageable. Three times a day is usually no problem, but it gets a little hard if I am travelling or working or out of the house for the day. Four times a day is nearly impossible. I would bet that most patients are non-compliant when prescribed medicine four times a day. For optimal compliance, two or three times a day is about all you can expect a patient to follow. The number of pills that must be taken is also a problem. As it is now, the greatest number of my pills can be attributed to mesalamine, one of the most commonly prescribed drugs. For something so well prescribed, couldn't there be a better way to administer it than 12–16 large pills a day? I also take mycophenolate, budesonide, and metronidazole. I take omeprazole because the mycophenolate can cause damage to the lining of the stomach, and a multivitamin and iron pill because I am so anaemic. Taking all of this can fill me up in a hurry! I am a pretty compliant patient, but even I have trouble swallowing all of these. By the time I am done taking all of my medicines, I am sometimes too full to eat properly. As someone who struggles to maintain her weight, this can be a problem. Compliance is easiest if the request is simple. One pill of any one kind is enough and should be the goal when formulating new or improved drugs. In addition, treatments that require injections or are used intravenously, such as infliximab, are extremely inconvenient and impractical for most patients. This means missed work time or scheduling family life around the treatments. All of this adds stress to the patient, which can adversely affect the disease.

In addition to being concerned about whether a treatment will work or not, and keeping up with all their pills, patients have to deal with some very frightening and serious side-effects. It is very intimidating and sobering to read the drug information included in prescriptions. Having taken most of the commonly prescribed drugs for Crohn's disease, I can vouch for the impact they have on your life. I suffered from pneumonia and various other infections while on 6-mercaptopurine, and eventually could not maintain my white cell count. I then switched to methotrexate, and during my time on that developed pneumonitis on multiple occasions and reactive airway disease, which required hospitalization and treatment by a pulmonologist. It also meant many weeks of not being able to function at full strength, and missed hours of work. Eventually I could no longer tolerate the methotrexate and had to move onto mycophenolate. Once we found the dose that would not depress my white cell count this has worked very well, and I haven't had any major side-effects that I know of, yet. Metronidazole affected my sense of taste for a very long time. It may seem like a minor problem, but it was very annoying to have everything taste metallic. Infliximab has been a great addition to my medications, but I did experience a rate-related transfusion reaction. Intravenous iron was a disaster. I had an anaphylactic transfusion reaction with the test dose despite being premedicated with benedryl and steroids. I have saved our old friend prednisone for last! It truly is a miracle drug that can turn a bad situation around in a hurry, but at a great price sometimes. I have been fortunate enough to have been switched to budesonide for my long-term steroid use, but am very familiar with all the nasty side-effects of prednisone.

Prednisone takes a toll both physically and emotionally. Some of the side-effects that seem the most minor to you as physicians are the very ones that drive your patients over the edge. The cosmetic changes (moon face, facial hair, back hump, and weight gain) can turn anyone into a recluse. You avoid social situations, and feel very self-conscious. The annoying side-effects of night sweats and leg cramps interrupt your sleep drastically. Not sleeping properly affects your whole attitude and emotional state. It is probably the one side-effect that drives me the craziest. The intense mood swings affect your entire family, including children. Other serious side-effects include muscle weakness (leading to falls, not being able to walk up stairs), elevated blood sugar, infections, osteoporosis (additional tests and treatments), and skin changes. I have had to have stitches on four separate occasions because my skin has torn from simply bumping into things. Whoever stated that sometimes the treatment can be worse than the disease itself must have had prednisone in mind. I think it is easy to forget how dramatically these medications can affect your patients' lives, and how even the smallest of side-effects impacts them. So, your job as a physician is to thoroughly and honestly explain the potential side-effects of medications, be empathetic to each patient's situation, give personal attention to each patient, LISTEN, and have a positive attitude yourself. Not all the responsibility lies with you the physician, though. Patients need to take their disease seriously, but not let it take over their lives. A positive attitude goes a long way in dealing with a chronic disease. We all complain sometimes, but when it becomes the norm, rather than the exception, it becomes a problem and can adversely affect a patient's disease.

While we're talking about stress, we need to mention costs. Certainly those on multiple medications are the most affected. I had my pharmacy calculate the cost of my medications for 1 month (Table 1). The grand total for 1 month, with no form of insurance prescription coverage, is $1055.15 US! That equals $12,661.80 per year! Not many people can afford that kind of money. Even with a good insurance plan the copays (a small fee required at the time of service by many US insurance companies) add up to $125 a month or $1500 a year. That figure does not include the cost of the multivitamin that I take or the cost of infliximab, which costs approximately $3500 per infusion, and is given every 8 weeks or six times a year. At these prices, patients with insurance risk reaching the limits of their policies. Those without insurance risk financial ruin or become a tax burden to the society. Needless to say, many patients make choices every day about whether to fill their prescriptions or spend their money on more pressing matters. If they do fill them, they make them last longer by not taking the correct dose. Obviously, this is a problem that can cause devastating results.

One important treatment for IBD that hasn't been mentioned yet is surgery. This has some very strong positives, as well as negatives. Positive results are that surgery is a cure for ulcerative colitis; it can increase local disease control in Crohn's by resecting obstructions, strictures and fistulas; and it can decrease the disease burden in patients who have one section of bowel that is more problematic than others. The negatives of surgery include emotional anxiety (How much

Table 1 Costs of medication

Drug	Monthly cost ($US)	Copay ($US)
Mesalamine	225	25
Mycophenolate	307	25
Budesonide	220	40
Metronidazole	18	10
Omeprazole	285	25

will this disfigure me? Will I survive surgery? Will I have limitations?), pain, prolonged recovery (patients already ill take longer to recover and medications such as prednisone make it more difficult to heal), family impact (will they be able to function without me for a while, financial implications), and long-term psychological impact (Do you tell people? Will dating be a problem?). Certainly sometimes the positives outweigh the negatives. Quality of life is an important goal and surgery is a way to accomplish that goal for patients with intractable disease.

One final issue that I wanted to address is the access to clinical trials and studies. As it is now, the neediest patients – those with ostomies and on multiple, long-term medications – are excluded. This is a personal crusade for me because I fit both categories. As you can see from my list of medications, I am taking all the latest, most advanced drugs available in the US. Infliximab is already not giving me the boost it once did. I need access to the newer, more advanced medications now. I know the scientific reasons behind not including these patients; they make terrible controls. I can tell you that patients with ostomies can quantify the way they are feeling and their ostomy output, as well as the number of times per day they are experiencing output. I can also tell you that patients on multiple medications can establish a baseline of activity of their disease and recognize if an added drug is making a difference or not. If a protocol can still not be developed to include these patients, perhaps compassionate need should be reason enough to allow them access to clinical trials.

Obviously, I have presented the ideal scenario to you. Patients want a few drugs that will work for everyone. They should have few side-effects and be easy to administer. They should be affordable and accessible. In return, patients should be expected to do their part by maintaining a positive attitude and actively participating in their treatment. It may be a lofty goal, but one that I will hold out hope for.

17
Measuring health-related quality of life: fad, fantasy or fruitful exercise?

E. J. IRVINE

INTRODUCTION

The impact of inflammatory bowel disease (IBD) has been measured traditionally by assessing symptom severity indices that examine stool frequency, bleeding, abdominal pain and well-being, together with the endoscopic appearance of the colonic mucosa. Radiology and laboratory inflammatory markers, such as erythrocyte sedimentation rate, C-reactive protein or other acute-phase reactants are helpful but do not always reflect therapeutic response. Moreover, these assessment methods, even when used collectively, still fail to reflect the functional status of some patients. Health-related quality of life (HRQOL) has emerged, therefore, as a clinically relevant measure of disease impact and treatment response.

HRQOL has been defined as the perceived functional effect of an illness and its therapy on an individual as described from the patient's own perspective. Several different domains determine HRQOL and these include physical and occupational function, emotional state, social interactions, and somatic sensation[1]. Clinicians may choose to consider the determinants as simply disease-related, including symptom severity, treatment efficacy, adverse effects of treatment, or disease-independent factors such as age, gender, education and knowledge, personality and coping skills, culture and beliefs[2].

Chronic illness is only one of the features that impacts on HRQOL in a bio-psychosocial model that was proposed by George Engel and applied more recently in functional gastrointestinal disorders as well as IBD[3]. Briefly, the model suggests that, in subjects with a biological predisposition to a particular condition, such as IBD, the presence of certain environmental or psychosocial factors (e.g. infection or stress), can trigger or modulate gut motility motor and sensory function. These changes are effected through complex interactions between the central, peripheral or enteric nervous systems producing a symptom and response pattern. Individual experiences and beliefs may also change these variables. This helps explain why no two individuals have identical biological function despite, in some cases, a rather similar clinical course.

HRQOL QUESTIONNAIRES

Evaluating HRQOL involves applying questionnaires that attempt to address the particular problems of chronic illness in a quantitative way. The types of instrument applied are utilities (global or summary scores), generic measures (multi-item profiles generated in a general population that can be applied to different diseases), and disease-specific instruments (developed in and for patients affected by a common condition) (reviewed in ref. 4). The main impetus supporting the use of a global assessment is the simple administration and scoring, while generic measures such as the SF-36[5] or Psychological Well Being Index (PGWBI)[6] permit comparisons between groups with different conditions. Disease-specific questionnaires are most likely to detect small but clinically important risks or benefits[4,7,8]. There are several ways to report the scores of the generic and disease-specific questionnaires. All items can be summed in a global or utility score, several similar items within a domain (such as physical function) can be clustered together in subscores, and individual items can also be considered as shown in Fig. 1. A considerable literature is available describing HRQOL assessment in gastrointestinal and liver disease and is reviewed in detail elsewhere[9]. The selection of which questionnaire to use at a particular time, should be determined by the particular application. For example, a clinician might prefer to use a global assessment, the health policy analyst a generic instrument and the clinical trial researcher a disease-specific instrument. Patients generally just hope to inform their caregivers about their areas of dysfunction to find solutions to their problems. It has become fashionable to combine the use of generic and disease-specific questionnaires in research to prevent missing important disease outcomes. However, selecting the best questionnaire(s) for a particular study should be based upon the research question and methodology. Users of these questionnaires should be cognizant of the need to use only well-evaluated tools that have established psychometric properties (*validity, reliability, responsiveness*)[4,7–12]. A list of HRQOL questionnaires[5,6,13–20] used in IBD patients and their psychometric properties is shown in Table 1.

Nordin *et al.*[21], in an almost population-based study, examining 492 patients registered in Sweden at the University of Uppsala hospital, demonstrated that the

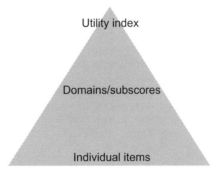

Fig. 1 The HRQOL pyramid

Table 1 HRQOL instruments used in inflammatory bowel disease

Global assessments
1. Utility (Standard Gamble or Time Trade Off; 0.0 death to 1.0 perfect health)
2. Visual analogue scale (feeling thermometer, 10 cm line)
3. Graded scale (excellent, very good, good, poor, extremely poor)

Generic instruments
1. Psychological General Well Being[6] (22 items; six subscales [anxiety, depression, well-being, self-control, health, vitality]; reliability 0.61–0.89; score 22–132, lower score better)
2. Short Form 36[5] (36 items, eight subscores; score 0, worst; 100, best)
3. Sickness Impact Profile[13] (136 items, 12 subscores; higher score = worse HRQOL)
4. Grogono and Woodgate[14] (20 items, 10 subscales)
5. Cleveland Clinic Questionnaire[15] (47 items, four subscores)
6. EuroQOL[16] (5 items-utility)

Disease-specific instruments
1. Inflammatory Bowel Disease questionnaire[17] (IBDQ; 32 items, four subscores, 32–224)
2. Rating Form of IBD Patient Concerns[18] (RFIPC) (25 items, four subscores, 0–100)
3. Cleveland Clinic Questionnaire[19] (18 items, four subscores, 0–100)
4. Pentasa Study instrument[20] (seven items, 0–100)

---

patients with Crohn's disease (CD) had significantly worse ($p < 0.05$) Physical Component Summary scores (PCS) (46.7 vs. 50.3) and Mental Component Summary scores (MCS) (43.0 vs. 50.1) for the SF-36 than did the normal population, while for the patients with ulcerative colitis (UC) only the PCS was significantly worse than the normal population (PCS 50.0, MCS 46.7). In addition, six of the eight subscores were poorer in UC patients (except physical function and bodily pain) while all eight subscores were significantly worse in those with CD than in the general population. An earlier study by Richards and Irving[22] was one of the first to examine the EuroQOL utility in patients with short bowel, most of whom had CD and were on home parenteral nutrition. The mean EuroQOL score for these patients was 0.51 (midway between death 0.0 and full health 1.0), compared to the background population score of 0.84. Interestingly, age was also an important predictor of self-rated health, being worse in the oldest (over age 55) compared to the youngest participants (under age 45 years). Respondents also scored worse in six of the eight subscores (not role emotional or mental health) of the SF-36 than the background population. Muir *et al.*[23] examined short-term outcomes in patients with UC preoperatively and post-colectomy with J pouch construction and observed that all eight of the SF-36 subscores were significantly worse than in the general population, but that these values 'normalized' after surgical therapy. In a Finnish study examining long-term outcome (median follow-up of 8 years post-colectomy) with a J pouch, all of the subscores of the SF-36 were similar to the 'normal' Finnish population[24]. However, only 65% of pouch patients were fully continent, 28% had some sleep disturbance, 25% had difficulty discriminating gas from stool and 71% had anal itching, that was chronic in 15%. In a small group with poor HRQOL there was a strong relationship between poor bowel function (if > 10 movements per day), chronic pouchitis, anal incontinence, and poor HRQOL. This, then, suggested a 'ceiling effect' of the generic questionnaire and demonstrated why a disease-specific instrument might be more relevant to a particular group of patients.

In a large study involving 13 countries, almost 2000 patients were surveyed to evaluate the determinants of HRQOL[25]. In both CD and UC the strongest determinant was disease severity, which explained 44% of the variance in HRQOL. This would suggest that effective therapy should definitely improve HRQOL status. Indeed, several clinical trials[26–29], examining anti-inflammatory drugs (5-aminosalicylates, corticosteroids, immunosuppressives and biological agents such as remicade) have shown significant improvements in HRQOL scores when the treatment administered effectively reduced disease severity. However, even patients in remission still appear to have residual impairment of HRQOL when compared to non-IBD subjects and healthy controls.

A recent review by Katon *et al.* has acknowledged comorbid medical and psychiatric illnesses as contributing substantially to poorer disease outcomes, higher mortality, greater use of health resources and poorer HRQOL in patients with chronic illness[30]. These patients often suffer from somatization disorders and multiple-organ system complaints, poorer adherence and also an increased mortality rate. The results of several studies (838 patients in 18 studies) have been combined in a Cochrane systematic review, to demonstrate a significant benefit from the use of antidepressant therapy using either a tricyclic or specific serotonin receptor inhibitor (odds ratio 0.37) in patients with depression together with a significant comorbid chronic illness[31].

Recent studies suggest that both depression and anxiety may be increased in patients with active IBD, and although some relationship exists between active disease and anxiety, depression appears to be an independent predictor of poor disease outcome, as measured by HRQOL instruments and health-care utilization[32,33]. In addition, work absenteeism and reduced productivity are also greater in patients with anxiety or depression. Until now, no effective mood-restoring interventions have been undertaken in IBD populations. One example of a study that attempted to address these issues was a randomized trial comparing medical therapy alone or combined with 10 verbal therapy sessions, which included instruction on relaxation, education and health-promoting behaviour aimed at improving coping skills and adjustment to disease[34]. The primary outcomes for that trial were remission and surgery rates, not the most relevant outcomes for a trial examining a psychosocial intervention. Although health status questionnaires were also applied during the trial, no significant improvements were noted after the intervention. It is likely that the main reason for the negative results was not identifying those patients who particularly needed such therapy. Other studies examining the use of patient support groups have had poor attendance and limited success, because of lack of selection of the patients in most need, and also because, at any given time, the majority of patients are coping with their illness. It is more likely that, at times of emotional stress (with or without active disease), when patients are coping poorly, short bursts of a supportive psychosocial intervention might have an important impact on HRQOL outcomes[35,36].

In summary, HRQOL is impaired in IBD patients and HRQOL status is worse in patients with active disease or more aggressive disease. Importantly, patients who have added depression or anxiety have poorer HRQOL than do patients without anxiety or depression. Interventions to reduce disease activity, whether medical or surgical, will ultimately improve HRQOL outcomes in the IBD population. The efficacy of psychosocial interventions is not yet proven and must be examined. Nevertheless, measuring HRQOL is an important part of assessing the burden of illness attributable to IBD, and should be a measured target for applied research.

References

1. Spilker B. Quality of Life and Pharmacoeconomics in Clinical Trials, 2nd edn. Philadelphia: Lippincott-Raven, 1996.
2. Garrett JW, Drossman DA. Health status in inflammatory bowel disease: Biological and behavioral considerations. Gastroenterology. 1990;99:90–6.
3. Engel GL. The clinical application of the biopsychosocial model. Am J Psychiatry. 1980;137: 535–44.
4. Guyatt GH, Feeny DH, Patrick DL. Measuring health-related quality of life. Ann Intern Med. 1993;118:622–9.
5. Ware JE, Sherbourne CD. The MOS 36 item Short Form Health Survey (SF-36).Conceptual framework and item selection. Med Care. 1992;30:473–83.
6. Dupuy HJ. The Psychological General Well Being Index. In: Assessment of Quality of Life in Clinical Trials of Cardiovascular Therapies. Wenger NK, Mattson ME, editors.
7. Furberg CF, Ellinson J. Le Jaq Publishing, 1984:170–83.
8. Patrick DL, Deyo RA. Generic and disease-specific measures in assessing health status and quality of life. Med Care. 1989; 27(Suppl. 3):S217–32.
9. Borgaonkar M, Irvine EJ. Quality of life measurement in gastrointestinal and liver disorders. Gut. 2000;47:444–54.
10. Ware JE. SF-36 Health Survey Manual and Interpretation Guide. Second printing 1997.
11. Deyo RA, Diehr P, Patrick DL. Reproducibility and responsiveness of health status measures: statistics and strategies for evaluation. Controlled Clin Trials. 1991;12:142–58S.
12. Guyatt GH, Walter S, Norman G. Measuring change over time: assessing the usefulness of evaluative instruments. J Chron Dis. 1987;40:171–8.
13. Bergner M, Bobbitt RA, Carter WB et al. The Sickness Impact Profile: Development and final revision of a health status measure. Med Care. 1981;19:787–805.
14. Grogono AW, Woodgate DJ. Index for measuring health. Lancet. 1971:1:1024–6.
15. Rudick RA, Miller D, Clough JD, Gragg LA, Farmer RG. Quality of life in multiple sclerosis. Comparison with inflammatory bowel disease and rheumatoid arthritis. Arch Neurol. 1992;49: 1237–42.
16. The EuroQOL Group. EuroQOL – a new facility for the measurement of health-related quality of life. Health Policy. 1990;16:199–208.
17. Guyatt GH, Mitchell A, Irvine EJ et al. A new measure of health status for clinical trials in IBD. Gastroenterology. 1989;96:804–10.
18. Drossman DA, Patrick DL, Mitchell CM et al. Health-related quality of life in inflammatory bowel disease: functional status and patient worries and concerns. Dig Dis Sci. 1989;34: 1379–86.
19. Farmer RG, Easley KA, Farmer JM. Quality of life assessment by patients with inflammatory bowel disease. Cleve Clin J Med. 1992;59:35–42.
20. Robinson M, Hanauer S, Hoop R et al. Mesalamine capsules enhance the quality of life for patients with ulcerative colitis. Aliment Pharmacol Ther. 1994;8:27–34.
21. Nordin K, Pahlman L, Larsson K et al. Health-related quality of life and psychological distress in a population-based sample of Swedish patients with inflammatory bowel disease. Scand J Gastroenterol. 2002;37:450–7.
22. Richards DM, Irving MH. Assessing the quality of life of patients with intestinal failure on home parenteral nutrition. Gut. 1997;40:218–22.
23. Muir AJ, Edwards LJ, Sanders LL et al. A prospective evaluation of health-related quality of life after ileal pouch–anal anastomosis for ulcerative colitis. Am J Gastroenterol. 2001;96:1480–5.
24. Tiainen J, Matikainen M. Health-related quality of life after ileal J-pouch–anal anastomosis for ulcerative colitis: long-term results. Scand J Gastroenterol. 1999;34:601–5.
25. Irvine EJ, Bolin T, Grace E et al. and the International Quality of Life Study Group. Geographic differences in health related quality of life in inflammatory bowel disease. Gastroenterology. 1997;A1003.

26. Martin F, Sutherland L, Beck IT *et al*. Oral 5ASA versus prednisone in short term treatment of Crohn's disease: a multicentre controlled trial. Can J Gastroenterol. 1990;4:452–8.
27. Greenberg GR, Feagan BG, Martin FM *et al*. Oral budesonide for active Crohn's disease. N Engl J Med. 1994;331:836–41.
28. Feagan BG, Rochon J, Fedorak RN *et al*. Methotrexate for the treatment of Crohn's disease. N Engl J Med. 1995;332:292–7.
29. Targan S, Hanauer SB, Van Deventer SJH *et al*. A short-term study of chimeric monoclonal antibody cA2 to tumor necrosis factor α for Crohn's disease. N Engl J Med. 1997;337:1029–35.
30. Katon W, Sullivan M, Walker E. Medical symptoms without identified pathology: relationship to psychiatric disorders, childhood and adult trauma, and personality traits. Ann Intern Med. 2001; 134:917–25.
31. Gill D, Hatcher S. Antidepressants for depression in medical illness. Cochrane Database Syst Rev. 2000(4):CD001312.
32. Guthrie E, Jackson J, Shaffer J *et al*. Psychological disorder and severity of inflammatory bowel disease predict health related quality of life in ulcerative colitis and Crohn's disease. Am J Gastroenterol. 2002;97:1994–9.
33. De Boer A, Sprangers MA, Bartlesman JF, de Haes HC. Predictors of health care utilization in patients with inflammatory bowel disease: a longitudinal study. Eur J Gastroenterol Hepatol. 1998;10:783–9.
34. Jantschek G, Zeitz M, Pritsch M *et al*. Effect of psychotherapy on the course of Crohn's disease. Results of the German prospective multicenter psychotherapy treatment study on Crohn's disease. German Study Group on Psychosocial Intervention in Crohn's disease. Scand J Gastroenterol. 1998;33:1289–96.
35. Moody GA, Bhakta P, Mayberry JF. Disinterest in local self-help groups amongst patients with inflammatory bowel disease in Leicester. Int J Colorect Dis. 1993;8:181–3.
36. Joachim G. The birth and dissolution of an inflammatory bowel disease support group: lessons in providing support. Gastroenterol Nurs. 1998;21:119–24.

Section VI
Specific targets

18
Specific targets of treatment: diarrhoea

W. KRUIS, R. M. HOFFMANN and D. J. ZIEGENHAGEN

INTRODUCTION

Diarrhoea is a leading symptom in patients with inflammatory bowel disease (IBD). At least 90% of patients with ulcerative colitis (UC) or those with Crohn's disease (CD) suffer intermittently or chronically from a form of diarrhoea.

In general, diarrhoea is thought to be a consequence of inflammatory reactions and damage to the intestinal mucosa. However, observations of diarrhoea in patients without active inflammation, as well as persistent diarrhoea in patients undergoing effective anti-inflammatory treatment, indicate causes of diarrhoea other than only inflammation. In addition one should keep in mind that not only IBD may exist in a patient, but there may also be other non-intestinal diseases such as hyperthyroidism which can cause diarrhoea.

In this chapter the multiple aetiologies of diarrhoea in patients with IBD, and appropriate therapeutic strategies, are reviewed.

INFLAMMATION CAUSING DIARRHOEA

Pathogenesis

Inflammation causes on the one hand decreased absorption of electrolytes and food ingredients, and on the other hand increased fluid secretion. Additional mechanisms leading to diarrhoea are a loss of plasma from damaged mucosa and altered motor activity[1]. As yet unknown stimuli from the intestinal lumen activate mucosal cells such as polymorphonuclear neutrophil leucocytes, macrophages and monocytes leading to production of arachidonic acid metabolites, histamine, platelet-activating factor, cytokines and other factors which are able to mediate and amplify inflammatory reactions. Inflammation results in a significant decrease of mucosal resistance (Isc) and transmural potential difference[2], which is associated with impaired sodium absorption. These alterations in intestinal functions may be a systemic effect of inflammation because of findings in active ulcerative colitis (UC) where electrolyte and water malabsorption was also found in unaffected jejunal segments[3].

At the cellular level a molecular pump, the $(Na^+ + K^+)$-ATPase, plays an important role in the regulation of electrolyte and water fluxes across the cell membrane. Colonic $(Na^+ + K^+)$-ATPase can be inhibited by arachidonic acid[4]. There exists an inverse relationship between colonic $(Na^+ + K^+)$-ATPase activity and the degree of mucosal inflammation in IBD[5].

Treatment

The aim of stopping diarrhoea in patients with active IBD is to control inflammatory processes. Thus, treatment is according to standard protocols. Basic therapy is aimed at compensating electrolyte and water losses as quickly and completely as possible. There is much controversy on the question of whether additional antidiarrhoeal drugs should be used in this situation. In the early years of the introduction of loperamide, case reports on worsening of active UC were published. This may be a result of antidiarrhoeal therapy but also of inappropriate standard treatment.

Corticosteroids, very effective anti-inflammatory drugs, also act directly on electrolyte and water fluxes. They induce sodium and potassium channels and they stimulate $(Na^+ + K^+)$-ATPase activity, resulting in improvement of diarrhoea in patients with UC prior to any effects on mucosal inflammation[6]. Most likely these antidiarrhoeal effects vary between different corticosteroids. In patients with collagenous colitis diarrhoea could be abolished with budesonide when the patients were refractory to prednisone[7].

NON-INFLAMMATORY CAUSES OF DIARRHOEA

In addition to a flare of the underlying IBD, diarrhoea in this patient group can be due to multiple aetiologies[8]. Table 1 comprises a list of non-inflammatory causes of diarrhoea in IBD. An attempt is made to include these different causes into a system which may help and guide differential diagnosis in a given patient.

Structural alterations

Though stenoses or strictures obstruct the regular passage, disintegration of solid and liquid bowel contents may lead to loose or even watery stools simulating diarrhoea. Fistula formation between proximal and distal bowel segments acts

Table 1 Non-inflammatory causes of diarrhoea in IBD

Structural alterations
Stenosis/stricture, fistula, resection/short bowel

Functional disorders
Rectosigmoid irritability, psychological

Varia
Infection, bacterial overgrowth, bile salt loss, lactose intolerance, drugs

---

like a short circuit, excludes the bowel contents from becoming thickened, and may produce softening of the stools.

Resection(s) of parts of the intestines may lead to diarrhoea either in a more global way or because of a loss of specific functions. Removal of a significant length of bowel(s) may result in short bowel syndrome. Apparently the frequency of this devastating situation is decreasing in recent years, most likely due to generally established tissue-saving surgical techniques and the development of superior medical treatment strategies. The symptoms and consequences of short bowel syndrome are complex and require a combined therapeutic approach. Diets and motility-modulating drugs such as loperamide or codeine play a major role in controlling diarrhoea. Somatostatin analogues may show beneficial effects in selected cases.

A still-existing clinical problem are the complications following ileal resection. Disruption of the enterohepatic cycling, and the subsequent exposure of the colonic mucosa to bile salts, can cause watery diarrhoea or steatorrhoea. Because bile acid malabsorption is not always related to ileal resection it is discussed in a later section of this chapter.

Functional disorders

Sometimes patients with inactive IBD, particularly with UC, resemble patients with irritable bowel syndrome. Indeed, early observations compared colonic motor activity between the two entities and in both diseases found an increase in the motility index[9]. Gastrointestinal motility disorders were also described in patients with inactive Crohn's disease[10]. Studies by Rao et al.[11] related diarrhoea in UC to increased rectosigmoid irritability rather than to rapid colonic transit, which may preferably contribute to diarrhoea in active pancolitis.

On the basis of these and similar data loperamide was proposed as a very valuable drug in the treatment of diarrhoea in UC if used after proper evaluation of the patient. Patients with inactive and more distal disease (not extended disease) should be considered for this treatment[12].

Another cause of non-organic diarrhoea in IBD may be psychological. To our knowledge there are no systematic studies in this area; but experienced clinicians can quote patients' comments such as: 'In contrast to travelling to work or to public events where I cannot go, or I'm not supposed to go, to the restrooms whenever I like to do so, at home in a familiar environment I feel much less urge, or no urge, to go to the toilet.' Such patients can sometimes be helped by simple relaxing exercises. Others need to have a feeling of using 'safe' antidiarrhoeals such as loperamide.

Other non-inflammatory causes of diarrhoea

Infection

Superimposed infection leading to diarrhoea can resemble a flare of IBD. Usually this type of infection is caused by a virus or by bacteria. Quite a number of studies have demonstrated a considerable frequency of superimposed infections concerning variable pathogens. In a given clinical situation the yield of positive microbiological tests depends not least on the skill and intensity of investigations performed, but results are often disappointing. Nevertheless, the consensus conference of the Deutsche Gesellschaft für Verdauungs- und Stoffwechselkrankheiten recommends microbiological testing at initial diagnosis and when deterioration or relapses occur[13]. A more practical, inexpensive and evidence-based approach to the accurate diagnosis of infectious disease is a detailed history. The sudden onset of maximal diarrhoea points towards infection, whereas a subacute onset with increasing diarrhoea is typical of a flare of IBD[14].

Particular attention should be paid to a patient who has recently received antibiotic therapy. In cases of rapid-onset diarrhoea a check for *Clostridium difficile* should be undertaken[8]. In general, less attention is paid to superimposed parasitic infection. The most frequent parasite in developed countries is *Giardia lamblia*, with a prevalence of 10–20% in the general population. A recent investigation in German IBD patients found significant giardiasis in more than 20% of patients. Of particular interest were results in patients treated for their giardiasis with metronidazole, demonstrating improved clinical activity and diarrhoea in most of the patients[15].

Treatment of superimposed infections follows general guidelines depending on the underlying microorganism.

Bile salt loss

Bile acid diarrhoea should be considered in patients with diseased or previously resected terminal ileum. In healthy subjects more than 90% of the cycling bile acid pool becomes reabsorbed through specific ileal function. Malabsorption leads to an increased load of bile acids in the colon, causing secretion of water and ions with subsequent diarrhoea. For therapeutic considerations it is important to distinguish between a compensated form of bile acid loss, where novel hepatic bile acid synthesis can compensate colonic loss, and a decompensated form, where the faecal loss exceeds the *de-novo* synthesis. Compensated bile acid loss causes watery diarrhoea, whereas the decompensated form is related to steatorrhoea. All degrees of bile acid loss and diarrhoea occur frequently in ileal IBD[16]. Today, diagnosis of bile acid loss is accurate and easy, determining 7α-hydroxy-4-cholesten-3-one in serum[17].

Treatment of compensated bile acid loss diarrhoea is by a diet restricted in fat and, in addition, cholestyramine before meals. The dose of cholestyramine should be titrated according to the quality of stools. In decompensated bile acid loss diarrhoea the mainstay of treatment is a strict diet with a fat content comprising exclusively middle-chain triglycerides (MCT). In some cases of not-too-advanced bile acid loss small doses of cholestyramine may be helpful.

Bacterial small bowel overgrowth

Mainly in patients with small bowel CD, stenoses/strictures or a history of laparotomy, bacterial overgrowth of the small intestines, particularly of proximal segments, should be considered when otherwise unexplained diarrhoea exists[8]. Functional alterations and structural destination cause impairment of the propulsive motor activity and promote ascending colonization of bacteria from the colon.

Though not definitely accurate bacterial overgrowth can easily be diagnosed by hydrogen breath testing using glucose as substrate[18].

Treatment has been demonstrated to be effective with norfloxacin and amoxycillin-clavulinic acid[19]. Because of otherwise reported therapeutic efficacy and tolerability in IBD quinolone antibiotics should be the choice.

Lactose intolerance

Lactose intolerance and subsequent diarrhoea occur frequently in IBD. Ileal CD is associated with a higher incidence of lactose intolerance than is Crohn's colitis. While UC patients may not suffer from lactose intolerance during inactive disease, malabsorption has been shown during acute colitis flares. It is notable that lactose malabsorption may be determined by factors other than lactase enzyme activity such as bacterial overgrowth and/or altered small bowel transit[8].

The diagnostic gold standard of lactose malabsorption and intolerance is hydrogen breath testing with lactose as substrate. In IBD patients with otherwise unexplained diarrhoea lactose intolerance should be either diagnosed or it should be treated empirically with lactose avoidance.

Drugs

Paradoxically, some of the medication for the treatment of IBD can also cause diarrhoea. Very rarely this may be due to allergic reactions, e.g. against amino-salicylates. Of more clinical relevance were early observations of an increased frequency of diarrhoea in patients treated with olsalazine, an azo-bond double molecule, consisting of two molecules of 5-aminosalicylic acid.

Animal studies have shown significant effects on water and electrolyte fluxes along the entire bowel resulting in netto fluid secretion[20]. Olsalazine as well as mesalazine were found to inhibit intestinal $(Na^+ + K^+)$-ATPase activity in humans[21]. The diarrhoeal effects of olsalazine may be more pronounced because of the direct exposure of the entire small and large intestinal mucosa to the double molecule. In contrast, because of delayed-release delivery formulations of mesalazine, the secretory effects are related only to the distal ileum and colon; thus the diarrhoeal potency may be less pronounced.

Treatment of drug-induced diarrhoea in IBD requires consideration of this possible adverse effect. Olsalazine in high doses is better tolerated when used in increasing doses, given in divided doses and applied strictly after meals[22]. Alternatively, mesalazine or sulphasalazine can be used.

CONCLUSIONS

Diarrhoea is a leading and debilitating symptom in patients with IBD. It can be due to multiple aetiologies. Most often it is related to a flare of the underlying IBD, but diarrhoea should always stimulate a thorough differential diagnosis of alternative causes other than inflammatory reaction (Fig. 1).

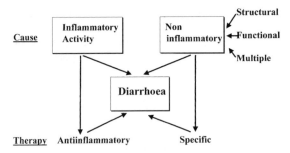

Fig. 1 Pathogenesis and treatment of diarrhoea in IBD

Acknowledgement

The authors gratefully appreciate the secreterial support of L. Sallhoff.

References

1. Sartor RB, Powell DW. Mechanism of diarrhea in intestinal inflammation and hypersensitivity: immune system modulation of intestinal transport. In: Field M, editor: Diarrheal Diseases. New York: Elsevier, 1991:75–114.
2. Hawker PC, McKay JS, Turnberg LA. Electrolyte transport across colonic mucosa from patients with inflammatory bowel disease. Gastroenterology. 1980;79:508–11.
3. Binder HJ, Ptak T. Jejunal absorption of water and electrolytes in inflammatory bowel disease. J Lab Clin Med. 1970;76:915–24.
4. Allgayer H, Brown L, Kruis W, Erdmann E, Paumgartner G. Inhibition of human colonic (Na$^+$+K$^+$)-ATPase by arachidonic and linoleic acid. Naunyn-Schmiedeberg's Arch Pharmacol. 1986;332:398–402.
5. Allgayer H, Kruis W, Paumgartner G, Wiebecke B, Brown L, Erdmann E. Inverse relationship between colonic (Na$^+$+K$^+$)-ATPase activity and degree of mucosal inflammation in inflammatory bowel disease. Dig Dis Sci. 1988;33:417–22.
6. Scheurlen C, Allgayer H, Kruis W, Hardt M, Sauerbruch T. Effect of a short term topical corticosteroid treatment on mucosal enzyme systems in patients with distal inflammatory bowel disease. Hepato-Gastroenterology. 1998;45:1539–45.
7. Lanyi B, Dries V, Dienes HP, Kruis W. Therapy of prednisone refractory collagenous colitis with budesonide. Int J Colorect Dis. 1999;14:58–61.
8. Gerson LB, Triadafilopoulos G. Palliative care in inflammatory bowel disease: an evidence-based approach. Inflamm Bowel Dis. 2000;6:228–43.
9. Chaudhary NA, Truelove SC. Human colonic motility: a comparative study of normal subjects, patients with ulcerative colitis and patients with irritable bowel syndrome. I. Resting patterns of motility. Gastroenterology. 1961;40:1–17.
10. Annese V, Bassotti G, Napolitano G, Usai P, Andriulli A, Vantrappen G. Gastrointestinal motility disorders in patients with inactive Crohn's disease. Scand J Gastroenterol. 1997;32:1107–17.
11. Rao SSC, Read NW, Brown C, Bruce C, Holdsworth CD. Studies on the mechanism of bowel disturbance in ulcerative colitis. Gastroenterology. 1987;93:934–40.
12. Heit HA. Use of antidiarrheals in ulcerative colitis. Gastroenterology. 1988;94:1520.
13. Stange EF, Riemann J, von Herbay A *et al.* Diagnostik und Therapie der Colitis ulcerosa – Ergebnisse einer evidenzbasierten Konsensuskonferenz der Deutschen Gesellschaft für Verdauungs und Stoffwechselkrankheiten. Z Gastroenterol. 2001;39:19–72.
14. Schumacher G, Sandstedt B, Kollberg B. A prospective study of first attacks of inflammatory bowel disease and infectious colitis. Clinical findings and early diagnosis. Scand J Gastroenterol. 1994;29:265–74.
15. Scheurlen C, Kruis W, Weinzierl M, Lamina J, Paumgartner G. Giardiasis in patients with Crohn's disease. Scand J Gastroenterol. 1988;23:833–9.

16. Kruis W, Kalek HD, Stellaard F, Paumgartner G. Altered fecal bile acid pattern in patients with inflammatory bowel disease. Digestion. 1986;35:189–98.
17. Sauter GH, Münzing W, von Ritter Ch, Paumgartner G. Bile acid malabsorption as a cause of chronic diarrhea. Diagnostic value of 7α-hydroxy-4-cholesten-3-one in serum. Dig Dis Sci. 1999;44:14–19.
18. Romagnulo J, Schiller D, Bailey RJ. Using breath tests wisely in a gastroenterology practice: an evidence-based review of indications and pitfalls in interpretation. Am J Gastroenterol. 2002;97: 1113–26.
19. Attar A, Flourie B, Rambaud JC et al. Antibiotic efficacy in small intestinal bacterial overgrowth-related chronic diarrhea: a crossover, randomized trial. Gastroenterology. 1999;117:794–7.
20. Scheurlen C, Wedel S, Kruis W, Zwiebel FM, Allgayer H, Scholz R. Olsalazine-related diarrhea: does rat intestine adapt in vivo? Scand J Gastroenterol. 1992;27:311–16.
21. Scheurlen C, Allgayer H, Kruis W, Erdmann E, Sauerbruch T. Effect of olsalazine and mesalazine on human ileal and colonic $(Na^+ + K^+)$-ATPase. A possible diarrhogenic factor? Clin Invest. 1993;71:286–9.
22. Kruis W, Brandes J-W, Schreiber S et al. Olsalazine versus mesalazine in the treatment of mild to moderate ulcerative colitis: a randomized double-blind multicentre trial. Aliment Pharmacol Ther. 1998;12:707–15.

19
Abdominal pain as a therapeutic target in inflammatory bowel disease

H. J. F. HODGSON

Lay literature contains numerous allusions to the belief that the mind cannot recollect pain. This is an interesting concept – to remember that one experienced pain is simple, to relive that pain in the imagination is indeed, perhaps fortunately, very hard. Such considerations remind us that, in considering pain as a therapeutic target – in inflammatory bowel disease or indeed in any other condition – pain has peculiar problems of its own. Notably, for example, the sensation of pain and the perception of pain are not identical; the assessment of the severity and description of type of pain is difficult; and, as already mentioned, recollection is imperfect.

The afferent innovation of the gastrointestinal tract is highly complex and remains ill-understood[1]. Conventional sensory afferents pass to the posterior columns of the spinal cord, their cell bodies lying in the dorsal root ganglia. Eventually they reach the thalamic area, and conscious appreciation may result. In general, all conscious appreciation of pathophysiological stimuli from the gut is attributed to this pathway. However, these ascending pathways also receive inputs from somatic areas, explaining both somatic radiation and/or referral of visceral pain. In contrast the vagal afferents pass via the nodose ganglia and are believed to be largely associated with physiological and non-pathological signalling. Patients with intact vagal tracts but transected spinal cords are said not to feel the pain of intestinal obstruction.

The receptors within the gut whence these afferent impulses come are complex – mechanoreceptors clearly, but also chemical receptors. Intrinsic gut neurones also have both afferent arms with chemical and mechanoreceptor function, with probably efferent actions on smooth muscle and vasculature[2,3]. Moreover the sensitivity of all these afferents is apparently modulatable – by interneuronal connections mediated by transmitters such as adenosine, adenosine diphosphate and adrenalin; by mediators from blood vessels such as bradykinin; by inflammatory mediators such as interleukin-1 and tumour necrosis factor-α, eicosanoids, histamine, and even proteolytic enzymes[4-7]. Thus the ancient correlations of colic with pain due to mechanoreceptor activation, and tenderness as pain receptors in the parietal peritoneum become sensitized, are only very abbreviated versions of a complex system.

Whilst events in the periphery, such as inflammation, can clearly alter the sensitivity of efferent nerve ending in the gut, there are also striking central-peripheral interactions. The sensitivity of stretch receptors, for example, can be modulated by stress – with pathways descending via the autonomic nervous system to affect baroreceptor sensitivity[8], mediated through factors such as substance P and neurokinin A[9,10]. Furthermore central modulation will affect an individual's appreciation of pain via, for example, opiate and serotonin receptors in the brainstem, and via modulation of cognition. The latter projection, with involvement of the limbic system, clearly highlights the whole area of personality and pain perception.

Gastroenterologists are prone to characterizing certain patients as having 'low pain thresholds' and 'supratentorial' or 'functional' overlay. How relevant is this to inflammatory bowel disease, and thus to pain as a therapeutic target? Gastroenterologists use functional bowel disease and the irritable bowel syndrome as the frame of reference for this. Well-characterized experimental systems have demonstrated increased neuronal sensitivity in irritable bowel and functional gut disease[11]. In non-ulcer dyspepsia, for example, gastric distension using an intraluminal balloon needs to be significantly less before pain is elicited, whilst the threshold to similar duodenal stimulation or to transcutaneous nerve stimulation is normal in the same patient[12,13]. When progressive inflation of an intrarectal balloon is performed in irritable bowel syndrome patients and healthy patients, with progressive discomfort leading to elicit pain, the curve of required volume is shifted significantly to the left in irritable bowel syndrome[14]. More strikingly, positron emission tomography scanning, which visualizes areas of increased cerebral blood flow in real time, demonstrates that a greater extent and distribution of increased vascular flow is induced by visceral pain in patients with irritable bowel syndrome, with relative hyperperfusion in the thalamic and anterior cingulate areas and the prefrontal cortex[9].

Given that up to 50% of patients with inflammatory bowel disease may have associated irritable bowel-type syndrome, does pain control remain an appropriate therapeutic goal, particularly in the context of seeking robust end-points for clinical trials? The question could be reformulated as: are patients with irritable bowel disease similarly hypersensitive to visceral pain? Lydiard characterized the psychological make-up of patients with irritable bowel syndrome, in which perhaps 50% of patients seek medical advice and 50% do not[15]. He concluded that, of those who did seek advice, 50–95% had some degree of psychiatric disturbance – panic disorders, anxiety, social phobia, post-traumatic stress or depression. The 50% defined as 'non-seekers' were psychiatrically normal. How do the patients in inflammatory bowel disease register in this regard?

Two studies have addressed the question. Bernstein *et al.* addressed the threshold for detecting first physiological distension and then pain in the rectum using progressive balloon dilatation in patients with Crohn's disease limited to the ileum, and found higher pain thresholds in Crohn's disease compared with either normal individuals or patients with the irritable bowel[16]. Furthermore skin conductance studies performed at the same time suggested a diminished systemic autonomic reflex in Crohn's disease. Mason *et al.* studied psychological and social morbidity, somatization and aspects of sexual satisfaction in patients with inflammatory bowel disease and normal individuals, in the context of a study primarily investigating women with chronic idiopathic constipation[17]. Whilst the latter group showed clear abnormalities, there were no differences between the inflammatory bowel disease patients and controls. Thus there is no scientific reason for assuming a greater propensity to suffer pain in patients with inflammatory bowel disease, and indeed perhaps reflecting some form of accommodation, this may be less.

Studies such as Bernstein *et al.*'s are of course highly artificial means of assessing pain – even though stimuli such as rectal distension can assess perception at both physiological and discomfort levels. Measuring pain in real life is significantly more different. The concepts that have emerged, particularly from instruments such as the McGill Pain Questionnaire[18], or the West Haven Yale Pain Inventory, emphasize the multi-dimensionality of pain[19]. McGill's score categorizes and describes pain under three headings – sensory, affective, and evaluative – from which is derived a pain rating index based on numerical scoring of severity in each category, and the number of descriptor words chosen. The Yale inventory uses three fields that more globally reflect the impact of pain on the patient's life, the responses of those to whom the patient communicates his/her pain, and the extent to which patients can participate in common daily activities. Clearly this appreciation of multi-dimensionality accords with approaches now current in inflammatory bowel disease such as the IBD Quality of Life Index.

Such complicated pain scores can be highly effective and surprisingly effectively allow statistical analysis of pain experiences. Physicians will probably appreciate the intuitive correctness of quantification of something as familiar as post-herpetic neuralgia which, using such a numerical approach, identifies the transition point of the subacute phase of pain as occurring at 11 ± 3 days after appearance of the rash and of 110 ± 11 days for the chronic phase[20]. With respect to abdominal pain, when a 100 mm visual analogue score was used to assess acute pain in an emergency-room setting, highly reproducible assessments of pain could be obtained when this was applied contemporaneously[21]. (Incidentally, the minimum clinically significant difference in pain that can be quantified is '16 mm'.) However, of course, such acute pains differ from those experienced in ulcerative colitis and Crohn's disease.

So – can the pain of inflammatory bowel disease be quantified to make this useful for a therapeutic trial. Well, of course, it can and is. Least quantitative but effective, certainly in individual patients, is the Present–Korelitz approach[22]. In this scheme, if in an individual patient pain is the dominant symptom, the aim of the trial in that individual is to ameliorate those symptoms, which is therefore simply 'better, worse or unchanged'. At a more quantitative level, in the Crohn's Disease Activity Index (CDAI), abdominal pain is one of the eight cardinal features – daily abdominal pain assessed over a week scored 0–3, given a range of 0–21; this is weighted $\times 5$ in the final index[23]. The Harvey Bradshaw index uses a simple unweighted score of 0–3[24]. Such figures can contribute 25% of a total activity score. One major problem arises when the information is gathered. I have referred to the validation of abdominal pain in an emergency room using a visual analogue score, and emphasized that this was a contemporaneous assessment. I have speculated elsewhere as to whether the majority of diary cards for the CDAI are filled in by patients as they wait in the outpatient waiting room. The issue of when pain is assessed, and thus the specific issue of the ability to recall pain, is very pertinent.

Interestingly, Feine *et al.* used the context of a randomized clinical trial of measures to treat chronic jaw pain, to prospectively assess memories of pain and perception of relief[25]. The conclusions are salutary.

1. Memory was inaccurate and recollect/recall errors worsened with time.
2. Subjects with low pretreatment pain exaggerated its severity afterwards, whilst it was underestimated by those with high pretreatment pain.
3. Memory of pain also varied with the pain experienced at the time of recall.
4. Finally almost all patients reported relief even when pain had increased.

The concept of different types of pain in inflammatory bowel disease also merits attention. Clinically pain may be acute and colicky, dull, nagging, with many subjective variations familiar to all. The quantification of such descriptions is very difficult, and not an area that has been extensively addressed. Of course there are certain types of pain that define particular therapeutic targets – but the most obvious is that of recurrent subacute obstruction, and here the syndrome is well understood clinically. Outside this simple example, pain is usually part of a symptom complex, and even simple colic may reflect a combination of inflammatory and fibrotic pathology.

In conclusion: is pain a relevant therapeutic target in inflammatory bowel disease? At the simplistic level the answer is obviously yes. Pain is a relevant and distressing symptom. In assessing pain prospectively, clinically but more particularly in clinical trials, it is reassuring that there is no reason to believe that an 'IBD personality' distorts pain perception. However, as a therapeutic target pain is but one part of a system complex. The relationships within an individual between physical and psychological factors, and the relationship of the sensation of pain to the wider aspects of human life, all suggest that a refined pain assessment on its own would be an oversensitive tool for gastroenterologists to develop.

References

1. Grundy D. Neuroanatomy of visceral nociception: vagal and splanchnic afferent Gut. 2002; 51(Suppl. 1):i2–5.
2. Furness JB, Kunze WA, Clere N. Nutrient tasting and signaling mechanisms in the gut. II. The intestine as a sensory organ: neural, endocrine and immuno responses. Am J Physiol. 1999;277:G922–8.
3. Szurszewski JH, Ermilov LG, Miller SM. Prevertebral ganglia and intestinofugal afferent neurones. Gut. 2002;51(Suppl. 1):i6–10.
4. Joshi SK, Gebhart GF. Visceral pain. Curr Rev Pain. 2000;4:499–506.
5. Berthoud B, Neuhuber WL. Functional and chemical anatomy of the afferent vagal system. Auton Neurosci. 2000;85:1–17.
6. Steranka LR, Manning DC, Dehaas CJ *et al.* Bradykinin as a pain mediator: receptors are localized to sensory neurones and antagonists have analgesic actions. Proc Natl Acad Sci USA. 1988;85:3245–52.
7. Gershon MD. Review article: Roles played by 5-hydroxytryptamine in the physiology of the bowel. Aliment Pharmacol Ther. 1999;13:15–30.

8. Julia V, Morteau O, Buéno L. Involvement of NK_1 and NK_2 receptors in viscerosensitive responses to rectal distension. Gastroenterology. 1994;107:94–102.
9. Mertz H. Role of the brain and sensory pathways in gastrointestinal sensory disorders in humans. Gut. 2002;51(Suppl. 1):i29–33.
10. Gue M, Del Rio-Lacheze C, Eutamene H et al. Stress-induced visceral hypersensitivity to rectal distension in rats: role of CRF and mast cells. Neurogastroenterol Motil. 1997;9:271–9.
11. Delvaux M. Role of visceral sensitivity in the pathophysiology of irritable bowel syndrome. Gut. 2002;51(Suppl. 1):i67–71.
12. Azpiroz F. Hypersensitivity in functional gastrointestinal disorders. Gut. 2002;51(Suppl. 1):i25–8.
13. Coffin B, Azpiroz F, Guarner F et al. Selective gastric hypersensitivity and reflex hyporeactivity in functional dyspepsia. Gastroenterology. 1994;107:1345–51.
14. Whitehead WE, Holtkotter B, Enck P et al. Tolerance for rectosigmoid distension in irritable bowel syndrome. Gastroenterology. 1990;98:1187–92.
15. Lydiard RB. Irritable bowel syndrome, anxiety, and depression: what are the links? J Clin Psychiatry. 2001;62(Suppl. 8):38–45.
16. Bernstein CN, Robert ME, Kodner A et al. Is there an irritable bowel syndrome (IBS) component in patients with ileal Crohn's disease (CD)? Gastroenterology. 1993;104:A477.
17. Mason HJ, Serrano-Ikkos E, Kamm MA. Psychological morbidity in women with idiopathic constipation. Am J Gastroenterol. 2000;95:2852–7.
18. Melzack R. The McGill Pain Questionnaire: major properties and scoring methods. Pain. 1975;1:277–99.
19. Kerns RD, Turk DC, Rudy TE. The West Haven–Yale Multidimensional Pain Inventory (WHYMPI). Pain. 1985;23:345–56.
20. Desmond RA, Weiss HL, Arani RB et al. Clinical applications for change-point analysis of herpes zoster pain. J Pain Symptom Manage. 2002;23:510–16.
21. Gallagher EJ, Bijur PE, Latimer C, Silver W. Reliability and validity of a visual analog scale for acute abdominal pain in the ED. Am J Emerg Med. 2002;20:287–90.
22. Present DH, Korelitz BI, Wisch N, Glass JL, Sachar DB, Pasternack BS. Treatment of Crohn's disease with 6-mercaptopurine. A long-term, randomized, double-blind study. N Engl J Med. 1980;302:981–7.
23. Best WR, Becktel JM, Singleton JW. Rederived values of the eight coefficients of the Crohn's Disease Activity Index (CDAI). Gastroenterology. 1979;77:843–6.
24. Harvey RF, Bradshaw JM. A simple index of Crohn's-disease activity. Lancet. 1980; i(8167); 514.
25. Feine JS, Lavigne GJ, Dao TT, Morin C, Lund JP. Memories of chronic pain and perceptions of relief. Pain. 1998;77:137–41.

20
Strictures in inflammatory bowel disease: are there differential indications for surgery or endoscopic dilation?

G. VAN ASSCHE, A. D'HOORE, F. PENNINCKX and P. RUTGEERTS

INTRODUCTION

Intestinal stenosis is a feared complication of Crohn's disease, which may lead to repeated bowel resection. Remission after surgical resection in Crohn's disease is only temporary since endoscopically more than 70% of patients will have new lesions within a year and 40% will be symptomatic within 4 years[1]. Even in the era of biological therapies and immunosuppressives which have been proven to induce complete mucosal healing, fibrostenosis remains a clinical challenge. In patients with a fibrostenotic disease behaviour symptomatic strictures also tend to return after surgically induced remission despite medical therapy, and this leads to repeated bowel resections and eventually to short-bowel syndrome. Therefore, in the past 20 years, both endoscopic and surgical strictureplasty techniques have been developed aimed at preserving valuable intestinal mucosa. The choice between endoscopic dilation and surgical strictureplasty is usually evident since the two techniques are indicated for different types of stricture.

TECHNICAL ASPECTS

Endoscopic balloon dilation

Through-the-scope (TTS) balloon dilation (Fig. 1) is a well-established technique in the upper gastrointestinal tract, but in the past 15 years this procedure has also come of age in the management of Crohn's disease-related ileocolonic strictures[2]. TTS balloons can be introduced through the stenosis under full endoscopic guidance, thus eliminating the need for fluoroscopy. The procedure involves a full colonoscopy, and thorough bowel preparation is essential. Once the stenosis is reached by the tip of the colonoscope a TTS balloon attached to a guiding catheter is passed through the biopsy channel (2.8 mm) of the scope. Balloon dilation should preferably be performed by an experienced endoscopist since maximal straightening of the scope is essential to facilitate balloon introduction. Low-compliance balloons with a diameter of 15–25 mm and a length of 3–8 cm are suitable. However, longer balloons are required to dilate strictures of a few centimetres since the balloon needs to extend beyond the stenosis while it is inflated for good fixation. We use a Rigiflex® balloon of 18 mm diameter and 8 cm length, which allows dilation of somewhat longer ileocolonic strictures. The guiding catheter of the balloon is attached to an inflation device. This device inflates the balloon with water under manometric control. The inflation pressure differs with the size and type of the balloon (maximum 7 atm for a 18 mm Rigiflex® balloon). Maximal inflation is maintained for 0.5–2 min and repeated inflation can be performed. Loss of pressure during inflation may indicate leaks or gradual dilation of the stricture. Inflation times over 20 s usually provoke pain due to local ischaemia and activation of afferent nerves; therefore, most centres will perform this procedure under general anaesthesia. During balloon inflation contact of the camera on the endoscope with the balloon will often allow inspection of the stricture. Most authors consider easy passage of the colonoscope through the dilation after inflation as an indication of successful strictureplasty. If this is not possible after a first inflation the balloon can be reinflated for up to four times, always attempting to pass the scope through the stenosis before a new inflation is commenced. The low compliance of the balloon protects against over-inflation since excessive pressure will lead to rupture of the balloon. Accessory techniques to balloon dilation have been described. In one series unsuccessful balloon dilation was supplemented by carving the stricture with a sphincterotome[3]. The incisions with the sphincterotome did not result in extra complications. More recently endoscopic stenting of ileocolonic stenoses has also been reported in a limited number of patients, with beneficial outcome[4].

The most likely causes for technical failure are: balloon or inflation-device dysfunction, excessive looping of the colonoscope which hinders balloon introduction and angulation of the ileocolonic anastomosis relative to the colon precluding balloon introduction. Complications of the procedure will be apparent within 4 h after the procedure; therefore TTS balloon dilation can be performed in a day clinic.

Surgical strictureplasty

Surgical strictureplasty was originally developed for stenoses after tuberculous ileitis, but the procedure was introduced in the surgical care of Crohn's disease patients by Lee and Papaioannou in 1982[5]. The surgical technique applied depends mainly on the length of the stricture. The Heineke–Mikulicz strictureplasty is the most widely performed; a recent meta-analysis showed that it comprised 85% of surgical strictureplasties[6]. This technique has been adapted from Heineke–Mikulicz pyloroplasty. A longitudinal incision is made extending 2 cm in macroscopically normal bowel (Fig. 2). The incision is then closed

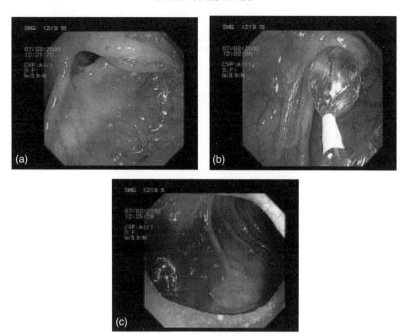

Fig. 1 Endoscopic view of a balloon dilation, showing: (**a**) the anastomotic stricture, (**b**) the inflated balloon inserted through the stenosis, (**c**) a view of the ileum through the dilated stricture

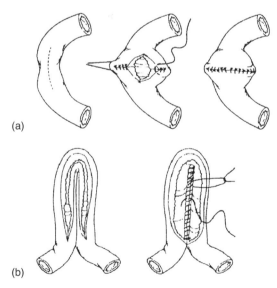

Fig. 2 Heineke–Mikulicz (**a**) and Finney (**b**) strictureplasty. Note that in the Heineke–Mikulicz strictureplasty a longitudinal incision is made that is closed with a transverse suture, whereas in the Finney procedure the strictured bowel is folded over onto itself. (Adapted from ref. 6)

195

transversely with absorbable sutures, which significantly widens the intestinal lumen. The Finney procedure is performed when strictures exceed 10–15 cm. In this technique a suture is placed in the middle of the narrowed segment and the bowel loop is folded over onto itself, allowing a second suture to be inserted between normal loops of bowel (Fig. 2b). Next a U-shaped incision over the strictured bowel loop will expose the lumen. The lining of the bowel in this incision is then sutured to reconstitute a bowel loop that will allow free passage of contents. For patients with long strictures, in whom maximal conservation of intestine is vital, side-to-side isoperistaltic strictureplasty has been proposed. The main purpose of this isoperistaltic loop is to avoid the formation of a blind loop that would allow bacterial stasis. Strictureplasty is often combined with resection of segments that are judged to be overtly inflamed and not suitable for bowel-conserving surgery. Most series mention that in 40–50% of surgical procedures strictureplasty and resection are combined. During surgery a careful assessment of possible strictured sites should be performed. Various techniques such as passing a Foley catheter or a glass marble have been proposed.

INDICATIONS

Endoscopic dilation

Careful patient selection is of paramount importance to optimize the outcomes of both endoscopic and surgical strictureplasty; therefore, a carefully performed barium meal with good visualization of the ileocolonic anastomosis is mandatory to allow proper prediction of successful outcome. Endoscopic balloon dilation is indicated for relatively short, symptomatic strictures of the ileocolonic anastomosis. These postoperative strictures are generally easily accessible. The ileocaecal valve in non-operated patients is usually too angulated to allow passage of the balloon. In the pre-procedure barium X-ray series prestenotic dilation of the neoterminal ileum usually suggests that the symptoms are caused by the stricture and not by mucosal inflammation or by postoperative adhesions. However, barium contrast X-rays can fail to demonstrate all strictures when there are multiple stenoses, and on the other hand may overestimate the severity of a stricture due to insufficient filling of the lumen. Concomitant medications such as steroids or immunosuppressives should not influence the decision towards dilation, although usually eligible patients have relatively quiescent inflammatory disease activity. Nevertheless, active ulcerative disease at the site of the anastomosis is frequent and is not a contraindication for dilation.

Apart from short stenoses of the ileocolonic anastomosis, colonic, duodenal and gastric stenoses are indications for endoscopic treatment in Crohn's disease patients. Dilation with enteroscopy for jejunal strictures has been reported[7], but we prefer surgical strictureplasty for these patients.

Strictureplasty

Distinct presentations of the disease in which strictureplasty should always be considered include diffuse ileocolonic disease with symptomatic strictures or patients at risk for short-bowel syndrome (e.g. previous small-bowel resection of more than 100 cm). However, since the concept that surgery does not cure Crohn's disease is now widely accepted, most surgeons will attempt to preserve as much bowel as possible at any procedure. Therefore a combination of bowel resection with bowel-conserving strictureplasties is commonly performed. Most studies mention that 40–50% of strictureplasties are performed during an operation with associated intestinal resection[6,8,9]. Although traditionally surgical strictureplasty was considered to be mainly indicated for patients with limited active small-bowel disease, a recent report demonstrated that patients with complications and recurrence rates of strictureplasties in patients with diffuse ileocolitis were comparable to those of patients with quiescent disease[10]. Presumably the restoration of a patent lumen decreases the faecal stasis in strictured bowel segments, which is highly beneficial for the local mucosal inflammation. The choice of surgical technique is mainly determined by the length of the stricture. The classical Heineke–Mikulicz procedure (Fig. 2) is reserved for short stenoses, whereas the Finney procedure can relieve longer stenoses up to 25 cm. A fistula in a strictured segment can be managed with a Judd strictureplasty, which is a modification of the Heineke–Mikulicz procedure[6].

OUTCOMES AND COMPLICATIONS

Endoscopic dilation

Generally immediate successful outcome is defined in most reported series as the ability to pass a normal colonoscope beyond the stricture after dilation. At least for dilations of the ileocolonic anastomosis this will allow faecal material to pass easily through the stenosis. Several series have been published in the past 10 years (Table 1) with immediate success rates varying between 71% and 100%[11–17]. In one of the largest studies published, our centre reported a success rate of 90%. In this study most dilations were performed for stenoses of the ileocolonic anastomosis (61%) and 85% of the patients had been operated before[12]. Similar results were obtained in a French study with 38 patients[13] and in studies with a more limited number of patients. Prominent angulation of the stricture preventing introduction of the TTS balloon is the most important reason for technical failure, as discussed above. In the long term success rates are lower and also more variable between different series. This can be partly explained by the variable follow-up period ranging from 0.6 to 3.8 years.

Symptom recurrence has been reported in 13–100% of patients (Table 1); however, not all of these patients need surgery. Repeated dilation is an option. This will imply each time that the patient is put under general anaesthesia, and the length of the symptom-free interval will be the main parameter used to decide between surgery and repeat endoscopic dilation. In our own experience, applying repeat dilation if necessary, 38% of patients needed surgery for stenotic disease with an interval of 5 years; 33% of patients had a second dilation for symptom recurrence[12].

Complications of endoscopic dilation occur usually within hours after the procedure. The two most common events are bowel perforation and major bleeding. Perforation has been reported to occur in 0–11% of patients or in 0–8% of

Table 1 Outcomes and complications of published series on endoscopic balloon dilation for Crohn's disease strictures

Reference	Number of patients	Percentage anastomotic	Short-term success rate (%)	Symptomatic recurrence (%) (mean follow-up, months)	Complications (perforations) (%)
Blomberg et al. (1991)[11]	27	100	85	33 (19)	15 (7)
Junge and Zuchner (1995)[16]	10	60	81	13 (11)	9
Ramboer et al. (1995)[14]	13	92	100	NS (45)	0
Couckuyt et al. (1995)[12]	55	87	90	62 (34)	11 (11)
Raedler et al. (1997)[17]	30	NS	NS	53 (12) 20 (budesonide)*	NS
Sabate et al. (2001)[13]	38	68	84	63 (60)	9
Dear and Hunter (2001)[15]	22	95	NS	NS	0

Only series with more than 10 patients were selected.
NS: not specified.
*Patients were randomized to azathioprine + budesonide 9 mg or placebo for 12 months.

procedures (Table 1). Symptoms will become apparent within 4 h from the dilation, allowing endoscopic dilation to be performed in a day-clinic setting. In our own experience more than two-thirds of the perforations are concealed and can be managed by bowel rest and antibiotics, and only one-third of patients need urgent surgery. Major bleeding episodes with noticeable decreases in haemoglobin levels or with a need for transfusion are rare (0–1.5% of procedures); however, minor bleeds occur in almost every procedure. In the first days following endoscopic dilation substantial oedema can develop at the site of the stenosis. This can lead to obstructive symptoms for a few days, and on barium contrast X-rays the stenoses will appear to have recurred. However, performing repeat endoscopy has taught us that these oedematous sites can be passed with the colonoscope and should be treated conservatively.

Surgical strictureplasty

Immediate relief of symptoms after strictureplasty is high (99% in one study) and this results in weight gain and improved food tolerance. Reports on outcomes of surgical strictureplasty for fibrostenosis in Crohn's disease have been numerous (Table 2). In a recent meta-analysis Tichansky et al. reported that 25% of patients experienced recurrence of symptoms that required repeat surgery[6]. The figure for symptomatic recurrence was also reported earlier by the Cleveland Clinic, but in this series only 15% of patients needed reoperation.

Interestingly, the Finney procedure was associated with a lower recurrence rate than the more commonly performed Heineke–Mikulicz technique. In most of the studies it is striking that the rate of so-called new stricture is much higher than that of restricture. These newly discovered strictures may have been already present at the first operation without being noticed by the surgeon, and without being symptomatic to the patient. As mentioned above, patients with diffuse jejunoileitis in between strictureplasties seem to have outcomes similar to patients

Table 2 Outcomes and complications of surgical strictureplasty in recently reported series

Reference	Number of patients	Number of stricture-plasties	Symptomatic recurrence (%)	Reoperation rate (%) (mean follow-up, months)	Complications (%)
Tichansky (2000) meta-analysis*[6]	506	1852	25	15 (23)	15
Ozuner et al. (1996)[18]	162	698	38	22 (42)	NS
Stebbing et al. (1995)[19]	52	241	36	36 (37)	NS
Alexander-Williams (1994)[20]	80	309	33	32 (72)	NS
Tonelli and Ficari (2000)[21]	44	174	45	23 (48)	7
Dietz et al. (2002)[10], diffuse disease	123	701	NS	29 (80)	20

Only the most recent series were selected.
NS: not specified.
Complications include all significant operation-related morbidity.
*Meta-analysis containing some of the series mentioned further.

with relatively quiescent disease. Combined strictureplasty with bowel resection and strictureplasty alone have similar reoperation rates.

Early postoperative complications have been reported to occur in approximately 13% of patients. Enterocutaneous fistulas, abdominal sepsis and obstruction occur most frequently. However, these complication rates are comparable to those reported for bowel resection in fibrostenotic Crohn's disease.

There have been concerns regarding the risk of small-bowel carcinoma in patients with long-standing jejunoileal Crohn's disease. Theoretically this risk may increase with bowel-conserving strictureplasty; however, to date there have been no reports of increased incidence of small-bowel cancers in patients followed up for strictureplasty.

CONCLUSION

Since surgical remission after curative resection for Crohn's disease is only temporary, and consecutive intestinal resection may lead to short-bowel syndrome, bowel-sparing alternatives are essential in the management of patients with fibrostenotic disease. Endoscopic balloon dilation and surgical strictureplasty have differential indications. Short strictures of the ileocolonic anastomosis or within the colon are good indications for balloon dilation if they are not too angulated. Surgical strictureplasty is indicated for single or multiple ileal or jejunal strictures of up to 20 cm in length, which are usually not accessible with an endoscope. The presence of diffuse disease is not a contraindication for strictureplasty since outcomes are similar to those obtained in patients with quiescent disease. Although indications for endoscopic and surgical strictureplasty are clearly different, the good overall outcomes and low complication rates of both procedures allow conserving valuable small bowel in patients with a history of repeated resection.

References

1. Rutgeerts P, Geboes K, Vantrappen G, Kerremans R, Coenegrachts JL, Coremans G. Natural history of recurrent Crohn's disease at the ileocolonic anastomosis after curative surgery. Gut. 1984;25:665–72.
2. Sabaté JM, Lemann M. Traitement endoscopique des sténoses dans la maladie de Crohn. Hépato-gastro enterologie. 2002;9:169–73.
3. Bedogni G, Ricci E, Pedrazolli C et al. Endoscopic dilation of anastomotic colonic stenosis by different techniques: an alternative to surgery? Gastrointest Endosc. 1987;33:21–4.
4. Matsuhashi N, Nakajima A, Suzuki A, Yakazi Y, Takazoe M. Long-term outcome of non-surgical strictureplasty using metallic stents for intestinal strictures in Crohn's disease. Gastrointest Endosc. 2000;51:343–5.
5. Lee EC, Papaioannou N. Minimal surgery for chronic obstruction in patients with extensive or universal Crohn's disease. Ann R Coll Surg Eng. 1982;64:229–33.
6. Tichansky D, Cagir B, Yoo E, Marcus S, Fry R. Strictureplasty for Crohn's disease: meta-analysis. Dis Colon Rectum. 2000;43:911–19.
7. Perez-Cuadrado E, Molina PE. Multiple strictures in jejunal Crohn's disease: push enteroscopy dilation. Endoscopy. 2001;33:194.
8. Sayfan J, Wilson DA, Allan A, Andrews H, Alexander-Williams J. Recurrence after strictureplasty or resection for Crohn's disease. Br J Surg. 1989;76:335–8.
9. Fazio VW, Tjandra JJ, Lavery IC et al. Long term follow-up of strictureplasty in Crohn's disease. Dis Colon Rectum. 1993;36:355–61.
10. Dietz D, Fazio V, Laureti S et al. Strictureplasty in diffuse Crohn's jejunoileitis: safe and durable. Dis Colon Rectum. 2002;45:764–70.
11. Blomberg B, Rolny P, Jarnerot G. Endoscopic treatment of anastomotic treatment in Crohn's disease. Endoscopy. 1991;23:195–8.
12. Couckuyt H, Gevers AM, Coremans G, Hiele M, Rutgeerts P. Efficacy and safety of hydrostatic balloon dilatation of ileocolonic Crohn's strictures: a prospective long term analysis. Gut. 1995;36:577–80.
13. Sabate JM, Villarejo J, Lemann M et al. Hydrostatic balloon dilatation of Crohn's strictures. Gastroenterology. 2001;120:A449 (abstract).
14. Ramboer C, Verhamme M, Dhondt E, Huys S, Van Eygen K, Vermeire L. Endoscopic treatment of stenosis in recurrent Crohn's disease with balloon dilation combined with local corticosteroid injection. Endoscopy. 1995;42:252–5.
15. Dear KL, Hunter JO. Colonoscopic hydrostatic balloon dilatation of Crohn's strictures. J Clin Gastroenterol. 2001;33:315–18.
16. Junge U, Zuchner H. Endoscopic balloon dilatation of symptomatic structures in Crohn's disease. Dtsch Med Wochenschr. 1994;119:1377–82.
17. Raedler A, Peters I, Schreiber S. Treatment with azathioprine and budesonide prevents reoccurrence of ileocolonic stenoses after endoscopic dilatation in Crohn's disease. Gastroenterology. 1997;112:A1067 (abstract).
18. Ozuner G, Fazio VW, Lavery IC, Church JM, Hull TL. How safe is strictureplasty in the management of Crohn's disease? Am J Surg. 1996;171:57–61.
19. Stebbing JF, Jewell DP, Kettlewell MG, Mortensen NJ. Long-term results of recurrence and reoperation after strictureplasty for obstructive Crohn's disease. Br J Surg. 1995;82:1471–4.
20. Alexander-Williams J. Surgical management of small intestinal Crohn's disease: resection or strictureplasty. Semin Colon Rectal Surg. 1994;30:135–8.
21. Tonelli F, Ficari F. Strictureplasty in Crohn's disease – surgical option. Dis Colon Rectum. 2000;43:920–6.

21
Spectrum of inflammatory bowel diseases-related arthropathy: are there differential treatment options?

M. DE VOS

INTRODUCTION

Inflammatory bowel diseases (IBD) are frequently associated with extraintestinal manifestations including articular involvement. The diagnosis of IBD-related arthropathy requires clinical symptoms of

1. Peripheral arthritis with an asymmetrical and oligoarticular involvement of joints principally of the lower limbs and frequently associated with inflammation of the Achilles tendon or the fascia plantaris. The synovitis is mostly self-limiting and only rarely chronic and destructive.
2. Axial involvement with an inflammatory back pain occurring at night or in rest and associated with a decreased mobility of the spine evident as morning stiffness.

Radiographic evaluations of the peripheral arthritis are mostly normal. Axial involvement is associated with sacroiliitis and/or spondylitis affecting the insertion of the collateral ligaments with syndesmophyte formation and the zygo-apophysial joints.

A prospective cross-sectional study showed evidence for peripheral arthritis in 10% of patients, inflammatory back pain in 30%, ankylosing spondylitis according to Rome criteria in 10% and asymptomatic sacroiliitis grade 2 or more in 18% of patients[1] (Fig. 1). This study confirmed that IBD-related arthropathy can be considered as spondylarthropathy (SpA).

ACTUAL STANDARD THERAPY

Optimal treatment of IBD-associated arthropathy is not established. Guidelines can only be extrapolated from studies in patients with other forms of SpA.

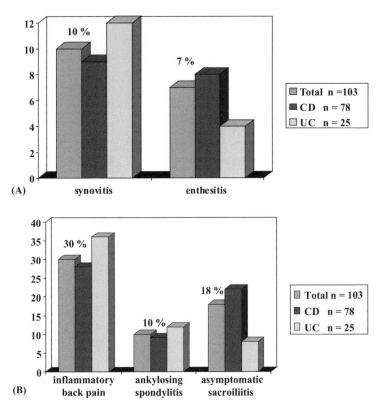

Fig. 1 Prevalences of IBD-related arthropathy. **A**: Peripheral arthropathy; **B**: Axial involvement; CD = Crohn's disease; UC = ulcerative colitis. (adapted from ref. 1)

The actual standard treatment for SpA is the combination of non-steroidal anti-inflammatory drugs (NSAIDs) with sulphasalazine and intensive physical training. In cases of persistent monoarthritis, intra-articular injection of corticosteroids is mandatory.

Clinical response to NSAIDs is rapid for both the peripheral arthritis and the axial disease but relapse is frequent after arrest of intake. However, NSAIDs may be associated with exacerbations of ulcerative colitis and Crohn's disease, although data are inconsistent. No prospective controlled trial of the effect of NSAIDs in IBD has been performed. A large case–control study including 200 patients admitted to hospital as emergencies with colitis demonstrated an association with current or recent NSAID use with adjusted odds ratios of respectively 1.35 and 1.76[2]. Since NSAID use was evaluated by a computerized database linking hospital admission and dispensed drug data, and since most NSAID use is as an over-the-counter medication, true NSAID use was probably underestimated. A second smaller case–control study including 60 consecutive IBD patients admitted to hospital because of exacerbation or onset of IBD demonstrated a possible relationship since 31% of those patients had taken

NSAIDs within the past month. In contrast, in only 2% of the control irritable bowel population NSAID use was recorded[3]. A recent large retrospective study of 1940 patients with IBD and a cohort study including 368 patients reported no significant differences in disease activity, but these results were reported only in abstract forms[4,5].

The question as to whether selective COX-2 inhibitors offer less risk for patients with IBD remains unanswered. In the colon there is evidence that COX-2 enzyme is activated in the inflamed mucosa and may be considered as part of a reparative process.

In animal models the use of selective COX-2 inhibitors leads to an increased severity of colitis induced by trinitrobenzene sulphonic acid[6], but ameliorates colitis induced by intracolonic administration of acetic acid[7]. In a small retrospective study including 11 patients treated with celecoxib and 16 patients treated with rofexocib, Mahadevan et al. reported an aggravation of IBD in 7.4%[8]. Since no control group was available interpretation of this flare rate is difficult.

The common association between spondylarthropathies and gut inflammation[9,10] and the well-known effect in rheumatoid arthritis was the stimulus to use sulphasalazine in the treatment of SpA. A number of randomized controlled trials confirmed the overall beneficial effect of the drug with improvement in clinical and laboratory markers[11–13]. Overall the observed beneficial effect was modest, and perceptible only for peripheral arthritis. Moreover, efficacy appeared to be restricted to early ankylosing disease.

Data concerning the effect of mesalamine are limited to two small open trials demonstrating a significant improvement in all clinical measures (pain, number of swollen joints, stiffness). Only measures of axial flexibility were not improved[14,15].

Recently effectiveness of infliximab was observed in spondylarthropathy patients associated or not with Crohn's disease. Infliximab or Remicade is a humanized chimaeric IgG1 anti-TNF-α monoclonal antibody capable of neutralizing soluble cytokine and blocking membrane-bound TNF. A small pilot study including five Crohn's patients with arthropathy demonstrated a very rapid disappearance of peripheral synovitis and axial inflammatory pain[16]. This effect on the arthropathy was confirmed in an open study and a placebo-controlled study[17,18].

The last study included 40 patients with active spondylarthropathy without evidence for Crohn's disease. In the group of patients treated with infliximab an early and sustained improvement of patient and physician assessments of global disease activity was observed, associated with a significant reduction in pain intensity, improvement of peripheral assessments and axial assessments. No improvement was observed in the ankylosing spondylitis metrology indices in this short-term trial. These results were confirmed in a second very similar study including 35 patients with active ankylosing spondylitis[19]. Infliximab was effective in every response criterion, even in the variable for spinal mobility. Moreover, NSAIDs could be reduced to more than 50% of the baseline value in 56% of patients on infliximab, but in only 19% of patients on placebo, and were completely stopped in respectively 41% and 13%. Whether infliximab can be considered as a disease-modifying drug and prevent ankylosis remains to be studied.

Recently another very similar trial was published with etanercept, a recombinant human TNF receptor (p75) fusion protein in patients with ankylosing spondylitis[20]. At 4 months 80% of patients in the etanercept group had a treatment response as compared to 30% in the placebo group. The effect on peripheral joint involvement was minimal. In contrast, morning stiffness, nocturnal pain and ankylosing spondylitis functionality index improved significantly. According to spinal mobility, only an improvement in chest expansion was observed. However, since evidence for efficacy in Crohn's disease is actually lacking[21], this molecule seems less suitable for IBD-related arthropathy.

Despite evidence that patients with SpA clearly benefit from treatments based on the inhibition of TNF-α activity, the precise mechanisms underlying these effects are not fully understood[22].

POSSIBLE FUTURE THERAPEUTIC PATHWAYS

Further elucidation of the immunocascade and genetic alterations explaining the chronic recurrent intestinal inflammation and associated extraintestinal manifestations can help in the development of new therapeutic strategies. Several aetiopathogenetic mechanisms can be considered:

1. Bacterial products, such as peptidoglycans and lipopolysaccharides, from a normal or altered intestinal flora can play a role either indirectly by affecting the immunological reaction or directly by the circulation of antigens from the gut to other sites. The most revealing evidence for this hypothesis comes from the HLA-B27/human β$_2$-microglobulin transgenic rat model developing intestinal and articular inflammation only after contact with luminal bacteria such as *Bacteroides* spp.[23]. Other bacteria thought to be involved in the pathogenesis of intestinal inflammation of Crohn's disease are *Escherichia coli*, and fusobacteria[24]. Although differences have been observed in the flora of Crohn's disease patients versus controls, no information is available concerning possible variations between patients with or without extraintestinal manifestations. Evidence for a circulation of bacterial antigens comes from studies in patients with SpA in which bacterial degradation products and bacterial DNA from *Yersinia, Chlamydia* and *Salmonella* were observed in synovium. An identification of so-called 'arthritogenic' bacterial strains and/or genetically susceptible hosts would support new strategies directed to these bacterial products or the use of probiotics and prebiotics in order to modify the bacterial flora.

2. Circulation between gut and joint involves macrophages and/or lymphocytes. The presence of intestinal peptidoglycan polysaccharide-positive dendritic cells in synovial tissues supports a circulation of monocytes/macrophages[25]. Macrophages play a crucial role in the local initiation and perpetuation of the inflammation by the production of a mix of inflammatory cytokines. Studies in patients with SpA demonstrated an increased expression of CD163$^+$ macrophages in the lamina propria and in synovium of patients with or without associated Crohn's disease[26]. This transmembrane protein belongs to the scavenger receptor cysteine-rich superfamily and plays a role

in the regulation of the immunological response by the production of IL-1 and TNF-α. Since CD163[+] are present in blood circulation they may represent potential candidates for the circulation of arthropathic products from intestinal flora.

3. Circulation of primed lymphocytes from the lamina propria to the synovial endothelium is also important. The sharing of homing receptors between gut and synovium with increased mononuclear cell adhesion and transmigration through synovial high endothelial venules during intestinal inflammation is a likely contributing factor[27]. An increased expression of αEβ7 integrin on T cell lines originating from gut and synovium of patients with Crohn's disease and patients with SpA has been observed[28]. This integrin is normally expressed on intraepithelial lymphocytes and lymphocytes migrating to the mucosa. Its presence on synovial lymphocytes suggests an intestinal origin. Monoclonal antibodies directed against adhesion molecules, in analogy to those developed against α4 integrins, may block the traffic not only between blood circulation and mucosal tissue but also between gut and extraintestinal locations.

A better understanding of the adherence phenomena and functional identification of the lymphocytes in gut and synovium, including cytokine profiles, may aid the development of new, very specific monoclonal antibodies.

4. Genetic factors may modulate the immunocascade. The NOD2/CARD15 gene has recently been recognized as a susceptibility gene for Crohn's disease[29]. The NOD2/CARD15 gene encodes a cytosolic protein restricted to monocytes/macrophages. This protein functions as an intracellular receptor for bacterial components. Although the presence of allelic variants in Crohn's disease seems not to be associated with a higher prevalence of articular symptoms[30], and the prevalence of mutations in SpA populations seems similar to those observed in control population[31], we were able to demonstrate a clear association between the presence of mutations and the presence of chronic inflammation in the intestine of spondylarthropathy patients (submitted). A genetically determined disturbed handling of bacterial products leading to an altered transport of antigens by macrophages is an attractive hypothesis.

References

1. De Vlam K, Mielants H, Cuvelier C et al. Spondyloarthropathy is underestimated in inflammatory bowel disease: prevalence and HLA association. J Rheumatol. 2000;27:2860–5.
2. Evans JMM, McMahon AD, Murray FE et al. Non-steroidal anti-inflammatory drugs are associated with emergency admission to hospital for colitis due to inflammatory bowel disease. Gut. 1997;40:619–22.
3. Felder JB, Korelitz BI, Rajapakse R et al. Effects of non-steroidal anti-inflammatory drugs on inflammatory bowel disease: a case control study. Am J Gastroenterol. 2000;95:1949–54.
4. Dominitz JA, Boyko EJ. Association between analgesic use and inflammatory bowel disease flares: a retrospective cohort study. Gastroenterology. 2000;118:A3024.
5. Bonner GF. Use of nonsteroidal anti-inflammatory drugs in outpatients with inflammatory bowel disease. Gastroenterology. 2001;120:A1393.
6. Reuter BK, Asfaha S, Buret A et al. Exacerbation of inflammation-associated colonic injury in rat through inhibition of cyclooxygenase-2. J Clin Invest. 1996;98:2076–85.
7. Karmeli F, Cohen P, Rachmilewitz D. Cyclooxygenase-2 inhibitors ameliorate severity of experimental colitis in rats. Eur J Gastroenterol Hepatol. 2000;12:223–31.

8. Mahadevan U, Loftus EV, Tremaine WJ *et al*. Safety of selective cyclooxygenase-2 inhibitors in inflammatory bowel disease. Am J Gastroenterol. 1997;4:910–14.
9. De Vos M, Cuvelier C, Mielants H *et al*. Ileocolonoscopy in seronegative spondylarthropathy. Gastroenterology. 1989;96:339–44.
10. Mielants H, Veys EM, Cuvelier C *et al*. Ileocolonoscopic findings in seronegative spondy-larthropathies. Br J Rheumatol. 1988;27(Suppl. II):95–105.
11. Clegg DO, Reda DJ, Weisman MH *et al*. Comparison of sulfasalazine and placebo in the treatment of ankylosing spondylitis. Arthritis Rheum. 1996;39:2004–12.
12. Clegg DO, Reda DJ, Weisman MH *et al*. Comparison of sulfasalazine and placebo in the treatment of reactive arthritis (Reiter's syndrome). Arthritis Rheum. 1996;39:2021–7.
13. Dougados M, van der Linden S, Leirisalo-Repo M *et al*. Sulfasalazine in the treatment of spondy-larthropathy. Arthritis Rheum. 1995;38:618–27.
14. Thomson GTD, Thomson BRJ, Thomson KS *et al*. Clinical efficacy of mesalamine in the treat-ment of the spondyloarthropathies. J Rheumatol. 2000;27:714–18.
15. Dekker-Saeys BJ, Dijkmans BAC, Tytgat GNJ. Treatment of spondyloarthropathy with 5-aminosalicylic acid (Mesalazine): an open trial. J Rheumatol. 2000;27:723–6.
16. Van den Bosch F, Kruithof E, De Vos M *et al*. Crohn's disease associated with spondy-loarthropathy: effect of TNF-α blockade with infliximab on the articular symptoms. Lancet. 2000;356:1821–2.
17. Van den Bosch F, Kruithof E, Baeten D *et al*. Effects of a loading dose regimen of three infusions of chimeric monoclonal antibody to tumour necrosis factor alpha (infliximab) in spondyloarthropathy: an open pilot study. Ann Rheum Dis. 2000;59:428–33.
18. Van den Bosch F, Kruithof E, Baeten D *et al*. Randomized double-blind comparison of chimeric monoclonal antibody to tumor necrosis factor alpha (infliximab) versus placebo in active spondylarthropathy. Arthritis Rheum. 2002;46:755–65.
19. Braun J, Brandt J, Listing J *et al*. Treatment of active ankylosing spondylitis with infliximab: a randomised controlled multicentre trial. Lancet. 2002;359:1187–93.
20. Gorman JD, Sack KE, Davis JC. Treatment of ankylosing spondylitis by inhibition of tumor necrosis factor α. N Engl J Med. 2002;346:1349–56.
21. Sandborn WJ, Hanauer SB, Katz S *et al*. Etanercept for active Crohn's disease: a randomised double-blind, placebo controlled trial. Gastroenterology. 2001;121:1088–94.
22. Dayer JM, Krane SM. Anti-TNF alpha therapy for ankylosing spondylitis: a specific or non-specific treatment? N Engl J Med. 2002;346:1399–400.
23. Rath HC, Herfarth HH, Ikeda JS *et al*. Normal luminal bacteria, especially *Bacteroides* species, mediate chronic colitis, gastritis, and arthritis in HLA-B27/human beta2 microglobulin trans-genic rats. J Clin Invest. 1996;98:945–53.
24. Neut C, Bulois P, Desreumaux P *et al*. Changes in the bacterial flora of the neoterminal ileum after ileocolonic resection for Crohn's disease. Am J Gastroenterol. 2002;97:939–46.
25. Hazenberg MP. Intestinal flora bacteria and arthritis: why the joints? Scand J Rheumatol. 1995;24(Suppl. 101):207–11.
26. Baeten D, Demetter P, Cuvelier C *et al*. Macrophages expressing the scavenger receptor CD163: a link between immune alterations of the gut and synovial inflammation in spondyloarthropathy. J Pathol. 2002;196:1–9.
27. Salmi M, Andrew DP, Butcher EC, Jalkanen S. Dual binding capacity of mucosal immunoblasts to mucosal and synovial endothelium in humans. J Exp Med. 1995;181:137–49.
28. Van Damme N, Elewaut D, Baeten D *et al*. Gut mucosal T cell lines from ankylosing spondylitis patients are enriched with αEβ7 integrin. Clin Exp Rheumatol. 2001;19:681–7.
29. Hugot JP, Chamaillard M, Zouali H *et al*. Association of NOD2 leucine-rich repeat variants with susceptibility to Crohn's disease. Nature. 2001;411:599–603.
30. Lesage S, Zouali H, Cezard JP *et al*. CARD15/NOD2 mutational analysis and genotype–phenotype correlation in 612 patients with inflammatory bowel disease. Am J Hum Genet. 2002;70:845–7.
31. Crane AM, Bradbury L, van Heel DA *et al*. Role of NOD2 variants in spondylarthritis. Arthritis Rheum. 2002;46:1629–33.

Section VII
Special problems

22
Magnetic resonance imaging in patients with inflammatory bowel disease: a new method to assess disease activity?

S. FEUERBACH, A. G. SCHREYER, J. SEITZ, H. HERFARTH
and J. SCHÖLMERICH

INTRODUCTION

For small bowel assessment several radiological techniques exist. First, classical conventional enteroclysis (using the 'Sellink modification') and the 'follow-through' examination, which can only assess intraluminal pathology directly. Using a sectional imaging technique, e.g. computerized tomography (CT) or magnetic resonance imaging (MRI) even segmental thickening of bowel wall, stenosis or pre-stenotic dilation can be appreciated. Additionally extraluminal lesions and complications such as fistula, abscess (Fig. 1) and local fatty infiltration can be seen. Consequently MRI has a better sensitivity to assess Crohn's lesions[1] than the 'classical' small bowel examinations with transnasal intubation combined with fluoroscopy.

MRI ENTEROCLYSIS, TECHNIQUE OF THE EXAMINATION, BOWEL CONTRAST

Fast imaging techniques and breath-hold techniques are prerequisites for adequate diagnostic image quality. To reduce bowel peristalsis, scopolamine (e.g. Buscopan®, Böhringer, Ingelheim) can be given intravenously. To gain fast imaging at least gradients with more than 20 mT/m in magnets with 1.0–1.5 Tesla are necessary. Using such equipment a short data acquisition time is feasible, which is important for breath-hold imaging and adequate patient cooperation. Additionally fat-saturation techniques are helpful. These sequences selectively suppress the fat signal and allow better differentiation and identification of fluid structures such as subtle wall oedemas or tiny extraluminal fluid collections.

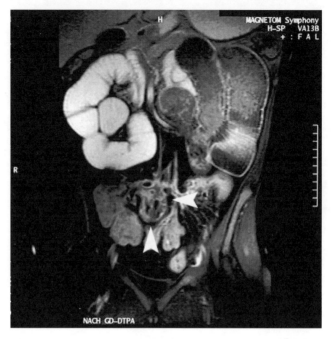

Fig. 1 MRI of a patient with a stenosis and an abscess (arrow) in the terminal ileum

Table 1 Individual brightness of different contrast media depending on the MRI sequence

	T1-weighted sequence	*T2-weighted sequence*
Water	Dark	Bright
Gd-DTPA	Bright	Dark
Juice (with manganese content)	Bright	Dark

A prerequisite to identify a stenosis or wall thickening is a sufficient contrast difference between the bowel lumen and the wall. Additionally a complete filling and distension of the small bowel is mandatory. There are several intraluminal contrast media for MRI bowel diagnosis:

1. regular water[2] (with or without methylcellulosis);
2. gadolinium (Gd-DTPA) mixture;
3. iron particles[3];
4. juices with high natural manganese content (e.g. pineapple juice, blueberry juice).

The contrast impression is dependent on T1- or T2-weighted image acquisition and the applied contrast media respectively. Table 1 describes the individual brightness of the different contrast media depending on the magnetic resonance sequence.

CROHN'S DISEASE – TYPICAL MRI FINDINGS

There are several typical MRI findings for bowel diagnosis in Crohn's disease:

1. segmental wall thickening;
2. consecutive stenosis and prestenotic dilatation;
3. wall oedema seen on T2-weighted sequences with enhancement of the inflamed bowel segment after Gd-DTPA application intravenously (T1-weighted sequence);
4. fistula, abscesses or inflammatory infiltration of the surrounding fatty tissue.

ASSESSMENT OF INFLAMMATORY BOWEL DISEASE ACTIVITY?

Basically the only criterion for disease activity is inflammation of the bowel. It is believed that an intense wall oedema or a strong signal enhancement after Gd-DTPA application indicates acute inflammatory disease. There are, however, no studies concerning the contrast behaviour of a scary stenosis, which does not respond to steroids.

Another problem is a missing reference method to assess disease activity, because currently the small bowel cannot be observed directly using endoscopic methods. The only way to assess parts are push enteroscopy or complete colonoscopy with intubation of the terminal ileum. Only using this method can histological specimens be obtained. There are only a few studies investigating the correlation of disease activity. These studies use other parameters such as the Crohn's Disease Activity Index (CDAI), C-reactive protein (CRP) or white cell count to assess disease activity.

Madsen et al.[4] studied eight patients with Crohn's disease using a low field scanner (0.1 T) to assess contrast enhancement and bowel wall thickening. All patients were examined again after 11–120 days after conservative therapy. In all patients with clinical response to the therapy there was a significant reduction in wall signal intensity and a significant reduction of wall thickening. The authors concluded that both criteria are suitable to assess disease activity.

An Italian study[5] is examining 20 patients with Crohn's disease, who were under therapy when they were scanned. Nineteen of these 20 patients had no clinical signs of their disease when they were scanned. Typical MRI appearance (wall thickening, contrast enhancement) was compared with white cell count and CRP. These authors concluded that there is a good correlation between the MRI criteria and the inflammation parameters. They suggest that MRI is a good parameter to assess disease activity.

In contrast to this group a study group from Mainz found no correlation between signal enhancement and bowel wall with the CDAI or CRP level. They suggest that signal intensity of the bowel wall compared with the CRP and white cell count is an adequate parameter to assess disease activity[2].

Neurath et al.[6], in a prospective study, compared fluorodeoxyglucose positron emission tomography (FDE-PET), MRI enteroclysis and immunoscintigraphy in 59 patients. Using PET 127 bowel segments with inflammation were assessed in 51 of 59 patients. Using MRI just 89 segments were identified as affected. Applying the nuclear medicine technique only 38 segments were identified. The authors conclude that FDG-PET is more sensitive than the other methods. In 28 patients a comparison with endoscopy was performed. Altogether 45 of the segments identified by PET, nine of the segments diagnosed using scintigraphy and 35 of the segments identified by MRI were correlated endoscopically. The evaluation of the data was based on the endoscopic findings of macroscopic inflammation. Based on these data there was an inhomogeneous group with a sensitivity for PET of 85%, 67% for MRI and 41% for scintigraphy. The specificity was 89.9% and 100%, respectively. Comparing only the localization of the inflamed segments, there was a minor difference in small bowel assessment between PET and MRI. Applying both techniques in 37 cases the terminal ileum was assessed as inflamed. PET imaging showed 24 inflamed areas whereas MRI identified only 20 lesions. The so-called 'hot spots' identified using PET imaging, which were not depicted using MRI, were predominantly in the colon. Is should be mentioned that the colon was not prepared for MRI examination, which explains the significant difference between PET and MRI. The study does not examine disease activity but leads to the conclusion that PET imaging was the most sensitive study to detect lesions; however, most of these lesions were in the colon, which was not prepared for MRI.

Schreyer et al.[7] studied 30 patients with Crohn's disease, applying virtual enteroscopy. In 90% a good image quality was achieved. In three cases fistulas and stenoses were depicted clearly. More information regarding disease activity was not assessed using this new technique. Mucosal assessment was not possible using this technique.

CONCLUSION

Currently there are no impressive data in the literature to confirm that using MRI is an adequate technique to assess disease activity in Crohn's disease. It is not clear if PET is a good method to diagnose lesions in Crohn's disease, because the method has fairly low spatial resolution. Image fusion with MRI and CT imaging could be a good approach to compensate for this disadvantage, but it is extremely difficult to perform because of bowel movement. High costs for this examination, and the low availability of this method, are further arguments against the application of this technique in disease assessment on a regular basis.

Acknowledgement

The studies performed at the University Hospital Regensburg were supported by DCCV e.V., Leverkusen, Germany (German Crohn's Disease and Ulcerative Colitis Association).

References

1. Rieber A, Wruk D, Potthast S et al. Diagnostic imaging in Crohn's disease: comparison of magnetic resonance imaging and conventional imaging methods. Int J Colorectal Dis. 2000; 15: 176–81.
2. Schunk K, Kern A, Oberholzer K et al. Hydro-MRI in Crohn's disease: appraisal of disease activity. Invest Radiol. 2000; 35:431–7.

3. Holzknecht N, Helmberger T, von Ritter C, Gauger J, Faber S, Reiser M. MRI of the small intestine with rapid MRI sequences in Crohn disease after enteroclysis with oral iron particles. Radiologe. 1998;38:29–36.
4. Madsen SM, Thomsen HS, Schlichting P, Dorph S, Munkholm P. Evaluation of treatment response in active Crohn's disease by low-field magnetic resonance imaging. Abdom Imag. 1999;24:232–9.
5. Maccioni F, Viscido A, Broglia L et al. Evaluation of Crohn disease activity with magnetic resonance imaging. Abdom Imag. 2000;25:219–28.
6. Neurath MF, Vehling D, Schunk K et al. Noninvasive assessment of Crohn's disease activity: a comparison of 18F-fluorodeoxyglucose positron emission tomography, hydromagnetic resonance imaging, and granulocyte scintigraphy with labeled antibodies. Am J Gastroenterol. 2002;97:1978–85.
7. Schreyer AG, Herfarth H, Kikinis R et al. 3D modeling and virtual endoscopy of the small bowel based on magnetic resonance imaging in patients with inflammatory bowel disease. Invest Radiol. 2002;37:528–33.

23
Cancer prevention in inflammatory bowel disease as a treatment goal

A. EKBOM

INTRODUCTION

There is an increased morbidity and mortality in cancer among patients with inflammatory bowel disease (IBD) in most follow-up studies published so far[1-5]. There are, however, exceptions and the most noteworthy is the follow-up studies conducted from Copenhagen, which indicate that there are strategies for cancer prevention in patients with IBD[6,7]. The excess morbidity and mortality is somewhat more pronounced in patients with ulcerative colitis than in patients with Crohn's disease. Colorectal cancer still remains the major reason for this excess risk[1] but there is also an excess risk for cholangiocarcinoma secondary to primary sclerosing cholangitis[8]. In patients with Crohn's disease there is also an excess risk for cancer of the small intestine[3] as well as an excess number of smoking-related cancers[3]. Recently there have also been indications that haematopoietic malignancies, i.e. leukaemias and lymphomas, could be a concern.

SMOKING-RELATED CANCERS

Smoking has consistently been associated with a decreased risk of ulcerative colitis in an abundance of aetiological studies[9]. A consistent finding is therefore that patients with ulcerative colitis will experience a decreased risk of respiratory cancers and other smoking-related cancers of a magnitude of 50%[1,4]. In the case of Crohn's disease smoking acts in the opposite direction, and it is therefore not surprising that there is an increased risk of smoking-related cancers in this patient group[3]. Thus, in addition to the beneficial effect of smoking cessation to the natural course of Crohn's disease, an intervention instigated by the treating physician aiming at a smoke-free life will have a major impact on the overall cancer risk in patients with Crohn's disease.

CANCER OF THE SMALL INTESTINE

The increased risk of cancer of the small intestine in patients with Crohn's disease is a consistent finding in most follow-up studies[3,7,10,11]. The relative risk estimate is often very high, two digits or more, but as the occurrence of cancer in the small intestine is a rarity, the impact on the overall cancer risk in patients with Crohn's disease is small. Moreover, Crohn's disease constitutes a major attributable fraction for these cancer forms, especially in the younger age groups[12]. Studies from Sweden and Israel have shown a substantially lower risk than in the United States[1,13]. This could be due to a more active surgical approach in Sweden and Israel compared to the United States, and the avoidance of the intestinal bypass procedure. It has also been shown that areas with long-standing chronic inflammation seem to carry the highest risk for malignant transformation as well as the presence of strictures[10]. It is therefore somewhat of a concern what sort of impact the introduction of surgery, including strictureplasty during the 1990s, will have on the long-term cancer risk. There are therefore reasons to continuously monitor to what extent such procedures will affect the cancer risk.

CHOLANGIOCARCINOMA

Approximately 4% of patients with extensive ulcerative colitis will eventually have a clinical overt primary sclerosing cholangitis[14]. There is also an excess risk for primary sclerosing cholangitis in patients with Crohn's disease but no risk estimates are available[15]. Patients with primary sclerosing cholangitis are at extremely high risk for a malignant transformation in the bile ducts. The cumulative incidence for such a malignant transformation 10 years after diagnosis of primary sclerosing cholangitis has been assessed to be as high as 10%[8]. There are no known strategies to avoid progression to cholangiocarcinoma, nor are there any known interventions that would decrease the risk of a primary sclerosing cholangitis. For instance, colectomy does not seem to affect the risk for cholangiocarcinoma[8,15] but there are some indications that patients with a prior malignancy of the colorectal tract are at an even higher risk for cholangiocarcinoma[8], which should be taken into account when discussing the venue of liver transplantation in this patient group.

HAEMATOPOIETIC MALIGNANCIES

The presence of a chronic inflammation has been postulated to increase the risk for malignant transformation in the lymphatic tissue[16]. This seems to be true for patients with rheumatoid arthritis where an increasing inflammatory activity is associated with an increased risk for lymphomas[16]. So far no such association has been shown for IBD. There are, however, reports of an increased risk of lymphomas in patients with IBD, originating almost exclusively from North America[17,18]. This could be due to the fact that use of immunosuppressive drugs in patients with IBD is more common in North America than in Europe. Lymphomas have also emerged as a major concern following the introduction of new therapeutic modalities in this patient group.

Leukaemias have been reported in a few case reports to be associated with IBD, but so far confined to longitudinal studies from referral centres[17,19]. However, there are presently in Sweden indications that patients with IBD during the 1990s are at an excess risk for leukaemias, especially myeloic leukaemias. This needs confirmation, but could be due to new treatment paradigms for this patient group. It is therefore presently of utmost importance to find good surveillance programmes in order to follow patients with IBD for the risk of haematopoietic malignancies in order to identify new patterns of cancer risk, possibly due to new treatments.

COLORECTAL CANCER

The long-term excess mortality in patients with ulcerative colitis is almost entirely due to colorectal cancer[2]. Colectomy as a preventive measure has been utilized for many decades. As early as 1973 Devroede *et al.*, from the Mayo Clinic, could demonstrate a substantially better long-term prognosis among paediatric patients who were subjected to proctocolectomy compared to those left with an intact colon[20]. Great efforts have been made to identify those patients at the highest risk for malignant transformation. Extent of disease[21], duration[22], family history of colorectal cancer but not IBD[23], presence of primary sclerosing cholangitis[24] and possibly young age at onset[21] have been identified as independent risk factors. However, proctocolectomy as a preventive measure is not always an option, and there is a growing reluctance among both clinicians and patients for such an approach. Colonoscopy surveillance in order to identify precursors such as dysplasia is another strategy[25], and there are indications that this will have an impact on cancer mortality[26]. However, there are still patients in surveillance programmes who will die from colorectal cancer.

There are reasons to believe that the excess risk of colorectal cancer presented in studies from the 1970s and 1980s is not entirely valid today. There are, for instance, indications from Sweden that there is a decrease in the number of cancers diagnosed in patients with ulcerative colitis[27]. The highest risk estimates for a malignant transformation were presented in earlier studies and the most recent ones, dealing with patients diagnosed during the 1970s with sufficient long-term follow-up, have shown lower risk estimates: most noteworthy are the results from Copenhagen where no excess risk could be demonstrated[6]. It is very unlikely that this decrease is entirely due to the surveillance programmes, as only a minority of patients with ulcerative colitis is enrolled in such programmes[26].

This decrease in risk could either be due to altered natural history or new treatment modalities. In the 1980s, researchers in Israel reported a lower incidence of colorectal cancer in patients with ulcerative colitis compared to other centres[28]. The authors attributed this to their maintenance therapy with sulphasalazine. A similar explanation has also been proposed from Copenhagen[6] where the patients are characterized by a consistent maintenance therapy, mainly with sulphasalazine. This finding is in accordance with a similar observation from the United Kingdom[29] when the effects of colonoscopy surveillance programmes were evaluated and the authors stated that a 'review of the notes of patients with colorectal cancer and ulcerative colitis suggested that virtually none of them were taking disease-suppressant drugs such as sulphasalazine regularly or at all'. The hypothesis that sulphasalazine acts as a protective factor against malignant transformation has been put to the test in some observational studies both from Sweden[30] and Great Britain[31,32] where similar findings have been presented with a substantially decreased risk among patients taking anti-inflammatory drugs such as sulphasalazine compared to those without. Similar findings were reported earlier from the United States, where sulpha allergy, i.e. patients who cannot be exposed to sulphasalazine, was associated with a substantial increase for malignant transformation[33]. The underlying biological mechanism for these findings still remains to be explained, but in the normal population exposure to salicylic acid has been shown to have a protective effect against sporadic colorectal cancer, perhaps also through anti-inflammatory mechanisms[34].

FOLATE DEFICIENCY

Folate deficiency has been reported to be associated with an increased risk of sporadic colorectal cancer as well as the risk for colorectal adenomas[35]. It has therefore been proposed that folate supplementation will be beneficial and prevent a malignant transformation in patients with ulcerative colitis. In two small studies in the United States there has been a consistent finding that folate use is associated with a non-significant reduction in the risk of dysplasia or colorectal cancer[33,36]. This is, of course, a very attractive alternative but there is a great need of further confirmatory studies before folate substitution can be recommended as a general preventive measure.

CROHN'S DISEASE IN PATIENTS WITH COLORECTAL CANCER

In the case of Crohn's disease and colorectal cancer, there seems to be an increased risk for colorectal cancer with similar risk patterns as for ulcerative colitis, i.e. extensive disease of the colon, long duration, family history of colorectal cancer and possibly young age at onset[37,38]. Prophylactic colectomy is, of course, a potential preventive measure, especially as no studies so far have addressed to what extent anti-inflammatory therapy will have any impact on this excess risk.

CONCLUSION

There is an excess risk of cancer among patients with IBD. Besides smoking cessation and prophylactic surgery, anti-inflammatory therapy in patients with ulcerative colitis is so far the only proven preventive measure against this excess morbidity and mortality. There are also reasons to monitor the long-term consequences of different immunosuppressant therapies and new pharmacological compounds and the impact on the cancer risk.

References

1. Ekbom A, Helmick C, Zack M, Adami HO. Extracolonic malignancies in inflammatory bowel disease. Cancer. 1991;67:2015–19.
2. Ekbom A, Helmick CG, Zack M, Holmberg L, Adami HO. Survival and causes of death in patients with inflammatory bowel disease: a population-based study. Gastroenterology. 1992;103:954–60.
3. Persson PG, Karlen P, Bernell O et al. Crohn's disease and cancer: a population-based cohort study. Gastroenterology. 1994;107:1675–9.
4. Prior P, Gyde SN, Macartney JC, Thompson H, Waterhouse JAH, Allan RN. Cancer morbidity in ulcerative colitis. Gut. 1982;23:490–7.
5. Gyde SN, Prior P, Macartney JC, Thompson H, Waterhouse JAH, Allan RN. Malignancy in Crohn's disease. Gut. 1980;21:1024–9.
6. Langholz E, Munkholm P, Davidsen M, Binder V. Colorectal cancer risk and mortality in patients with ulcerative colitis. Gastroenterology. 1992;103:1444–51.
7. Munkholm P, Langholz E, Davidsen M, Binder V. Intestinal cancer risk and mortality in patients with Crohn's disease. Gastroenterology. 1993;105:1716–23.
8. Kornfeld D, Ekbom A, Ihre T. Survival and risk of cholangiocarcinoma in patients with primary sclerosing cholangitis – a population-based study. Scand J Gastroenterol. 1997;32:1042–5.
9. Lindberg E, Tysk C, Andersson K, Järnerot G. Smoking and inflammatory bowel disease. A case control study. Gut. 1988;29:352–7.
10. Senay E, Sachar DB, Keohane M, Greenstein AJ. Small bowel carcinoma in Crohn's disease. Distinguishing features and risk factors. Cancer. 1989;63:360–3.
11. Greenstein AJ, Sachar DB, Smith H, Janowitz HD, Aufses AH Jr. A comparison of cancer risk in Crohn's disease and ulcerative colitis. Cancer. 1981;48:2742–5.
12. Chen CC, Neugut, AI, Rotterdam H. Risk factors for adenocarcinomas and malignant carcinoids of the small intestine: preliminary findings. Cancer Epidemiol Biomarkers Prev. 1994;3:205–7.
13. Fireman Z, Grossman A, Lilos P et al. Intestinal cancer in patients with Crohn's disease. A population study in central Israel. Scand J Gastroenterol. 1989;24:346–50.
14. Olsson R, Danielsson A, Jarnerot G et al. Prevalence of primary sclerosing cholangitis in patients with ulcerative colitis. Gastroenterology. 1991;100:1319–23.
15. Broome U, Olsson R, Loof L et al. Natural history and prognostic factors in 305 Swedish patients with primary sclerosing cholangitis. Gut. 1996;38:610–15.
16. Baecklund E, Ekbom A, Sparén P, Feltelius N, Klareskog L. Disease activity and risk of lymphoma in patients with rheumatoid arthritis: nested case–control study. Br Med J. 1998;317:180–1.
17. Greenstein AJ, Gennuso R, Sachar DB et al. Extraintestinal cancers in inflammatory bowel disease. Cancer. 1985;56:2914–21.
18. Greenstein AJ, Mullin GE, Stracuhen JA et al. Lymphoma in inflammatory bowel disease. Cancer. 1992;69:1119–23.
19. Mir-Madjlessi SH, Farmer RG, Easly KA, Beck GJ. Colorectal cancer and extra-colonic malignancies in ulcerative colitis. Cancer. 1986;58:1569–74.
20. Devroede GJ, Taylor WF, Saucer WG, Jackman RJ, Stickler GB. Cancer risk and life expectancy of children with ulcerative colitis. N Engl J Med. 1971;285:17–21.
21. Ekbom A, Helmick C, Zack M, Adami HO. Ulcerative colitis and colorectal cancer; a population-based study. N Engl J Med. 1990;323:1228–33.
22. Gyde SN, Prior P, Allan RN et al. Colorectal cancer in ulcerative colitis: a cohort study of primary referrals from three centres. Gut. 1988;29:206–17.
23. Askling J, Dickman PW, Karlen P et al. Family history as a risk factor for colorectal cancer in inflammatory bowel disease. Gastroenterology. 2001;120:1356–62.
24. Broome U, Lindberg G, Löfberg R. Primary sclerosing cholangitis in ulcerative colitis: a risk factor for the development of dysplasia and DNA aneuploidy? Gastroenterology. 1992;102: 1877–80.
25. Löfberg R, Bröstrom O, Karlen P, Tribukait B, Ost A. Colonoscopic surveillance in long-standing total ulcerative colitis – a 15-year follow-up study. Gastroenterology. 1990;99:1021–31.
26. Karlén P, Kornfeld D, Broström O, Löfberg R, Persson PG, Ekbom A. Is colonoscopic surveillance reducing colorectal cancer mortality in ulcerative colitis? A population-based case-control study. Gut. 1998;42:711–14.

27. Rubio CA, Befrits R, Ljung T, Jaramillo E, Slezak P. Colorectal carcinoma in ulcerative colitis is decreasing in Scandinavian countries. Anticancer Res. 2001;21:2921–4.
28. Odes HS, Fraser D. Ulcerative colitis in Israel: epidemiology, morbidity, and genetics. Public Health Rev. 1989–90;17:297–319.
29. Lynch DA, Lobo AJ, Sobala GM, Dixon MF, Axon AT. Failure of colonoscopic surveillance in ulcerative colitis. Gut. 1993;34:1075–80.
30. Pinczowski D, Ekbom A, Baron J, Yuen J, Adami HO. Risk factors for colorectal cancer among patients with ulcerative colitis – a case–control study. Gastroenterology. 1994;107:117–20.
31. Moody GA, Jayanthi V, Probert CS, Mac Kay H, Mayberry JF. Long-term therapy with sulphasalazine protects against colorectal cancer in ulcerative colitis: a retrospective study of colorectal cancer risk and compliance with treatment in Leicestershire. Eur J Gastroenterol Hepatol. 1996;8:1179–83.
32. Eaden J, Abrams K, Ekbom A, Jackson E, Mayberry J. Colorectal cancer prevention in ulcerative colitis: a case–control study. Aliment Pharmacol Ther. 2000;14:145–53.
33. Lashner BA, Heidenreich PA, Su GL, Kane SV, Hanauer SB. Effect of folate supplementation on the incidence of dysplasia and cancer in chronic ulcerative colitis. A case–control study. Gastroenterology. 1989;97:255–9.
34. Thun M, Namboodiri N, Heath CJ. Aspirin use and reduced risk of fatal colon cancer. N Engl J Med. 1991;325:1593–6.
35. Giovannucci E, Rimm EB, Ascherio A, Stampfer MJ, Colditz GA, Willett WC. Alcohol, low-methionine–low-folate diets, and risk of colon cancer in men. J Natl Cancer Inst. 1995;87:265–73.
36. Lashner BA, Provencher KS, Seidner DL, Knesebeck A, Brzezinski A. The effect of folic acid supplementation on the risk for cancer or dysplasia in ulcerative colitis. Gastroenterology. 1997;112:29–32.
37. Ekbom A, Helmick C, Zack M, Adami HO. Increased risk of large bowel cancer in Crohn's disease with colonic involvement. Lancet. 1990;336:357–9.
38. Sachar D. Cancer in Crohn's disease: dispelling the myth. Gut. 1994;35:1507–8.

Section VIII
Quality of care

24
Quality of care: the impact of age and social environment on therapeutic concepts

C. GASCHÉ

INTRODUCTION

Most of our current knowledge on the therapy of inflammatory bowel disease is based on the results of controlled clinical trials. These trials focus on the effects of anti-inflammatory therapies and on lowering the clinical activity indexes of Crohn's disease or ulcerative colitis. In recent years the outcome measures have been improved by implementing quality-of-life scores; however, the influence of psychosocial factors and the age of the patient have not been well studied in such controlled trials. When facing real life in clinical medicine such factors, however, strongly influence our therapeutic strategies. In addition, it is evident that only a small percentage of patients in our daily practice fit into protocols of controlled clinical trials. The majority of patients do not meet the rigorous inclusion criteria. This is why we need to tailor the treatment to the specific problems of the patient. This tailoring is typically done outside of the evidence-based-medicine world.

Before prescribing therapy for individual patients we need to consider several dimensions of the individual in front of us. First of all, we have to understand who is our individual patient; second, we need to identify the therapeutic target; and third we need to define the therapeutic goal. General and specific therapeutic targets are already covered in other chapters of this book. After identifying such targets, we need to define the therapeutic goals for individual outcomes. Interestingly, when focusing on common targets such as strictures or fistulas, only a few data are available from controlled trials in literature. The therapeutic target may not only be a complication of inflammatory bowel disease but it may also be the prevention of such complications. This chapter will focus on the primary question: Who is my individual patient?

MY INDIVIDUAL PATIENT

Whenever physicians have contact with patients they interact with individuals. In a case of inflammatory bowel diseases such individuals should not only be placed into one or the other inflammatory bowel disease boxes (ulcerative colitis or Crohn's disease), but need to be understood as personalities with multiple dimensions (Fig. 1). These dimensions should be appreciated and understood before therapeutic advice is given. We have to know the disease phenotype, not only the major group but also the certain subtype. In Crohn's disease this relates to the phenotypic classification of Crohn's disease (Vienna classification)[1], and in ulcerative colitis to the extent of disease (pouchitis, left-sided colitis, extended colitis or pancolitis). In addition it is important to understand the disease history. Disease history relates to the number and type of operations in the past, and to the response or unresponsiveness to certain medications.

These two dimensions are generally taken care of. I would like to indicate further dimensions which are rather neglected. When dealing with inflammatory bowel diseases certain nutritional deficits such as vitamins or iron also need to be explored. It is a fact that iron-deficiency anaemia is present in one-third of patients[2]. A major emphasis during the individual exploration should be on the smoking history or smoking habits of the patient. Even in the era of genetics, smoking is still the most important factor that has impact on the clinical course of Crohn's disease and, rather than genetic mutations, this factor can be avoided! The fifth and possibly most important dimension of our patient relates to psychosocial factors.

The burden of inflammatory bowel diseases is strongly influenced by psychosocial factors. Stressful life events such as the daily aspects of working life have been shown to affect bowel symptoms[3]. Emotional disturbances such as the loss of a family member or separation from the partner may cause similar effects. The disease itself causes anxiety regarding future health, future ability to work, and future ability to maintain relationships. In a questionnaire the fear of having an ileostomy operation scored highest on the anxiety scale[4]. When dealing with individual inflammatory bowel disease patients it may be more important to know about these psychosocial factors, the fears, excitements and emotions, than to know about certain disease subgroups of a patient.

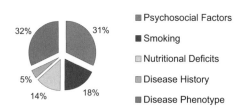

Fig. 1 Different aspects of my individual patient. Each patient is a composition of various individual dimensions of disease. These aspects include, but are not limited to, disease phenotype, disease history, nutritional deficits, smoking habits and psychosocial factors. Before prescribing therapy for inflammatory bowel diseases we need to understand each patient in an individual way. The anticipation of our patient's specific problems is the key to patient-tailored medicine

INFLAMMATORY BOWEL DISEASE AND PSYCHIATRIC DISEASE

The myth still persists in some areas that ulcerative colitis and Crohn's disease are specific expressions of certain pathological personality types. This 'inflammatory bowel disease personality' idea has mostly been fuelled by anecdotal experiences. Larger epidemiological studies, however, have demonstrated a higher incidence of major psychiatric illness in patients with inflammatory bowel disease than in patients with other chronic diseases. This is specifically true for depression. It has been argued that depression is a causal factor of inflammatory bowel diseases. Controlled studies point to the fact that depression may rather be a consequence of chronic intestinal inflammation than the cause[5]. Chronic diarrhoea is associated with social isolation, and a lack of human interactions. The chronicity and severity of bowel symptoms in the course of inflammatory bowel diseases was argued as a cause of depression[5]. A third possibility, which has not been addressed in the past, is a common genetic susceptibility to inflammatory bowel diseases and depression. Little is known regarding the overlap of genetic susceptibility regions in these two disorders. Our own studies on the interleukin-10 receptor 1 polymorphisms showed that such an overlap might exist. When the frequency of certain loss-of-function alleles of the interleukin-10 receptor 1 was studied in colonic Crohn's disease, we found twice as many homozygous mutants compared with controls, and even more homozygous mutants were found in unipolar depression samples. This points to the possibility that colonic Crohn's disease and unipolar depression may share a common genetic background. The pathophysiological role of the interleukin-10 pathway in inflammatory bowel diseases has been clearly identified by various knockout models[6]. The pathophysiological role of interleukin-10 receptor variants for susceptibility to unipolar depression is not yet clear. It has been observed, however, that interleukin-10 therapy for inflammatory bowel diseases also improved the depression scale in affected patients.

In any case, psychosocial factors can directly affect the progression of the underlying inflammatory bowel disease through psychoimmunological effects (see chapter by Dr Collins) and affect the quality of life of patients (see chapter by Dr Irving). The psychosocial dimension of disease therefore needs specific attention. It may not be enough to ask our patients how they are doing. Doctors need to open up their minds and need to listen to the patients' individual concerns, whether these are related to disease or not. The doctor's anticipation of the patient's personal problems is the key to better medical care.

Let me give a specific example of such a doctor–patient interaction. The doctor asked the patient after he had entered his office: 'How are you doing today Mr Smith?' And Mr Smith answered that he hadn't felt that good in months. It is likely that the doctor's perception would be that Mr Smith is feeling really good. When Mr Smith was asked to fill in a specific questionnaire regarding his physical activity, cognitive function, social activity, and work performance, he mostly scored at the very low end of the scale. When he was asked again after his condition, he stated that it had improved during recent months; however, it is still far from what he used to call normal. Such physician misperceptions are frequent in patient–physician interactions, and this has recently been studied in oncology units. I encourage performing such studies also in the setting of inflammatory bowel disease.

SMOKING CESSATION

The social environment also plays a certain role regarding smoking. It has been known for a long time that smoking relates to socioeconomic status; the higher the educational level the more unlikely it is that people smoke. This has also recently been addressed in a prospective smoking cessation trial[7]. The French group investigated 474 smokers with Crohn's disease and tested the hypothesis that smoking cessation improves the clinical course of disease. Smoking cessation was successful in only 12% of their population; indeed cessation was associated with an improvement in the clinical course of Crohn's disease similar to patients who had never smoked. Interestingly the study identified four factors which were associated with successful smoking cessation: first was the particular physician; second was higher socioeconomic status; third was previous bowel surgery; and last was concomitant use of oral contraceptives. In my opinion it is the first goal in patients with Crohn's disease to have them quit smoking. The effects of smoking cessation might be regarded to be as strong as the effects of steroids on the clinical course, but without any side-effects. Patient's education and physician's credibility are most fundamental to achieve this goal.

THE AGE FACTOR

There are only a few studies that stratified for patients' age as a factor defining therapy outcome. Obviously, some therapies cannot be applied to elderly patients, such as enemas. The age is also a category to classify patients with Crohn's disease. This has been established within the Vienna classification of Crohn's disease. Two subgroups were separated: first, patients with age at diagnosis under 40 years, and second, those above 40 years. Studies from the 1990s showed that patients with age at diagnosis above 40 are phenotypically different from those under 40[8]. It was found that they have a lower likelihood of positive family history, less small bowel disease and more colonic disease involvement. In addition, they have less stricturing disease and more inflammatory disease. Colonic Crohn's disease has also been known not to respond to steroids[9]. The age factor does determine the therapeutic concept: the older the patient, the more likely one is to find concomitant diseases such as osteoporosis, diabetes, or hypertension. This may specifically influence the use of steroids in elderly women.

PATIENT-TAILORED MEDICINE

The general practice of inflammatory bowel disease therapy includes a stepwise approach to more effective and more toxic drugs (Fig. 2). Such a stepwise approach may also be called a 'method of trial and error'. At the bottom of such a stepwise approach stand dietary changes. These are followed by mesalamine, then local or systemic steroids, continuing on to immunosuppression and ending with surgery. It is provocative to claim that the identification of specific therapeutic targets and of individual disease problems may help to better direct inflammatory bowel disease therapy. I do not want to push for top-down therapy with infliximab; I rather claim that the identification of individual disease

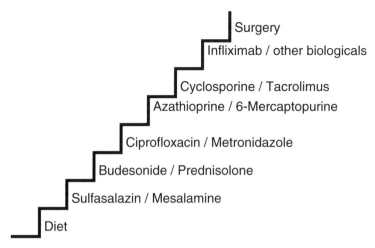

Fig. 2 Common practice of inflammatory bowel disease therapy. It is a general rule to prefer therapies with few side-effects. This leads to the common practice of starting therapy with mostly ineffective drugs and stepping up the therapeutic pyramid. If such an approach is to be successful we could implement a computer program for treating patients with inflammatory bowel diseases. I may call this the 'method of trial and error'. Good IBD therapy, however, should target a specific patient's problems, such as anaemia, or strictures, or maintenance of remission

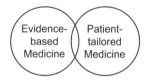

Fig. 3 Evidence-based medicine vs. patient-tailored medicine. These two philosophies of patient care have been used as 'opponents' in the past. The integration of the two concepts is for the good of our patients

problems such as strictures or fistulas should lead to appropriate therapies for reaching the therapeutic goal. With regard to strictures there is no published control trial regarding the therapeutic options. It is a physical rule, however, that mechanical problems such as bowel obstruction need mechanical relief such as endoscopic dilation or, if this is not possible, strictureplasty or resection. This indicates that evidence-based medicine fails to help with the common therapeutic decision. The only controlled data available concerning the treatment of fistulas come from trials that were testing infliximab[10]. Again, the level of evidence regarding other therapies for fistulas is low. In any case there is no evidence that steroids are effective in treating strictures or fistulas.

I suggest that future clinical research should address the question of targeting inflammatory bowel disease therapy. Placebo-controlled trials are needed to identify active drugs or treatment options for common inflammatory bowel disease problems such as strictures or fistulas. The improvement of the general symptoms measured by the Crohn's Disease Activity Index or by the Ulcerative

Colitis Activity Index is not adequate for the majority of our patients. It is anticipated that both concepts, evidence-based medicine and patient-tailored medicine, can be integrated into optimized medical care for our inflammatory bowel disease patients (Fig. 3). The physician will still need to identify each patient as an individual person, with individual concerns, worries, and disease problems. Only after the physician becomes part of the patient's case can treatment alter the disease course for the good of the patient.

References

1. Gasche C, Scholmerich J, Brynskov J *et al*. A simple classification of Crohn's disease: report of the Working Party for the World Congresses of Gastroenterology, Vienna, 1998. Inflamm Bowel Dis. 2000;6:8–15.
2. Gasche C. Anemia in IBD: the overlooked villain. Inflamm Bowel Dis. 2000;6:142–50.
3. Moser G, Tillinger W, Sachs G *et al*. Disease-related worries and concerns: a study on out-patients with inflammatory bowel disease. Eur J Gastroenterol Hepatol. 1995;7:853–8.
4. Levenstein S, Li Z, Almer S *et al*. Cross-cultural variation in disease-related concerns among patients with inflammatory bowel disease. Am J Gastroenterol. 2001;96:1822–30.
5. North CS, Alpers DH, Helzer JE, Spitznagel EL, Clouse RE. Do life events or depression exacerbate inflammatory bowel disease? A prospective study. Ann Intern Med. 1991;114:381–6.
6. Rennick DM, Fort MM. Lessons from genetically engineered animal models. XII. IL-10-deficient (IL-10(−/−)) mice and intestinal inflammation. Am J Physiol Gastrointest Liver Physiol. 2000;278:G829–33.
7. Cosnes J, Beaugerie L, Carbonnel F, Gendre JP. Smoking cessation and the course of Crohn's disease: an intervention study. Gastroenterology. 2001;120:1093–9.
8. Polito JM, Childs B, Mellits ED, Tokayer AZ, Harris ML, Bayless TM. Crohn's disease: influence of age at diagnosis on site and clinical type of disease. Gastroenterology. 1996;111:580–6.
9. Summers RW, Switz DM, Sessions JTJ *et al*. National Cooperative Crohn's Disease Study: results of drug treatment. Gastroenterology. 1979;77:847–69.
10. Present DH, Rutgeerts P, Targan S *et al*. Infliximab for the treatment of fistulas in patients with Crohn's disease. N Engl J Med. 1999;340:1398–405.

25
Avoiding side-effects: a therapeutic goal?

W. J. SANDBORN

INTRODUCTION

The general principles to be followed when new medical or surgical therapies are accepted into clinical practice include the following. First, therapies should be both effective and safe. Second, demonstration of efficacy usually requires two adequate and well-controlled trials for drugs (regulatory requirements may be less for devices and procedures). Third, demonstration of safety usually requires exposure of 500–1000 patients (requirements may be less for devices and procedures). The approaches that can be taken to avoid side-effects of therapy in general include: (1) improving the safety profile of a drug known to be effective through pharmacogenetics; (2) altering the chemical structure or delivery system or surgical approach of an agent or surgical technique known to be effective in order to improve the safety profile; (3) identifying a novel mechanism of action targeted towards specific receptors, enzymes, etc.; and (4) administering a second drug to block the adverse effects of the therapeutic agent. The specific approaches that have been used to avoid side-effects in patients with inflammatory bowel disease include the use of: (1) pharmacogenetics (sulphasalazine, azathioprine, 6-mercaptopurine); (2) alteration of the structure or delivery system (mesalamine, olsalazine, balsalazide, budesonide, CDP 571, etanercept, D2E7); (3) identifying a novel mechanism of action (infliximab, natalizumab, etc.); and (4) blocking the adverse effects of medications (concomitant treatment with immunosuppressives or pretreatment with steroids in infliximab-treated patients). Each of these approaches will be discussed further below.

PHARMACOGENOMICS

N-acetyltransferase 2 (NAT 2) – sulphasalazine

The NAT 2 slow acetylator genotype, as well as free and total serum sulphapyridine, have been associated with side-effects in patients with ulcerative colitis treated with sulphasalazine. A slow acetylator genotype/phenotype has been associated with sulphasalazine side-effects including: nausea, vomiting, cyanosis, haemolysis, leukopenia, agranulocytosis, fever, headache, and dizziness[1,2]. N-acetyltransferase 2 activity and the rapid acetylator phenotype correlate inversely with plasma sulphapyridine but not with total sulphapyridine in patients treated with sulphasalazine[1,2]. A study of NAT 2 acetylation capacity as measured by ability to acetylate caffeine demonstrated that a smaller number of patients were homozygous for slow acetylation ($n = 39$), about half of the patients were heterozygous with respect to NAT 2 acetylation ($n = 312$), and about half of the patients were homozygous for rapid NAT 2 acetylation ($n = 444$)[3]. A recent population-based study of sulphasalazine therapy in patients with ulcerative colitis demonstrated the following toxicity profile: (1) rash 20%, (2) nausea and vomiting 8%, (3) headache 6%, (4) agranulocytosis 3%, (5) arthralgias 3%, (6) fever 2%, (7) dyspnoea 2%, (8) diarrhoea 2%[4]. The patients were genotyped for NAT 2 and divided into slow or rapid acetylator status. Thirty-four per cent of patients with slow acetylator NAT 2 genotypes developed sulphasalazine-associated toxicity compared to 45% of rapid acetylator NAT 2 genotypes (odds ratio not significant)[4]. Thus, although in theory pharmacogenetics could be helpful in identifying patients at risk for sulphasalazine toxicity, in practice studies have not demonstrated that NAT 2 genotyping is clinically useful.

Thiopurine methyltransferase (TPMT) – azathioprine and 6-mercaptopurine

Azathioprine is a prodrug which is non-enzymatically converted to 6-mercaptopurine after absorption by glutathione or other sulphahydryl containing proteins. 6-Mercaptopurine is subsequently metabolized to active metabolites, the 6-thioguanine nucleotides (6-TGN) or through two alternate pathways to what have been considered inactive metabolites, 6-thiouric acid (via metabolism by xanthine oxidase) or 6-methylmercaptopurine (6-MMP) (via metabolism by TPMT)[5]. TPMT enzyme activity is generally mediated with approximately 89% of patients having two high activity alleles (normal enzyme activity), 11% of patients being heterozygotes with one high and one low activity allele, and 0.3% of patients having homozygote low activity with two low activity alleles[6]. Patients who have low or intermediate TPMT activity are more likely to experience clinical efficacy on the one hand, and myelotoxicity on the other hand. There are at least eight genetic polymorphisms that contribute to intermediate or low TPMT enzyme activity[7,8].

In a recent study 41 patients with Crohn's disease who developed severe myelosuppression (white blood cell count < 3000 or platelet count <100000) during treatment with azathioprine or 6-mercaptopurine were evaluated for TPMT genotype[8]. Four of 41 patients (10%) had low enzyme activity and seven of 41 (17%) had intermediate activity. Early leukopenia was noted in subjects with low or intermediate TPMT enzyme activity genotypes, whereas normal TPMT enzyme activity genotypes were noted in patients with late leukopenia. This study suggests that baseline determination of TPMT activity (phenotype) or genotype could predict the occurrence of early leukopenia in approximately 27% of patients with Crohn's disease who are treated with azathioprine or 6-mercaptopurine.

ALTER STRUCTURE OR DELIVER SYSTEM

Mesalamine and 5-ASA prodrugs

Sulphasalazine is effective for the treatment of ulcerative colitis and Crohn's disease. Sulphasalazine is a prodrug that passes to the colon where bacterial azoreductase enzymes cleave the azo bond, releasing free 5-aminosalicylate and sulphapyridine[9,10]. Studies have demonstrated that 5-aminosalicylate is the active component for treatment of ulcerative colitis[11], and that sulphapyridine, which is well absorbed from the colon, leads to the majority of side-effects[1]. A variety of strategies were subsequently undertaken to deliver 5-aminosalicylate directly to the colon, without linking it to sulphapyridine. Administered orally, 5-aminosalicylate is well absorbed in the proximal small bowel and is thus not available to the colon for topical therapy[12]. In order to 'protect' orally administered 5-aminosalicylate, a variety of oral formulations have been developed including the creation of a 5-aminosalicylate dimer (olsalazine) and linking 5-aminosalicylate to an inert carrier (balsalazide) as well as creation of delayed-release and sustained-release formulations[13–17]. Both olsalazine and balsalazide are prodrugs which, like sulphasalazine, are activated in the colon by azo-reductase enzyme activity from colonic bacteria. Asacol is a delayed-release formulation of 5-aminosalicylate coated with Eudragit-S that dissolves in the terminal ileum and right colon at pH 7. Salofalk is a delayed-release formulation coated with Eudragit-L which releases in the mid small bowel at pH 6–6.5. Pentasa is a sustained-release formulation composed of ethylcellulose-coated granules which begins releasing in the duodenum with completion of release in the rectum. Delivery of 5-aminosalicylate directly to the colon via olsalazine or balsalazide prodrugs, or through delayed release or sustained release with Asacol, Salofalk, or Pentasa, markedly improves the toxicity profile. Toxicity associated with sulphasalazine includes headache, epigastric pain, nausea and vomiting, skin rash, fever, hepatitis, autoimmune haemolysis, aplastic anaemia, leukopenia, agranulocytosis, folate deficiency, pancreatitis, lupus, pneumonitis, Stevens-Johnson syndrome, and male infertility[18]. Up to 30% of patients who take sulphasalazine will experience some form of toxicity. Toxicity associated with olsalazine, balsalazide, and mesalamine includes headache, rash, alopecia, interstitial nephritis, pericarditis, pneumonitis, hepatitis, pancreatitis, worsening diarrhoea and abdominal pain (hypersensitivity reaction), and worsening diarrhoea (secretory diarrhoea with olsalazine only). These reactions are relatively infrequent, and in clinical trials the frequency of side-effects with olsalazine, balsalazide, and mesalamine is comparable to placebo.

Ileal release budesonide

Corticosteroids such as prednisone and prednisolone are highly effective for the treatment of active ulcerative colitis and Crohn's disease. However, side-effects occur frequently. Budesonide is a potent corticosteroid with a high receptor-binding affinity in tissue that undergoes extensive first-pass hepatic metabolism in the liver[19]. A controlled ileal release formulation of budesonide has been developed which consists of hard gelatin capsules containing microgranules of budesonide sprayed with an insoluble polymer, allowing time-dependent controlled release. Each microgranule is then coated with Eudragit-L, an acrylic resin that dissolves above pH 5.5. First-pass inactivation of budesonide is 90%, resulting in 10% systemic bioavailability, with the majority of absorption occurring in the distal small bowel and right colon. The efficacy of budesonide at a dose of 9 mg is comparable to prednisolone 40 mg for active Crohn's disease. From the perspective of side-effects the frequency of side-effects with budesonide is substantially lower than with prednisolone in the setting of Crohn's disease: moon face 17% versus 35%; acne 6% versus 23%; swollen ankles 2% versus 11%; easy bruising 2% versus 7%; hirsutism 2% versus 2%; buffalo hump 1% versus 3%; skin striae 0% versus 0%; other side-effects 9% versus 16%; and total steroid-related side-effects 40% versus 98%[20].

Humanization of monoclonal antibodies to tumour necrosis factor

The mouse–human chimaeric monoclonal antibody against tumour necrosis factor (TNF), infliximab, is effective for the treatment of Crohn's disease (see below). However, the murine portion of the chimaeric antibody leads to immunogenicity, which in turn has been associated with infusion reactions, delayed hypersensitivity reactions, and loss of efficacy. Attempts to address this problem have included humanization of the antibody, whereby complementary determining regions (CDRs) are grafted into a human antibody, creating a humanized antibody, or fusion proteins which are composed of a human antibody FC portion and a soluble receptor to TNF fusion proteins in which a fully human FC portion of an antibody is linked to a fully human soluble receptor for TNF, or the creation of fully human monoclonal antibodies. An example of a humanized anti-TNF antibody is CDP 571 which is an IgG4 humanized monoclonal antibody to TNF[21]. Initial clinical trials suggested that CDP 571 was more effective than placebo for the treatment of active Crohn's disease[22]; however, this result was not confirmed in large phase III trials. Thus, although CDP 571 has a low rate of immunogenicity, it is not clearly effective. Etanercept is a p75 receptor fusion protein[21]. This fully human fusion protein again has a low rate of immunogenicity but was not effective for the treatment of active Crohn's disease[23], probably because it does not induce T-cell apoptosis. Adalimumab (D2E7) is a fully human IgG1 monoclonal antibody to TNF. It has a very low rate of immunogenicity, and is just beginning phase II trials in Crohn's disease.

IDENTIFY A NOVEL MECHANISM OF ACTION

Infliximab

TNF is elevated in the stool, blood, and gastrointestinal tissue in patients with Crohn's disease. Infliximab, a mouse–human chimaeric monoclonal antibody to TNF, is effective for the induction and maintenance of remission in patients with inflammatory luminal disease, as well as for the reduction in the number of draining enterocutaneous fistulas and maintenance of that reduction[24–27]. Infliximab is an IgG1 antibody that leads to complement fixation, antibody-dependent cytotoxicity, and T-cell apoptosis in addition to binding TNF[21,28]. These novel and specific mechanisms of action appear to be linked to the efficacy of infliximab for Crohn's disease.

Natalizumab

VCAM-1 and MAdCAM-1 expression is increased in the mucosa of patients with inflammatory bowel disease. Inhibition of leucocyte homing by blocking the adhesion molecule alpha 4 has resulted in decreased disease activity in animal models of inflammatory bowel disease. Natalizumab is a humanized IgG1 monoclonal antibody against alpha 4 integrins[29,30]. Two studies have demonstrated that natalizumab is effective for the induction of remission in patients with Crohn's disease[31,32].

BLOCK ADVERSE EFFECTS

Concomitant treatment with immunosuppressives or steroids and infliximab

As noted above, the murine portion of infliximab leads to an immunogenic reaction. In data from an integrated safety data set, 28% of patients were human anti-chimaeric antibody (HACA)-positive[33–35]. The highest incidence of HACA appeared to occur at lower infliximab doses (1 mg/kg). Concomitant immunosuppressive therapy with methotrexate, azathioprine, or 6-mercaptopurine reduced the incidence of HACA by 2–3-fold[33–35]. In another study the occurrence of HACA was evaluated in 125 patients with refractory Crohn's disease who were treated with infliximab on demand to control symptoms[36,37]. HACA developed in 61% of patients. HACA concentrations greater than 8 μg/L predicted shorter duration of response (35 days versus 71 days) and greater risk of infusion reactions (relative risk 2.4). Infliximab concentrations were nearly undetectable (1.21 μg/ml) in patients with infusion reactions as compared to 14.09 at 4 weeks after an infusion. Infusion reactions shortened the duration of response from 65 days down to 38.5 days. Concomitant therapy with azathioprine, 6-mercaptopurine, or methotrexate was a significant predictor for low HACA titres and high infliximab concentrations 4 weeks after infusion. Finally, Farrell and colleagues demonstrated that pretreatment with 200 mg of intravenous hydrocortisone prior to administration of infliximab reduced the frequency of HACA-positive status at week 16 from 47% down to 21%[38,39]. Interestingly, for the subset of patients pretreated with placebo who are receiving other immunosuppressives, the rate of HACA-positivity was low, so that the elevated HACA rates were really limited to those patients who did not receive hydrocortisone pretreatment and were not receiving a concomitant immunosuppressive.

CONCLUSIONS

The results of pharmacogenetic testing to improve the side-effect profile of sulphasalazine therapy (NAT 2 genotype testing) and azathioprine/6-mercaptopurine (TPMT phenotype or genotype testing) have been disappointing. Altering the structure or delivery system of drugs that are known to be efficacious has generally resulted in an improvement in toxicity, albeit sometimes at the loss of efficacy. The identification of novel mechanisms of action can occasionally lead to very good results, but there are many failures. Finally, blocking the adverse effects of a medication by concomitant therapy with other medications can also be very helpful, but this strategy usually is not uniformly reliable.

References

1. Das KM, Eastwood MA, McManus JP, Sircus W. Adverse reactions during salicylazosulphapyridine therapy and the relation with drug metabolism and acetylator phenotype. N Engl J Med. 1973;289:491–5.
2. Azad Khan AK, Nurazzaman M, Truelove SC. The effect of the acetylator phenotype on the metabolism of sulphasalazine in man. J Med Genet. 1983;20:30–6.
3. Cascorbi I, Brockmoller J, Mrozikiewicz PM, Muller A, Roots I. Arylamine N-acetyltransferase activity in man. Drug Metab Rev. 1999;31:489–502.
4. Ricart E, Taylor WR, Loftus EV et al. N-acetyltransferase 1 and 2 genotypes do not predict response or toxicity to treatment with mesalamine and sulphasalazine in patients with ulcerative colitis. Am J Gastroenterol. 2002;97:1763–8.
5. Lennard L. The clinical pharmacology of 6-mercaptopurine. Eur J Clin Pharmacol. 1992;43:329–39.
6. Weinshilboum RM, Sladek SL. Mercaptopurine pharmacogenetics: monogenic inheritance of erythrocyte thiopurine methyltransferase activity. Am J Human Genet. 1980;32:651–62.
7. Otterness D, Szumlanski C, Lennard L et al. Human thiopurine methyltransferase activity pharmacogenetics: gene sequence polymorphisms. Clin Pharmacol Ther. 1997;62:60–73.
8. Colombel JF, Ferrari N, Debuysere H et al. Genotypic analysis of thiopurine S-methyltransferase in patients with Crohn's disease and severe myelosuppression during azathioprine therapy. Gastroenterology. 2000;118:1025–30.
9. Das KM, Dubin R. Clinical pharmacokinetics of sulphasalazine. Clin Pharmacokinet. 1976;1:406–25.
10. Klotz U. Clinical pharmacokinetics of sulphasalazine, its metabolites and other prodrugs of 5-aminosalicylic acid. Clin Pharmacokinet. 1985;10:285–302.
11. Azad Khan AK, Piris J, Truelove SC. An experiment to determine the active therapeutic moiety of sulphasalazine. Lancet. 1977;2:892–5.
12. Bondesen S, Hegnhoj J, Larsen F, Hansen SH, Hansen CP, Rasmussen SN. Pharmacokinetics of 5-aminosalicylic acid in man following administration of intravenous bolus and per os slow-release formulation. Dig Dis Sci. 1991;36:1735–40.
13. Wadworth AN, Fitton A. Olsalazine. A review of its pharmacodynamic and pharmacokinetic properties, and therapeutic potential in inflammatory bowel disease. Drugs. 1991;41:647–64.
14. Prakash A, Spencer CM. Balsalazide. Drugs. 1998;56:83–9; discussion 90.
15. Ragunath K, Williams JG. Review article: Balsalazide therapy in ulcerative colitis. Aliment Pharmacol Ther. 2001;15:1549–54.
16. Prakash A, Markham A. Oral delayed-release mesalazine: a review of its use in ulcerative colitis and Crohn's disease. Drugs. 1999;57:383–408.
17. De Vos M. Clinical pharmacokinetics of slow release mesalazine. Clin Pharmacokinet. 2000;39:85–97.
18. Taffet SL, Das KM. Sulphasalazine. Adverse effects and desensitization. Dig Dis Sci. 1983;28:833–42.
19. Spencer CM, McTavish D. Budesonide. A review of its pharmacological properties and therapeutic efficacy in inflammatory bowel disease. Drugs. 1995;50:854–72.
20. Rutgeerts P, Lofberg R, Malchow H et al. A comparison of budesonide with prednisolone for active Crohn's disease. N Engl J Med. 1994;331:842–5.
21. Sandborn WJ, Hanauer SB. Antitumor necrosis factor therapy for inflammatory bowel disease: a review of agents, pharmacology, clinical results, and safety. Inflamm Bowel Dis. 1999;5:119–33.
22. Sandborn WJ, Feagan BG, Hanauer SB et al. An engineered human antibody to TNF (CDP571) for active Crohn's disease: a randomized double-blind placebo-controlled trial. Gastroenterology. 2001;120:1330–8.

23. Sandborn WJ, Hanauer SB, Katz S *et al.* Etanercept for active Crohn's disease: A randomized, double-blind, placebo-controlled trial. Gastroenterology. 2001;121:1088–94.
24. Targan SR, Hanauer SB, van Deventer SJ *et al.* A short-term study of chimaeric monoclonal antibody cA2 to tumor necrosis factor alpha for Crohn's disease. Crohn's Disease cA2 Study Group. N Engl J Med. 1997;337:1029–35.
25. Hanauer SB, Feagan BG, Lichtenstein GR *et al.* Maintenance infliximab for Crohn's disease: the ACCENT I randomised trial. Lancet. 2002;359:1541–9.
26. Present DH, Rutgeerts P, Targan S *et al.* Infliximab for the treatment of fistulas in patients with Crohn's disease. N Engl J Med. 1999;340:1398–405.
27. Sands B, Van Deventer S, Bernstein C *et al.* Long-term treatment of fistulizing Crohn's disease: response to infliximab in the ACCENT II trial through 54 weeks. Gastroenterology. 2002;122:A81.
28. Lugering A, Schmidt M, Lugering N, Pauels HG, Domschke W, Kucharzik T. Infliximab induces apoptosis in monocytes from patients with chronic active Crohn's disease by using a caspase-dependent pathway. Gastroenterology. 2001;121:1145–57.
29. van Assche G, Rutgeerts P. Antiadhesion molecule therapy in inflammatory bowel disease. Inflamm Bowel Dis. 2002;8:291–300.
30. Sandborn WJ, Targan SR. Biologic therapy of inflammatory bowel disease. Gastroenterology. 2002;122:1592–608.
31. Gordon FH, Lai CW, Hamilton MI *et al.* A randomized placebo-controlled trial of a humanized monoclonal antibody to alpha4 integrin in active Crohn's disease. Gastroenterology. 2001;121:268–74.
32. Ghosh S, Goldin E, Malchow H *et al.* A randomised, double-blind, placebo-controlled, pan-European study of a recombinant humanised antibody to alpha 4 integrin (Antegren) in moderate to severely active Crohn's disease. Gastroenterology. 2001;120:A127–8.
33. Remicade (infliximab). Prescribing information. Physicians Desk Reference. 2001:1085–88.
34. Remicade (infliximab) for IV injection. Package Insert. 2002.
35. Schaible TF. Long term safety of infliximab. Can J Gastroenterol. 2000;14 (Suppl. C):29–32C.
36. Norman M, Baert F, D'Haens G *et al.* HACA formation after infliximab (Remicade) treatment in Crohn's disease is clearly associated with infusion reactions. Gastroenterology. 2001;120:A261.
37. Norman M, Baert F, Vermeire S, Van Assche G, Carbonez A, Rutgeerts P. Post-infusion infliximab levels determine duration of response in Crohn's disease and are directly related to infusion reactions. Gastroenterology. 2002;122:A-100.
38. Farrell R, Alsahli M, Falchuk K, Peppercorn M, Michetti P. A randomized, double-blind, placebo-controlled trial of intravenous hydrocortisone in reducing human anti-chimaeric antibody following infliximab therapy. Gastroenterology. 2001;120:A618–19.
39. Alsahli M, Jeen YTJ, Peppercorn MA, Michetti P, Farrell RJ. A randomized, double-blind, placebo-controlled trial of intravenous hydrocortisone in reducing human anti-chimaeric antibody following infliximab therapy. Gastroenterology. 2002;122:A-100.

Index

Falk Symposium Series

43. Reutter W, Popper H, Arias IM, Heinrich PC, Keppler D, Landmann L, eds.: *Modulation of Liver Cell Expression.* Falk Symposium No. 43. 1987   ISBN: 0-85200-677-2*
44. Boyer JL, Bianchi L, eds.: *Liver Cirrhosis.* Falk Symposium No. 44. 1987
ISBN: 0-85200-993-3*
45. Paumgartner G, Stiehl A, Gerok W, eds.: *Bile Acids and the Liver.* Falk Symposium No. 45. 1987   ISBN: 0-85200-675-6*
46. Goebell H, Peskar BM, Malchow H, eds.: *Inflammatory Bowel Diseases – Basic Research & Clinical Implications.* Falk Symposium No. 46. 1988   ISBN: 0-7462-0067-6*
47. Bianchi L, Holt P, James OFW, Butler RN, eds.: *Aging in Liver and Gastrointestinal Tract.* Falk Symposium No. 47. 1988   ISBN: 0-7462-0066-8*
48. Heilmann C, ed.: *Calcium-Dependent Processes in the Liver.* Falk Symposium No. 48. 1988   ISBN: 0-7462-0075-7*
50. Singer MV, Goebell H, eds.: *Nerves and the Gastrointestinal Tract.* Falk Symposium No. 50. 1989   ISBN: 0-7462-0114-1
51. Bannasch P, Keppler D, Weber G, eds.: *Liver Cell Carcinoma.* Falk Symposium No. 51. 1989   ISBN: 0-7462-0111-7
52. Paumgartner G, Stiehl A, Gerok W, eds.: *Trends in Bile Acid Research.* Falk Symposium No. 52. 1989   ISBN: 0-7462-0112-5
53. Paumgartner G, Stiehl A, Barbara L, Roda E, eds.: *Strategies for the Treatment of Hepatobiliary Diseases.* Falk Symposium No. 53. 1990   ISBN: 0-7923-8903-4
54. Bianchi L, Gerok W, Maier K-P, Deinhardt F, eds.: *Infectious Diseases of the Liver.* Falk Symposium No. 54. 1990   ISBN: 0-7923-8902-6
55. Falk Symposium No. 55 not published
55B.Hadziselimovic F, Herzog B, Bürgin-Wolff A, eds.: *Inflammatory Bowel Disease and Coeliac Disease in Children.* International Falk Symposium. 1990 ISBN 0-7462-0125-7
56. Williams CN, eds.: *Trends in Inflammatory Bowel Disease Therapy.* Falk Symposium No. 56. 1990   ISBN: 0-7923-8952-2
57. Bock KW, Gerok W, Matern S, Schmid R, eds.: *Hepatic Metabolism and Disposition of Endo- and Xenobiotics.* Falk Symposium No. 57. 1991   ISBN: 0-7923-8953-0
58. Paumgartner G, Stiehl A, Gerok W, eds.: *Bile Acids as Therapeutic Agents: From Basic Science to Clinical Practice.* Falk Symposium No. 58. 1991   ISBN: 0-7923-8954-9
59. Halter F, Garner A, Tytgat GNJ, eds.: *Mechanisms of Peptic Ulcer Healing.* Falk Symposium No. 59. 1991   ISBN: 0-7923-8955-7
60. Goebell H, Ewe K, Malchow H, Koelbel Ch, eds.: *Inflammatory Bowel Diseases – Progress in Basic Research and Clinical Implications.* Falk Symposium No. 60. 1991
ISBN: 0-7923-8956-5
61. Falk Symposium No. 61 not published
62. Dowling RH, Folsch UR, Löser Ch, eds.: *Polyamines in the Gastrointestinal Tract.* Falk Symposium No. 62. 1992   ISBN: 0-7923-8976-X
63. Lentze MJ, Reichen J, eds.: *Paediatric Cholestasis: Novel Approaches to Treatment.* Falk Symposium No. 63. 1992   ISBN: 0-7923-8977-8
64. Demling L, Frühmorgen P, eds.: *Non-Neoplastic Diseases of the Anorectum.* Falk Symposium No. 64. 1992   ISBN: 0-7923-8979-4
64B.Gressner AM, Ramadori G, eds.: *Molecular and Cell Biology of Liver Fibrogenesis.* International Falk Symposium. 1992   ISBN: 0-7923-8980-8

*These titles were published under the MTP Press imprint.

Falk Symposium Series

65. Hadziselimovic F, Herzog B, eds.: *Inflammatory Bowel Diseases and Morbus Hirschprung.* Falk Symposium No. 65. 1992   ISBN: 0-7923-8995-6
66. Martin F, McLeod RS, Sutherland LR, Williams CN, eds.: *Trends in Inflammatory Bowel Disease Therapy.* Falk Symposium No. 66. 1993   ISBN: 0-7923-8827-5
67. Schölmerich J, Kruis W, Goebell H, Hohenberger W, Gross V, eds.: *Inflammatory Bowel Diseases – Pathophysiology as Basis of Treatment.* Falk Symposium No. 67. 1993
    ISBN: 0-7923-8996-4
68. Paumgartner G, Stiehl A, Gerok W, eds.: *Bile Acids and The Hepatobiliary System: From Basic Science to Clinical Practice.* Falk Symposium No. 68. 1993
    ISBN: 0-7923-8829-1
69. Schmid R, Bianchi L, Gerok W, Maier K-P, eds.: *Extrahepatic Manifestations in Liver Diseases.* Falk Symposium No. 69. 1993   ISBN: 0-7923-8821-6
70. Meyer zum Büschenfelde K-H, Hoofnagle J, Manns M, eds.: *Immunology and Liver.* Falk Symposium No. 70. 1993   ISBN: 0-7923-8830-5
71. Surrenti C, Casini A, Milani S, Pinzani M , eds.: *Fat-Storing Cells and Liver Fibrosis.* Falk Symposium No. 71. 1994   ISBN: 0-7923-8842-9
72. Rachmilewitz D, ed.: *Inflammatory Bowel Diseases – 1994.* Falk Symposium No. 72. 1994   ISBN: 0-7923-8845-3
73. Binder HJ, Cummings J, Soergel KH, eds.: *Short Chain Fatty Acids.* Falk Symposium No. 73. 1994   ISBN: 0-7923-8849-6
73B.Möllmann HW, May B, eds.: *Glucocorticoid Therapy in Chronic Inflammatory Bowel Disease: from basic principles to rational therapy.* International Falk Workshop. 1996
    ISBN 0-7923-8708-2
74. Keppler D, Jungermann K, eds.: *Transport in the Liver.* Falk Symposium No. 74. 1994
    ISBN: 0-7923-8858-5
74B.Stange EF, ed.: *Chronic Inflammatory Bowel Disease.* Falk Symposium. 1995
    ISBN: 0-7923-8876-3
75. van Berge Henegouwen GP, van Hoek B, De Groote J, Matern S, Stockbrügger RW, eds.: *Cholestatic Liver Diseases: New Strategies for Prevention and Treatment of Hepatobiliary and Cholestatic Liver Diseases.* Falk Symposium 75. 1994.
    ISBN: 0-7923-8867-4
76. Monteiro E, Tavarela Veloso F, eds.: *Inflammatory Bowel Diseases: New Insights into Mechanisms of Inflammation and Challenges in Diagnosis and Treatment.* Falk Symposium 76. 1995.   ISBN 0-7923-8884-4
77. Singer MV, Ziegler R, Rohr G, eds.: *Gastrointestinal Tract and Endocrine System.* Falk Symposium 77. 1995.   ISBN 0-7923-8877-1
78. Decker K, Gerok W, Andus T, Gross V, eds.: *Cytokines and the Liver.* Falk Symposium 78. 1995.   ISBN 0-7923-8878-X
79. Holstege A, Schölmerich J, Hahn EG, eds.: *Portal Hypertension.* Falk Symposium 79. 1995.   ISBN 0-7923-8879-8
80. Hofmann AF, Paumgartner G, Stiehl A, eds.: *Bile Acids in Gastroenterology: Basic and Clinical Aspects.* Falk Symposium 80. 1995   ISBN 0-7923-8880-1
81. Riecken EO, Stallmach A, Zeitz M, Heise W, eds.: *Malignancy and Chronic Inflammation in the Gastrointestinal Tract – New Concepts.* Falk Symposium 81. 1995
    ISBN 0-7923-8889-5
82. Fleig WE, ed.: *Inflammatory Bowel Diseases: New Developments and Standards.* Falk Symposium 82. 1995   ISBN 0-7923-8890-6

Falk Symposium Series

82B. Paumgartner G, Beuers U, eds.: *Bile Acids in Liver Diseases*. International Falk Workshop. 1995   ISBN 0-7923-8891-7
83. Dobrilla G, Felder M, de Pretis G, eds.: *Advances in Hepatobiliary and Pancreatic Diseases: Special Clinical Topics*. Falk Symposium 83. 1995.   ISBN 0-7923-8892-5
84. Fromm H, Leuschner U, eds.: *Bile Acids – Cholestasis – Gallstones: Advances in Basic and Clinical Bile Acid Research*. Falk Symposium 84. 1995   ISBN 0-7923-8893-3
85. Tytgat GNJ, Bartelsman JFWM, van Deventer SJH, eds.: *Inflammatory Bowel Diseases*. Falk Symposium 85. 1995   ISBN 0-7923-8894-1
86. Berg PA, Leuschner U, eds.: *Bile Acids and Immunology*. Falk Symposium 86. 1996
                                                                            ISBN 0-7923-8700-7
87. Schmid R, Bianchi L, Blum HE, Gerok W, Maier KP, Stalder GA, eds.: *Acute and Chronic Liver Diseases: Molecular Biology and Clinics*. Falk Symposium 87. 1996
                                                                            ISBN 0-7923-8701-5
88. Blum HE, Wu GY, Wu CH, eds.: *Molecular Diagnosis and Gene Therapy*. Falk Symposium 88. 1996   ISBN 0-7923-8702-3
88B. Poupon RE, Reichen J, eds.: *Surrogate Markers to Assess Efficacy of TReatment in Chronic Liver Diseases*. International Falk Workshop. 1996   ISBN 0-7923-8705-8
89. Reyes HB, Leuschner U, Arias IM, eds.: *Pregnancy, Sex Hormones and the Liver*. Falk Symposium 89. 1996   ISBN 0-7923-8704-X
89B. Broelsch CE, Burdelski M, Rogiers X, eds.: *Cholestatic Liver Diseases in Children and Adults*. International Falk Workshop. 1996   ISBN 0-7923-8710-4
90. Lam S-K, Paumgartner P, Wang B, eds.: *Update on Hepatobiliary Diseases 1996*. Falk Symposium 90. 1996   ISBN 0-7923-8715-5
91. Hadziselimovic F, Herzog B, eds.: *Inflammatory Bowel Diseases and Chronic Recurrent Abdominal Pain*. Falk Symposium 91. 1996   ISBN 0-7923-8722-8
91B. Alvaro D, Benedetti A, Strazzabosco M, eds.: *Vanishing Bile Duct Syndrome – Pathophysiology and Treatment*. International Falk Workshop. 1996
                                                                            ISBN 0-7923-8721-X
92. Gerok W, Loginov AS, Pokrowskij VI, eds.: *New Trends in Hepatology 1996*. Falk Symposium 92. 1997   ISBN 0-7923-8723-6
93. Paumgartner G, Stiehl A, Gerok W, eds.: *Bile Acids in Hepatobiliary Diseases – Basic Research and Clinical Application*. Falk Symposium 93. 1997   ISBN 0-7923-8725-2
94. Halter F, Winton D, Wright NA, eds.: *The Gut as a Model in Cell and Molecular Biology*. Falk Symposium 94. 1997   ISBN 0-7923-8726-0
94B. Kruse-Jarres JD, Schölmerich J, eds.: *Zinc and Diseases of the Digestive Tract*. International Falk Workshop. 1997   ISBN 0-7923-8724-4
95. Ewe K, Eckardt VF, Enck P, eds.: *Constipation and Anorectal Insufficiency*. Falk Symposium 95. 1997   ISBN 0-7923-8727-9
96. Andus T, Goebell H, Layer P, Schölmerich J, eds.: *Inflammatory Bowel Disease – from Bench to Bedside*. Falk Symposium 96. 1997   ISBN 0-7923-8728-7
97. Campieri M, Bianchi-Porro G, Fiocchi C, Schölmerich J, eds. *Clinical Challenges in Inflammatory Bowel Diseases: Diagnosis, Prognosis and Treatment*. Falk Symposium 97. 1998   ISBN 0-7923-8733-3
98. Lembcke B, Kruis W, Sartor RB, eds. *Systemic Manifestations of IBD: The Pending Challenge for Subtle Diagnosis and Treatment*. Falk Symposium 98. 1998
                                                                            ISBN 0-7923-8734-1

Falk Symposium Series

99. Goebell H, Holtmann G, Talley NJ, eds. *Functional Dyspepsia and Irritable Bowel Syndrome: Concepts and Controversies.* Falk Symposium 99. 1998
ISBN 0-7923-8735-X

100. Blum HE, Bode Ch, Bode JCh, Sartor RB, eds. *Gut and the Liver.* Falk Symposium 100. 1998
ISBN 0-7923-8736-8

101. Rachmilewitz D, ed. *V International Symposium on Inflammatory Bowel Diseases.* Falk Symposium 101. 1998
ISBN 0-7923-8743-0

102. Manns MP, Boyer JL, Jansen PLM, Reichen J, eds. *Cholestatic Liver Diseases.* Falk Symposium 102. 1998
ISBN 0-7923-8746-5

102B. Manns MP, Chapman RW, Stiehl A, Wiesner R, eds. *Primary Sclerosing Cholangitis.* International Falk Workshop. 1998.
ISBN 0-7923-8745-7

103. Häussinger D, Jungermann K, eds. *Liver and Nervous System.* Falk Symposium 102. 1998
ISBN 0-7924-8742-2

103B. Häussinger D, Heinrich PC, eds. *Signalling in the Liver.* International Falk Workshop. 1998
ISBN 0-7923-8744-9

103C. Fleig W, ed. *Normal and Malignant Liver Cell Growth.* International Falk Workshop. 1998
ISBN 0-7923-8748-1

104. Stallmach A, Zeitz M, Strober W, MacDonald TT, Lochs H, eds. *Induction and Modulation of Gastrointestinal Inflammation.* Falk Symposium 104. 1998
ISBN 0-7923-8747-3

105. Emmrich J, Liebe S, Stange EF, eds. *Innovative Concepts in Inflammatory Bowel Diseases.* Falk Symposium 105. 1999   ISBN 0-7923-8749-X

106. Rutgeerts P, Colombel J-F, Hanauer SB, Schölmerich J, Tytgat GNJ, van Gossum A, eds. *Advances in Inflammatory Bowel Diseases.* Falk Symposium 106. 1999
ISBN 0-7923-8750-3

107. Špičák J, Boyer J, Gilat T, Kotrlik K, Mareček Z, Paumgartner G, eds. *Diseases of the Liver and the Bile Ducts – New Aspects and Clinical Implications.* Falk Symposium 107. 1999   ISBN 0-7923-8751-1

108. Paumgartner G, Stiehl A, Gerok W, Keppler D, Leuschner U, eds. *Bile Acids and Cholestasis.* Falk Symposium 108. 1999   ISBN 0-7923-8752-X

109. Schmiegel W, Schölmerich J, eds. *Colorectal Cancer – Molecular Mechanisms, Premalignant State and its Prevention.* Falk Symposium 109. 1999
ISBN 0-7923-8753-8

110. Domschke W, Stoll R, Brasitus TA, Kagnoff MF, eds. *Intestinal Mucosa and its Diseases – Pathophysiology and Clinics.* Falk Symposium 110. 1999
ISBN 0-7923-8754-6

110B. Northfield TC, Ahmed HA, Jazwari RP, Zentler-Munro PL, eds. *Bile Acids in Hepatobiliary Disease.* Falk Workshop. 2000   ISBN 0-7923-8755-4

111. Rogler G, Kullmann F, Rutgeerts P, Sartor RB, Schölmerich J, eds. *IBD at the End of its First Century.* Falk Symposium 111. 2000   ISBN 0-7923-8756-2

112. Krammer HJ, Singer MV, eds. *Neurogastroenterology: From the Basics to the Clinics.* Falk Symposium 112. 2000   ISBN 0-7923-8757-0

113. Andus T, Rogler G, Schlottmann K, Frick E, Adler G, Schmiegel W, Zeitz M, Schölmerich J, eds. *Cytokines and Cell Homeostasis in the Gastrointestinal Tract.* Falk Symposium 113. 2000   ISBN 0-7923-8758-9

114. Manns MP, Paumgartner G, Leuschner U, eds. *Immunology and Liver.* Falk Symposium 114. 2000   ISBN 0-7923-8759-7

Falk Symposium Series

Falk Symposium Series

130. Holtmann G, Talley NJ, eds. *Gastrointestinal Inflammation and Disturbed Gut Function: The Challenge of New Concepts*. Falk Symposium 130. 2003
ISBN 0-7923-8783-X

131. Herfarth H, Feagan BJ, Folsch UR, Schölmerich J, Vatn MH, Zeitz M, eds. *Targets of Treatment in Chronic Inflammatory Bowel Diseases*. Falk Symposium 131. 2003
ISBN 0-7923-8784-8

132. Galle PR, Gerken G, Schmidt WE, Wiedenmann B, eds. *Disease Progression and Carcinogenesis in the Gastrointestinal Tract*. Falk Symposium 132. 2003
ISBN 0-7923-8785-6